CRITICAL CARE MEDICINE MANUAL

CRITICAL CARE MEDICINE MANUAL

MAX HARRY WEIL
PROTASIO L. DALUZ

SPRINGER-VERLAG
NEW YORK HEIDELBERG BERLIN

Max Harry Weil, M.D., Ph.D.
Chairman and Clinical Professor
Division of Critical Care Medicine and
Director of the Institute of Critical Care Medicine
University of Southern California
Schools of Medicine and Engineering
1300 North Vermont Avenue
Los Angeles, California 90027

Protasio L. DaLuz, M.D.
Hospital das Clinicas da Faculdade de Medicine da Univ. de Sao Paulo
Cairia Postal 8091
Sao Paulo, Brazil

Library of Congress Cataloging in Publication Data

Main entry under title:

Critical care medicine manual.

Includes bibliographical references and index.
1. Critical care medicine. I. Weil, Max Harry.
II. DaLuz, Protasio L. [DNLM: 1. Critical care—Congresses. 2. Intensive care units—Congresses. WX218 C936]
RC86.7.C74 616 77-24959

Softcover reprint of the hardcover 1st edition 1978

9 8 7 6 5 4 3 2 1

ISBN 978-1-4612-9934-9 ISBN 978-1-4612-9932-5 (eBook)
DOI 10.1007/978-1-4612-9932-5

Preface

During the past twelve years, a course on critical care medicine has been sponsored by the Post Graduate Division of the University of Southern California School of Medicine in association with its Center for the Critically Ill. The content of each of the symposia has paralleled the evolution of critical care medicine as a recognized service specialty.

The annual program was planned as a teaching session for physicians and allied medical personnel who sought to advance their involvement in this rapidly advancing field. A panel of highly regarded authorities on subjects bearing on critical care medicine, faculty members of the USC School of Medicine, and staff members of our own Center for the Critically Ill at the Hollywood Presbyterian Medical Center serve as faculty of these symposia.

Although the primary commitment of the organizers to maintain this as a teaching and demonstration session was not abandoned, the number of annual registrants progressively increased from fewer than 100 to more than 1200, gradually outstripping local hotel facilities in central Los Angeles. The symposium for the past two years has been held in the large and attractive Anaheim Convention Center adjacent to Disneyland.

In response to the request of many of those who had attended these sessions over the years, a monograph summarizing the content of the presentations was first evolved in 1974. Although the intent was to create a volume primarily for those who had attended this course, there was substantial interest on the part of practitioners, internists, anesthesiologists, surgeons, nurse specialists, and technical specialists for this compilation. This provided the incentive for publication of a more comprehensive monograph which would simultaneously serve as a permanent record of the presentations for those who attended the symposium and as a ready reference for those who may seek current information directly applicable to the care of the critically ill quite independently of the course itself.

The orientation of critical care specialists is necessarily multidisciplinary. This is reflected in the Table of Contents. The critical care specialist has a major commitment to respiratory care for respiratory crises, which constitute the largest single problem confronted by the critical care specialist. Current concepts on respiratory monitoring, methods of mechanical ventilation, and the specific problem of pulmonary embolism are addressed.

Shock and trauma are viewed as multisystemic injuries with multisystemic failure. Perhaps no more important technique has come to the fore than that of systemic fluid challenge guided by measurement of intravascular pressures and, more recently, colloid osmotic pressure. The roles of vasopressors and vasodilator drugs for the treatment of shock states have been reappraised. Vasopressor agents have largely been abandoned but vasodilator agents have secured a substantial place in the treatment of cardiogenic shock.

Giant strides have been made in neurological monitoring of the critically ill since brain salvage is now an important commitment. We also seek to promptly identify brain death, less there be futile and extremely costly prolongation of life in the absence of brain viability. In this context the critical care team has an important obligation to secure organ donations after brain death is identified.

Oxygen availability to the myocardium is likely to be the critical factor to survival after acute myocardial infarction. Therapeutic procedures by which preload, afterload, and diastolic coronary perfusion pressure are favorably altered form the basis for fluid therapy, pharmacological interventions, and mechanical assist devices.

Only within the last five years, the selective risk of alkalosis due to either or both respiratory and electrolyte management of critically ill patients has been recognized. Nutritional support of patients has been greatly improved by evolution of parenteral alimentation especially in patients during gastrointestinal crises. More general applicability of parenterally administered nutrients is now recognized for the sustenance of the acutely ill patient with overwhelming infections, renal failure, and respiratory failure.

Neonatalogy has evolved as a specialty of pediatrics, obstetrics, and critical care medicine.

Organ transplantation and implantation and chemotherapy of neoplasma have greatly altered host susceptibility to disease substantially increasing the risk of and the frequency of iatrogenic infections.

The facilities available for management of the critically ill, including laboratory support, electrical safety, and arrangements that favor the psychosocial welfare of patients have all been greatly improved.

The practical demands for early publication have precluded detailed editing for style and even content. We have made no effort to edit potentially different points of view, recognizing the importance of exposing various points of view on issues which may be considered controversial. We also made every effort to include all of the presentations at the 13th Annual Symposium, however, a very few manuscripts were not available, and were not included for this reason.

Most sadly we must record the untimely death on June 29, 1975 of Doctor Herbert Shubin. He was Co-Director of these symposia since their inception in 1962 and a uniquely treasured colleague. His attributes were not only those of the superior physician-scientist but also of the concerned, loving human. To have known him is to have loved him.

Finally, we would like to express our sincere gratitude for each of the faculty participating in this effort and especially to the Post Graduate Division of our School of Medicine directed by Doctor Phil Manning. We are also very much indebted to each of our associates in the USC Shock Research Unit and the Center for the Critically Ill and particularly to our dedicated secretaries, Mrs. Sharman Davis Jamison, Mrs. Ferne Ginewsky, and Ms. Lynne Pinsky.

Max Harry Weil, M.D., Ph.D.

Protasio L. DaLuz, M.D.

Contents

Contributors

J. Ali
Health Sciences Centre, Winnipeg, Manitoba, Canada

John De Angelis
University of California at Los Angeles, Cedars-Sinai Medical Center, Los Angeles, California

Stephen M. Ayres
St. Louis University, St. Louis, Missouri

Betty Bernard
The Los Angeles County/University of Southern California Medical Center, Los Angeles, California

Jose Bisera
University of Southern California School of Medicine and the Center for the Critically Ill, Hollywood Presbyterian and LAC/USC Medical Centers, Los Angeles, California

Doreen R. G. Browne
Harvard Medical School, Boston, Massachusetts

Christopher W. Bryan-Brown
Mount Sinai School of Medicine, City University of New York, New York

Rev. Jack Calhoun
Hollywood Presbyterian Medical Center, Los Angeles, California

Richard W. Carlson
University of Southern California School of Medicine and the Center for the Critically Ill, Hollywood Presbyterian and LAC/USC Medical Centers, Los Angeles, California

J. Howard Carrington
University of Southern California School of Medicine and the Center for the Critically Ill, Hollywood Presbyterian and LAC/USC Medical Centers, Los Angeles, California

Potter Chang
University of California at Los Angeles, School of Public Health, Los Angeles, California

Protasio L. DaLuz
Universidade de Sao Paulo, Sao Paulo, Brazil

William French
University of Southern California School of Medicine and the Center for the Critically Ill, Hollywood Presbyterian and LAC/USC Medical Centers, Los Angeles, California

Uri Freund
University of Southern California School of Medicine and the Center for the Critically Ill, Hollywood Presbyterian and LAC/USC Medical Centers, Los Angeles, California

William Ganz
University of California at Los Angeles, Cedars-Sinai Medical Center, Los Angeles, California

Arthur Gordon
University of California at Los Angeles, Los Angeles, California

William J. Grace
St. Vincent's Hospital and Medical Center; New York University School of Medicine, New York, New York

Robert M. Hardaway, III
William Beaumont Army Medical Center, El Paso, Texas

Roger W. Jelliffe
University of Southern California School of Medicine, Los Angeles, California

William F. Kiely
The Los Angeles County/University of Southern California Medical Center, Los Angeles, California

B. W. Kirk
Health Sciences Centre, Winnipeg, Manitoba, Canada

Francis Y. K. Lau
The Los Angeles County/University of Southern California Medical Center, Los Angeles, California

W. L. MacKeen
Health Sciences Centre, Winnipeg, Manitoba, Canada

Phil R. Manning
University of Southern California School of Medicine, Los Angeles, California

John McRae
University of Southern California School of Medicine, Los Angeles, California

Sybil Michaels
University of Southern California Center for the Critically Ill, Los Angeles, California

Arnold C. G. Platzker
Children's Hospital of Los Angeles, Los Angeles, California

Henning Pontoppidan
Harvard Medical School, Boston, Massachusetts

Lawrence Portigal
University of Southern California School of Medicine and the Center for the Critically Ill, Hollywood Presbyterian and LAC/USC Medical Centers, Los Angeles, California

Angela Ramos
Children's Hospital of Los Angeles, Los Angeles, California

Peter Safar
University of Pittsburgh School of Medicine, Pittsburgh, Pennsylvania

Richard C. Schaeffer
University of Southern California School of Medicine and the Center for the Critically Ill, Hollywood Presbyterian and LAC/USC Medical Centers, Los Angeles, California

William Schumer
University of Health Sciences/The Chicago Medical School, Chicago, Illinois

William C. Shoemaker
Harbor General Hospital, Torrance, California; University of California at Los Angeles School of Medicine, Los Angeles, California

Herbert Shubin
University of Southern California School of Medicine and the Center for the Critically Ill, Hollywood Presbyterian and LAC/USC Medical Centers, Los Angeles, California

H. J. C. Swan
University of California at Los Angeles, Cedars-Sinai Medical Center, Los Angeles, California

Teruo Takano
Cedars-Sinai Medical Center, Los Angeles, California

John K. Vyden
Cedars-Sinai Medical Center; University of California at Los Angeles, Los Angeles, California

Paul F. Wehrle
The Los Angeles County/University of Southern California Medical Center, Los Angeles, California

Max Harry Weil
University of Southern California School of Medicine and the Center for the Critically Ill, Hollywood Presbyterian and LAC/USC Medical Centers, Los Angeles, California

Milford G. Wyman
San Pedro Community Hospital, San Pedro, California

Abbreviations

ADH	Antidiuretic hormone
a Pco_2	Arterial carbon dioxide pressure, torr
a Po_2	Arterial oxygen pressure, torr
ARF	Acute respiratory failure
ATP	Adenosine triphosphate
BBB	Blood brain barrier
CBF	Cerebral blood flow
CMRG	Cerebral metabolic rate for glucose
CMRL	Cerebral metabolic rate for lactate
$CMRO_2$	Cerebral metabolic rate for oxygen
CNS	Central nervous system
COP	Colloid osmotic pressure
CPP	Cerebral perfusion pressure, torr
CSF	Cerebrospinal fluid
CVP	Central venous pressure
$\overline{CV}$ Po_2	Mixed cerebral venous oxygen pressure, torr
CVR	Cerebrovascular resistance (i.e., CPP/CBF)
DIC	Disseminated intravascular coagulation
EACA	Epsilon-amino caproic acid
ECF	Extracellular fluid
EEG	Electroencephalogram
EKG	Electrocardiogram (-kardiogram)
FIo_2	Inhaled oxygen concentration
FRC	Functional residual capacity
ICF	Intracellular fluid
ICP	Intracranial pressure, torr
IMV	Intermittent mandatory ventilation
IPPB	Intermittent positive pressure breathing
LGI	Lactate–glucose index
mEq/1	Milliequivalents per liter
MV	Mandatory ventilation
OGI	Oxygen–glucose index
PADP	Pulmonary artery diastolic pressure
PAWP	Pulmonary artery wedge pressure
PCWP	Pulmonary capillary wedge pressure
PEEP	Positive end expired pressure
SAP	Mean systemic arterial pressure, torr
torr	Toricelli unit (i.e., mm Hg pressure)

I

RESPIRATORY CRISES

Respiratory Monitoring

B. W. KIRK, M.D.
Department of Medicine, University of Manitoba, Intensive Care Unit, Health Sciences Centre, Winnipeg, Manitoba, Canada

Respiratory monitoring should provide information that safeguards a patient with respiratory failure on and off the ventilator. The information should both prevent disasters and allow control over the levels of oxygen and carbon dioxide in the blood. There are four levels of respiratory monitoring discussed in this paper: (a) disaster prevention, (b) mechanics monitoring, (c) blood-gas monitoring, and (d) derived-parameters monitoring.

This chapter begins with a review of the basics of respiratory monitoring and attempts to show how new developments fit into the systems that have evolved since ventilators first saw widespread use in the 1950s.

The philosophy behind the respiratory monitoring system is to provide adequate warning when something which could lead to death of the patient has occurred. Informal surveys still suggest that the most common cause of sudden death across North America during mechanical ventilation is mechanical failure and disconnect.

One of the most crucial components of respiratory monitoring is the alarm unit. The first alarm systems were set up to warn of disconnect or major leaks [1,7]. Every ventilator obviously should be equipped with an alarm that will sound if the ventilator, tubing, or patient mechanically malfunctions. The most satisfactory alarm currently available is the Bennett spirometer alarm modified to prevent someone inadvertently turning it off (Fig. 1). Inspired line pressure alarms (Emerson, Ohio 560) are useful as a backup for the volume alarm (Fig. 2). Ganging alarms can be used to increase the reliability of the system. For example, if the probability of alarm (not human) failure is 1/1000 hr, by using two noninterdependent alarms (e.g., $V + P$) the failure rate will be once in one million hours (1000×1000). Discipline in the setting, disabling, and reenabling alarms has been proven extremely important since most "alarm failures" are due to human error. Most intensive care units have a policy of never leaving patients on ventilators alone since the best disaster alarm available is still the nurse.

MECHANICS MONITORING

Tidal Volume

On the ventilator, tidal volume (V_T) is the most important parameter to monitor because it usually falls with the common disasters. Using a volume ventilator, a decrease in volume usually means a leak, pressure cycling from an obstruction, or minute ventilation beyond the capacity of the ventilator. Tidal volume on a pressure-cycled ventilator provides an index of changes in impedance of the lung and chest wall. The Bennett spirometer with alarm has been the most widely used device across North America and new developments are often compared to this spirometer in terms of simplicity and reliability.

MINUTE VENTILATION AND ITS RELATION TO a P_{CO_2}

Considering the patient-ventilator system, the P_{CO_2} is expressed as:

$$\text{a } P_{CO_2} = \frac{V_{CO_2}}{V_A} \times .863$$

where V_{CO_2} is metabolically determined carbon dioxide production and V_A is alveolar ventilation. V_{CO_2} is usually a slowly changing parameter, therefore, a P_{CO_2} is inversely proportional to V_A. Minute ventilation, V_E, consists of V_A and physiologic deadspace ventilation V_D. Thus,

$$V_A = V_E \left(1 - \frac{V_D}{V_T}\right)$$

where V_D/V_T is the ratio of deadspace ventilation to the total ventilation. The V_D/V_T ratio is usually a slowly changing parameter as well. It follows that at any value of a P_{CO_2} at a given minute ventilation, for example, a

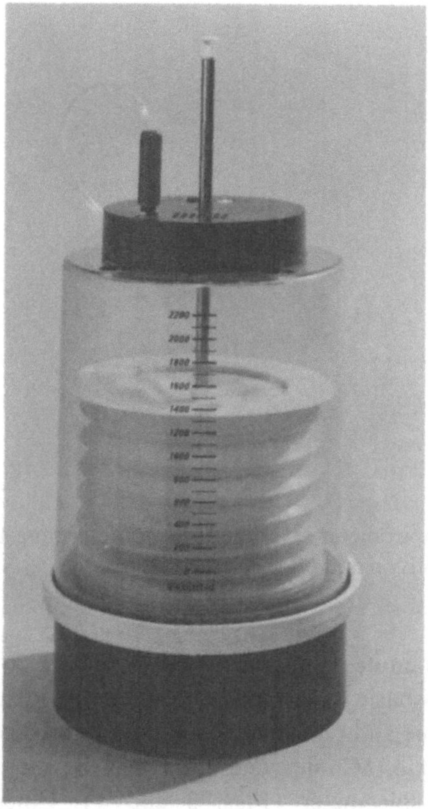

FIGURE 1 Modified Bennett spirometer with alarm. Placing the red plug in the phono jack disables the alarm visibly.

FIGURE 2 Emerson disconnect alarm. Responds to a drop in inspired line pressure or failure to cycle.

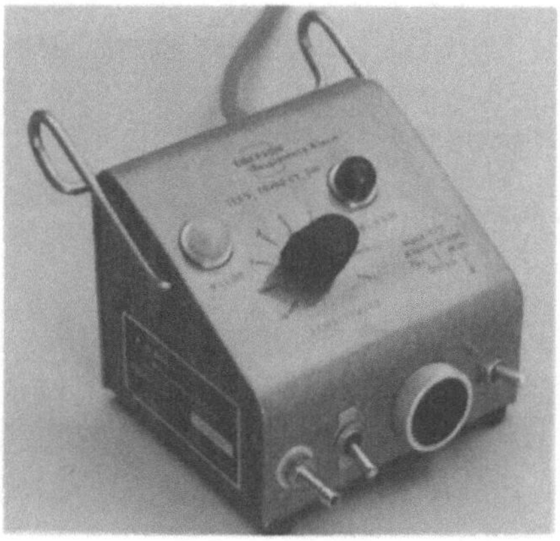

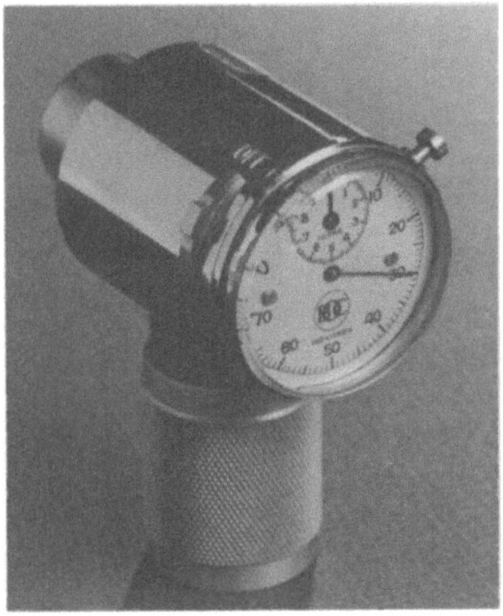

FIGURE 3 Wright spirometer. May be used to determine tidal volume or minute ventilation both on and off the ventilator.

25% increase in minute ventilation, will result in a 25% decrease in a P_{CO_2}. This logic is basic to systems of continuous or discontinuous monitoring of tidal volume and rate since the minute ventilation is the product of rate and tidal volume. Minute ventilation may be monitored using many devices, a Wright spirometer (Figs. 3 and 4), Emerson or Engstrom

FIGURE 4 Electronic Wright spirometer. Provides continuous readout of either tidal volume or minute ventilation. Current models are sensitive to prolonged wetting.

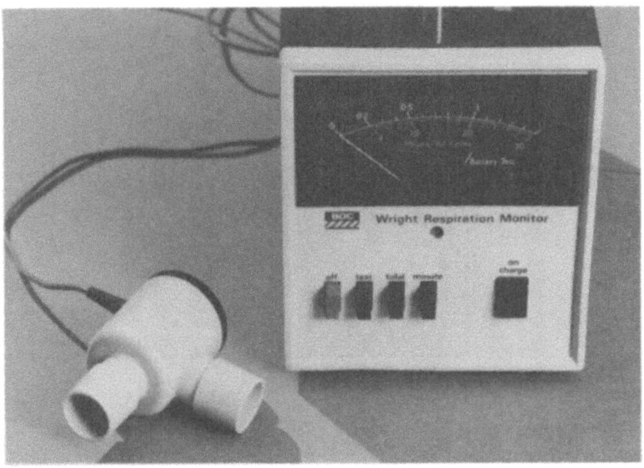

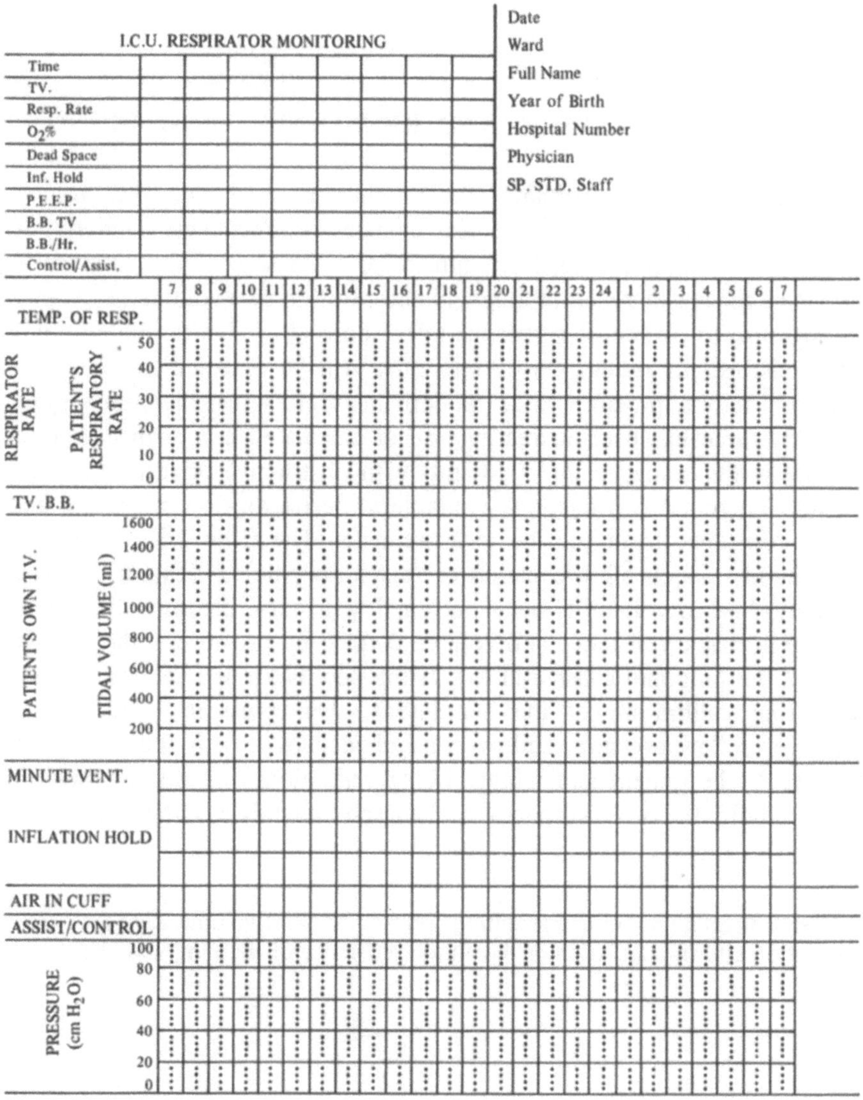

FIGURE 5 Respirator monitoring sheet used in Intensive Care Unit, Health Sciences Centre, Winnipeg. Changes in orders are recorded at top left. Analog charting allows changes to be seen at a glance.

spirometer, Bennett spirometer, or one of the newer pneumotachograph monitors (Cavitron, Monaghan, or Hewlett-Packard).

Changes in minute ventilation of > 15–20% should result in some physician response in terms of another arterial blood-gas sample, change in ventilator settings and/or acceptance of the new V_E and therefore a new set of alarm limits. Figure 5 shows the respiratory monitoring sheet used in the unit. Analog rather than digital charting allows changes to be spotted rapidly.

PRESSURE, COMPLIANCE, AND RESISTANCE MONITORING

On a pressure-limited ventilator the pressure is fixed and tidal volume varies, along with inspired time during changes in impedance. Similarly, on a volume ventilator the peak pressure reflects the sum of the pressure to overcome the elastic recoil of lung and chest wall to that volume (P_{el}), plus the pressure to overcome resistance to air flow (P_R). Unfortunately, only major changes in patient elastic resistance will be reflected in noticeable changes in total pressure since modern ventilators use high flow rates. Recently there has been increasing use of calculated compliance and resistance in the management of patients with obstructive or restrictive lung disease. There are two methods available to derive air-flow resistance and elastic resistance from bedside measurements. The Ohio 560, Engstrom, and Phillips models allow a period of "inspiratory hold," (Fig. 6). During the period when volume is held, but air flow is zero, pressure divided by volume is elastic resistance and volume divided by pressure is the compliance of the lung and chest wall [5]. If the flow is known at peak volume (requiring calibration of the ventilator), then pressure minus elastic pressure = flow pressure, and pressure divided by flow is the airflow resistance of the patient and tubing. Using ventilators that do not have an inflation hold, the two resistances can be approximately calculated as shown

FIGURE 6 Inflation hold. The static pressure and tidal volume at end inspiration allows calculation of the elastic resistance of the lung and chest wall.

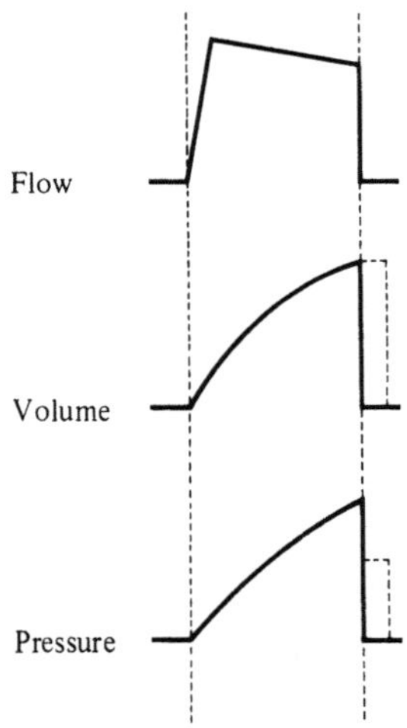

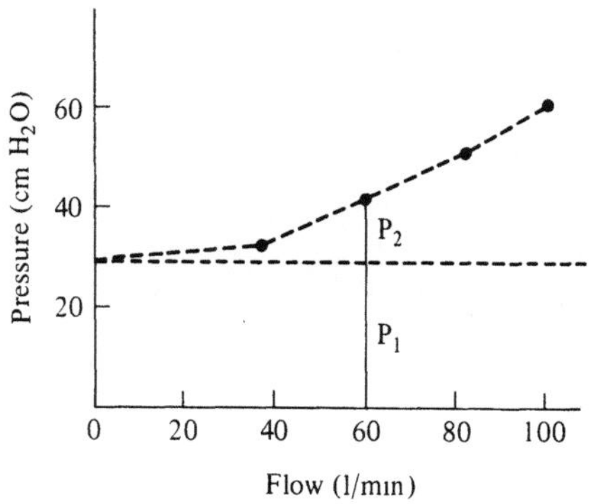

FIGURE 7 Method of calculating elastic resistance by extrapolating pressures to zero flow. If the flow is also known, nonelastic resistance may be calculated as well.

in Fig. 7. Several manufacturers are currently developing equipment that will give direct readout of the flow and volume resistance. When available, these should be useful in respiratory care. A number of manufacturers have developed electronic spirometers designed for use during either mechanical ventilation or weaning. There are two general types: (a) those using a turbine similar to the familiar Wright spirometer and (b) those employing a pneumotachograph which senses flow.

Turbine spirometers. These include the new Wright electronic spirometer and the Phillips spirometer (Fig. 8). In these devices the turbines have the advantage of being relatively insensitive to water droplets, a major problem with the pneumotachographs. Each allow either tidal volume or minute volume to be read on an analog meter. The electronic Wright spirometer has no alarms, fails if wet for too long, and is not suitable for continuous monitoring. The Phillips spirometer has alarm settings for tidal volume that work satisfactorily. There are no published data available on accuracy but we have observed this device to be both reasonably accurate and reliable. The inclusion of monitoring equipment on a ventilator is an important new development in respiratory care.

Pneumotachograph spirometers. Two of these units, the Monaghan and the Cavitron, use a heated wire to sense flow. The electrical signal proportional to flow is integrated to volume electronically. Great care must be taken to avoid water droplets or sputum on the wire. We have found that the most satisfactory arrangement is to mount the pneumotachograph transducer on the top end of an upright metal tube filled with loose copper mesh. Of the monitors currently available, the Monaghan is the most sophisticated (Fig. 9). A respiratory monitor marketed by Hewlett-Packard uses a Fleisch

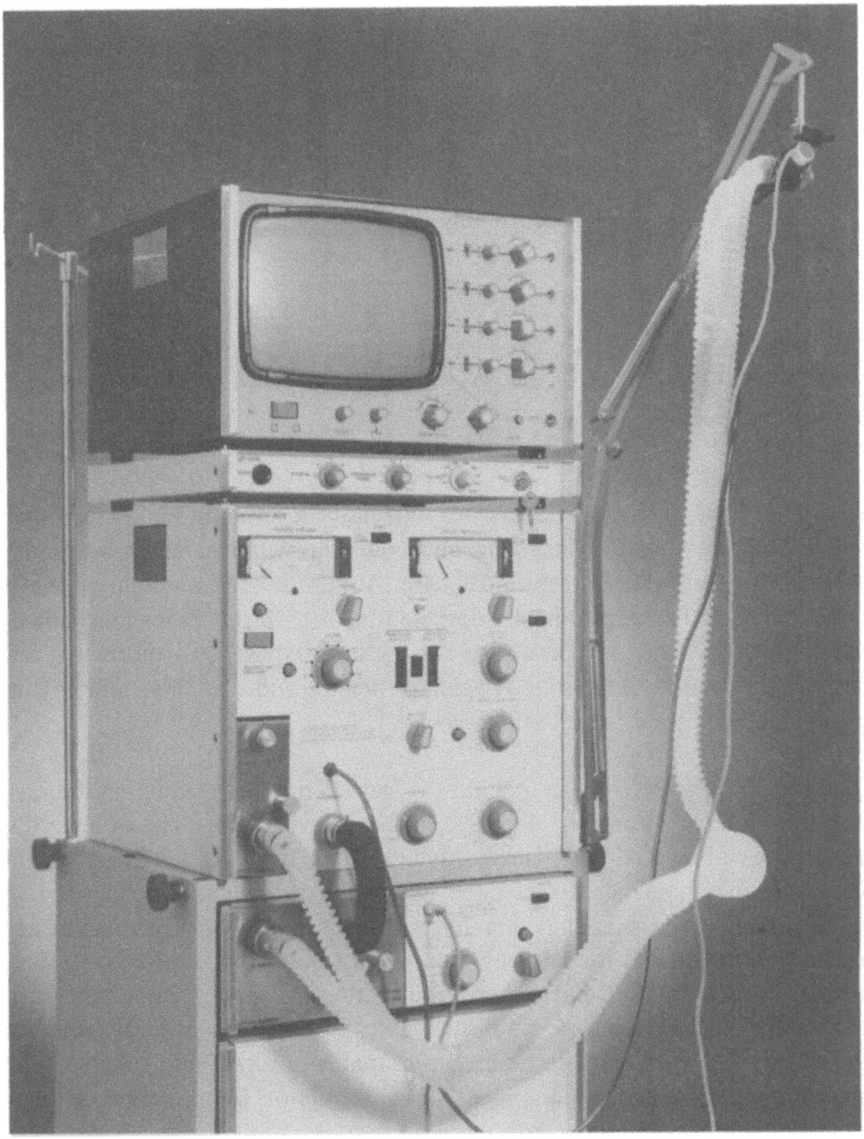

FIGURE 8 Philips AV-3 ventilator with built-in turbine spirometer. Combining ventilators and monitoring equipment is a desirable trend.

differential pressure-flow sensor mounted in the cabinet. It too is somewhat sensitive to water and particles. All of these monitors currently suffer from a variety of problems that sometimes make their use awkward. However, use of electronic monitors during weaning will undoubtedly become increasingly widespread, especially as the technical problems are solved.

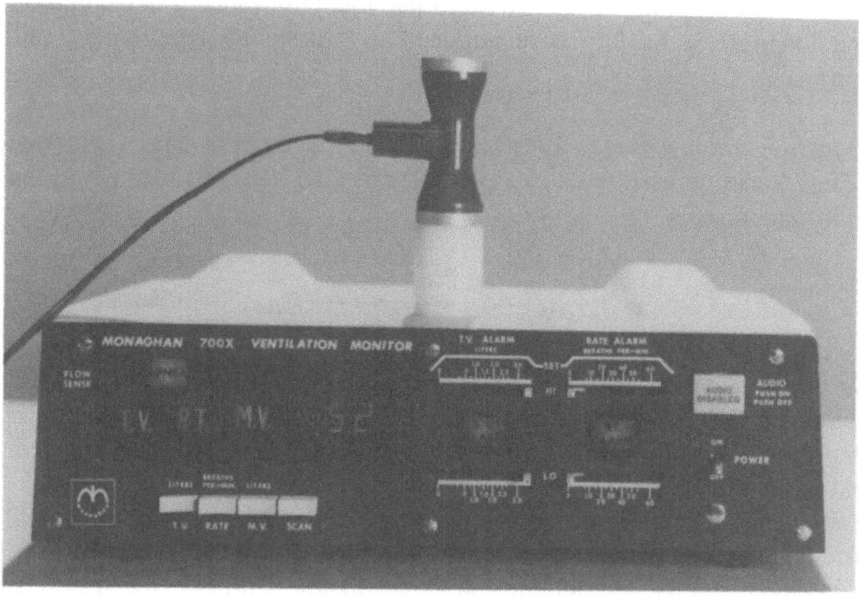

FIGURE 9 Monaghan Model 700 respiration monitor (modified). Although there are some difficulties in its use (see text), this type of apparatus allows monitoring both on and off the ventilator.

MONITORING INSPIRED AND EXPIRED GASES

Sampling of the inspired and expired gases on a ventilator provides additional information about the ventilator and the patient. The data serve as a base for calculations of other parameters [3]. In most centers the current approach is to collect gas with a syringe or bag and carry it to a central blood gas analyzer. In a few units a central mass spectrometer has been used to analyze gas drawn from each cubicle through metal tubing but this is expensive [7].

Oxygen. It is desirable to monitor the $FI_{O_2}\%$ (fractional concentration inspired $O_2\%$) or the FE_{O_2} (% expired O_2) to prevent oxygen toxicity, especially when using ventilators which have back pressure sensitive Venturi oxygen–air mixing (Bird). In addition, the partial pressure of expired O_2 (PE_{O_2}) can be used to approximately calculate the alveolar–arterial O_2 partial-pressure gradient ($A\text{–}aD_{O_2}$). To calculate aP_{O_2}, the following equation is used:

$$aP_{O_2} = (PE_{O_2} + PE_{CO_2}) - aP_{CO_2},$$

assuming $RQ = 1$. We have found gas sampling with a syringe is satisfactory for PE_{O_2} in the Bennett system at the bellows. A number of small oxygen meters are now available for in-line use, but problems in calibration and long-term reliability have not lead to widespread adoption of this approach.

Expired carbon dioxide. Mixed expired carbon dioxide partial pressure (PE_{CO_2}) can be used to calculate deadspace tidal volume ratio. Using the following formula:

$$\frac{V_D}{V_T} = \frac{a\,P_{CO_2} - PE_{CO_2}}{a\,P_{CO_2}}$$

the expired gas is collected in a syringe at the bellows of a Bennett spirometer or, better, in a Douglas bag. Accuracy of V_D/V_T calculations is improved if the effect of gas compressed within the ventilator is subtracted, but this is seldom done in practice.

End-expired P_{CO_2}. In normal subjects, this value is close to alveolar and arterial P_{CO_2} and theoretically should be useful as a guide to constancy of ventilation and in determining initial ventilation settings. Unfortunately, end-expired P_{CO_2} becomes inaccurate for this purpose in the presence of obstructive lung disease and thus is seldom used clinically.

BLOOD-GAS MONITORING

In most respiratory care situations, blood is obtained from an artery by direct puncture. Arterial catheters are used when frequent samples over a prolonged period may be required and/or when arterial pressure is directly monitored. The preferred sites are the femoral, radial, and brachial arteries. We prefer the femoral site, using a 15-cm handmade Teflon catheter. For continuous monitoring in vivo, indwelling P_{O_2} electrodes have been developed and used alone or in combination with electrodes for P_{CO_2} and pH. The mass spectrometer can also be used to continuously measure P_{O_2} and P_{CO_2} in blood and in expired gases as well. However, in vivo techniques at present are too complex and costly for routine use in the intensive care unit, having a current role in some clinical research. Thus for the present we must rely on samples of arterial and mixed venous blood taken discontinuously and interpolate between the values obtained. In our unit syringes of blood and expired gas are obtained simultaneously and analyzed together. This approach allows calculation of a number of physiologic parameters.

Blood and Gas Calculations

Some simple calculations allow the maximum information to be extracted from the blood and gas data. The calculations may include: (a) temperature correction, bicarbonate and/or base excess, and oxygen saturation and content, (b) V_D/V_T ratio, A–aD_{O_2}, and estimated shunt, and (c) arteriovenous oxygen content difference, calculated shunt, %.

Group (a) requires arterial blood only, (b) requires arterial blood and a syringe of mixed expired gas, (c) requires arterial and venous bloods and mixed expired gas [6]. Group (a) calculations can be done with a nomogram, Severinghaus slide rule, or calculator integrated into the blood-gas machine. Groups (b) and (c) calculations are most easily done with a desk top or phone-access digital computer [4]. We use the last approach in our unit, displaying the results on a cathode-ray terminal. The cost is low and the information is extremely useful in monitoring of the critically ill patient.

Large-scale integration of mechanical monitoring, gas sampling, blood-gas calculations and other respiratory calculations has not been attempted at more than a few centers because of the complexity of such systems and the high cost involved. The IBM system, which originated at Pacific Medical Center, San Francisco, has been in operation for more than 5 years and represents the state of the art in this area at the present time [2].

MONITORING OFF THE VENTILATOR

At the present time in most intensive care units, patients carefully monitored throughout mechanical ventilation are tested only infrequently during weaning, and most off-ventilator monitoring is done by "eyeball instrumentation" by the bedside nurse. Satisfactory methods of monitoring ventilatory parameters have only recently become available with the newer electronic spirometers for intubated patients. In nonintubated patients, respiratory data are available only with the use of either a nasal thermistor or transthoracic impedance monitoring through ECG-type electrodes. Ideally, the same respiratory monitor, humidifier, and FI_{O_2} gauge should be used during weaning both on and off the ventilator. The introduction of complex weaning programs such as intermittent mandatory ventilation or (IMV) has made this integration almost inevitable.

FUTURE DEVELOPMENTS

What has been striking in the last 2–3 years is the growing interest in respiratory monitoring, in both Europe and North America. Digital circuitry has made it economically feasible to perform many measurements and calculations not possible a few years ago. The future will undoubtedly see respiratory monitors integrated into ventilators. Ventilator-monitors will also provide for weaning and monitoring during weaning. Calculation and display of compliance and resistance should be available in a year or two. Programs for desk-top calculators now allow routine calculation of A–a D_{O_2}, shunt, andV_D/V_T ratio, even in small hospitals. The larger hospitals may opt for integrated systems in communication with a larger digital computer. Although this vision may be exciting to many people, including equipment manufacturers, there will be problems. Understanding of the process is often inversely proportional to the degree of automation. Finally, we should not lose sight of the fact that the challenge in health-care delivery systems in North America today is to make the important basics equally available to all who need them.

References

1. **Bendixen, H. H., Egbert, L. D., Hedley-Whyte, J., Laver, M. B.,** and **Pontoppidan, H.** (1965). *Respiratory Care*, New York: Mosby.
2. **Osborn, J. J., Beaumont, J. O., Raison, J. C. A., Russel, J.,** and **Gerbode, F.** (1968). Measurement and monitoring of acutely ill patients by digital computer. *Surg. 64:*1057–1070.
3. **Pontoppidan, H., Geffin, B.,** and **Lowenstein, E.** (1973). *Acute Respiratory Failure in the Adult.* Boston: Little, Brown.
4. **Ruiz, B. C., Tucker, W. K.,** and **Kirby, R. R.** (1975). A program for calculation of intra pulmonary shunts, blood gas and acid base values with a programmable calculator. *Anesthesiol. 42:*88–95.
5. **Suter, P. M., Fairley, H. B.,** and **Isenberg, M. D.** (1975). Optimum end-expiratory pressure in patients with acute pulmonary failure. *N. Engl. J. Med. 292:*284–289.
6. **Swan, H. J. C., Ganz, W., Forrester, J., Marcus, H., Diamond, G.,** and **Chonette, D.** (1970). Catheterization of the heart in man with use of a flow directed balloon tip catheter. *N. Engl. J. Med. 283:*447.
7. **Webb, W. R.** (1974). Symposium on pulmonary problems in surgery. *Surg. Clin. N. Am. 54* (5).

Management of Acute Hypoxia and Hypercarbia in the Patient with Advanced Obstructive Airway Disease

STEPHEN M. AYRES, M.D.
Department of Medicine, St. Louis University, St. Louis, Missouri

The treatment of acute respiratory failure in advanced chronic airways obstruction is strikingly different from that where the lungs are relatively normal and failure develops following some acute nonspecific insult. It is now realized that the patient with underlying chronic airway obstruction rarely requires intubation and can usually be treated successfully with carefully controlled oxygen administration. In contrast, the patient with the "adult respiratory distress syndrome" usually requires early intubation with controlled ventilation. Various differences between these two types of acute respiratory failure are shown in Table 1.

MORPHOLOGIC BASIS FOR ABNORMAL DISTRIBUTION OF VENTILATION AND PERFUSION

Chronic airways obstruction is a descriptive clinical term applied to a group of pathologic abnormalities. Most patients have elements of both chronic bronchitis and emphysema. Chronic bronchitis is characterized by hypertrophy of the mucus-secreting glands and inflammatory changes in the bronchial wall; emphysema is characterized by enlargement of air spaces

TABLE 1 Comparison between Two Types of Respiratory Failure

	CHRONIC AIRWAYS OBSTRUCTION	NONOBSTRUCTIVE FAILURE
Previous status of lungs	Abnormal	Usually normal
Cause of hypoxemia	V/Q inequality	Shunting
Response to low O_2 concentrations	Increase in Pa_{O_2}	Little effect
Minute ventilation	Normal or low	May hyperventilate
Ventilatory response to CO_2	Reduced	Normal or increased
"Pulmonary" diagnosis	Usually	Rare
Body buffer stores	Increased	Normal or decreased
Blood flow	High, normal, or low	Normal or low
Need for intubation	Rare	Frequent

distal to the terminal bronchiole due to destruction of alveolar septa and hyperinflation of surviving alveolar units. Narrowing of the small airways by inflammatory changes and accumulation of mucus produces obstruction to airflow and leads to hypoventilation of alveolar units; loss of alveolar tissue reduces the area for gas exchange and also decreases the retractive force of the lung parenchyma, further decreasing ventilation.

Whole-lung sections show areas of bronchitis and emphysema scattered throughout the entire lung; this random dispersion of pathologic lesions constitutes the morphologic basis for the nonuniformity of ventilation that characterizes chronic airways obstruction. Exertional dyspnea occurs when more than 20–30% of the total lung becomes involved in the emphysematous process, although the relationship between amount of emphysematous lung and symptoms of chronic airways obstruction is modified by the degree of small-airway disease. Abnormalities of gas exchange are not related directly to the maldistribution of ventilation but to the matching of ventilation to perfusion. In many patients, blood vessels within alveolar septa are destroyed along with alveolar tissue; since capacities for ventilation and perfusion are both lost, this matching of alveolar and capillary gas exchange remains normal. In other patients, blood flow through poorly ventilated regions is preserved, and extreme ventilation–perfusion mismatching evolves.

Oxygen and Carbon Dioxide Transfer in Chronic Airways Obstruction

The ventilation–perfusion mismatching is reflected by considerable variation in oxygen and carbon dioxide tensions (P_{O_2} and P_{CO_2}) in patients with chronic airways obstruction. Gilbert, Keighley, and others [5] studied the mechanism underlying chronic carbon dioxide retention in 30 patients and observed hypercapnia to be concomitant almost exclusively with severe airway obstruction. When studied during exercise, 15 of 19 patients with an $FEV_{1.0}$ below 1.3 l had a P_{CO_2} above 45 mm Hg; at rest 12 of 20 patients had a P_{CO_2} over 45 mm Hg. Those authors concluded that abnormal distribution of alveolar ventilation relative to perfusion was responsible for both retention of carbon dioxide and hypoxemia. Increasing carbon dioxide retention with exercise indicated that factors tending to increase the amount of metabolic carbon dioxide presented to the lung could also lead to an increase in P_{CO_2}.

Subsequent investigators recognized that the broad spectrum of chronic airway obstruction had two recognizable extremes: (a) the patient with severe airway obstruction but relatively normal arterial and oxygen tensions and (b) the patient with equally severe airway obstruction but markedly abnormal gas exchange.

West [11] has presented computer-simulated quantitative data showing that oxygen tension falls linearly while carbon dioxide rises in hyperbolic fashion with increased ventilation–perfusion inequality. Hyperventilation of unaffected regions maintains carbon dioxide tension at normal levels but is unable to raise arterial oxygen tension because of the shape of the oxyhemoglobin-dissociation curve.

A. C. Dornhorst described these two recognizable extremes by unforgettable names, the "pink puffer" and the "blue bloater." The pink puffer exhibits parallel reduction in ventilation and perfusion. Carbon dioxide tension is usually normal, oxygen tension is modestly reduced, and the patient is extremely dyspneic. Perfusion continues through poorly ventilated areas in the blue bloater; very low ventilation–perfusion ratios are found leading to severe hypoxemia, hypercapnia, and evidence of pulmonary artery hypertension. Filley, Beckwith, and others [4] showed that the pink puffer frequently had lower peripheral blood flow than the blue bloater and thus might actually have less oxygen available for peripheral utilization than the cyanotic blue bloater. It is significant in all cases that injudicious therapy with oxygen and sedatives, as well as pulmonary inflammation, may reduce regional ventilation and transform the pink puffer into a blue bloater.

The remarkable increase in arterial oxygen tension following administration of low concentrations of oxygen to the patient with chronic airway obstruction is due to the presence of large lung volumes with low ventilation–perfusion ratios. Figure 1 shows variation in response to oxygen administration between areas with low ventilation–perfusion ratios and totally unventilated areas—the true venoarterial shunt. Note that even small increments in oxygen concentration are effective in areas of reduced ventilation because of improvement in regional alveolar oxygen tension. If the region is completely unventilated, gas transfer does not occur and venous blood mixes with the arterial circulation regardless of the inspired oxygen concentration.

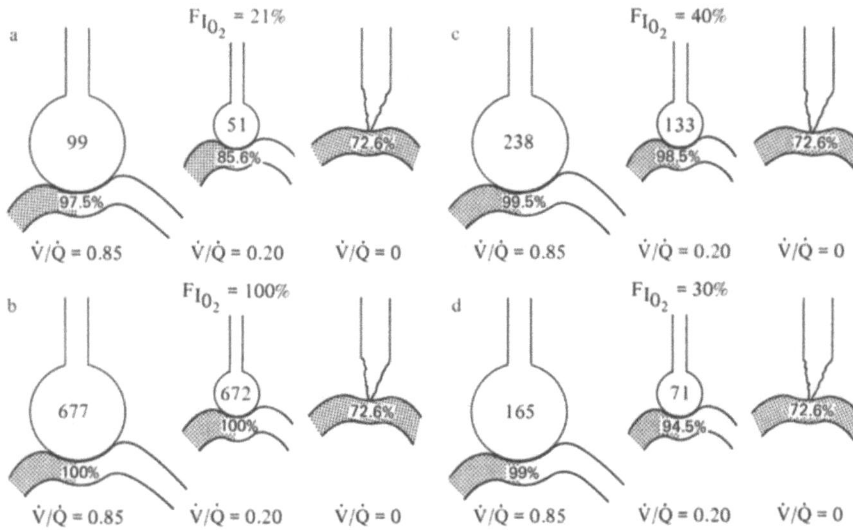

FIGURE 1 Effect of increasing inspired oxygen concentration. At the left is a normally ventilated alveolar unit with a V/Q ratio of 0.85. In the center is a poorly ventilated lung unit with a V/Q ratio of 0.20. On the right is a completely collapsed alveolar unit with a V/Q ratio of zero. (a) Capillary saturation breathing room air. (b) Breathing 100% oxygen. (c) Breathing 40% oxygen. (d) Breathing 30% oxygen. From *Care of the Critically Ill*, Second Edition, 1974. Courtesy of Appleton-Century-Crofts.

Respiratory Failure in Chronic Airways Obstruction

A sudden decrease in alveolar ventilation ushers in acute respiratory failure; carbon dioxide tension rises further, oxygen tension falls precipitiously. Viral or bacterial respiratory infections are almost always responsible for episodes of acute respiratory failure. Mucus and infected secretions obstruct the smaller airways, bronchial mucous glands hypertrophy, goblet cells occlude bronchioles and active bronchospasm further impedes airflow [7]. Increasing expiratory force produces airway collapse during expiration. Increasing airway obstruction increases the work of breathing (Fig. 2). More oxygen is required by the respiratory muscles and more carbon dioxide is produced, further intensifying hypercapnia and hypoxemia. Hypoxemia and acidosis lead to active constriction of the pulmonary vascular bed [3]. Pulmonary arterial and right ventricular systolic pressures rise; ultimately the right ventricle fails and right atrial and central venous pressure rise. Hypoxic stimulation of the bone marrow leads to polycythemia increasing blood viscosity and further increasing the workload on the right ventricle.

Severe acidosis is much less common when acute respiratory failure follows chronic airways obstruction than in other forms of acute respiratory failure. The buffer stores of the body determine the hydrogen ion response to acute elevations of carbon dioxide (Fig. 3). Note that a carbon dioxide

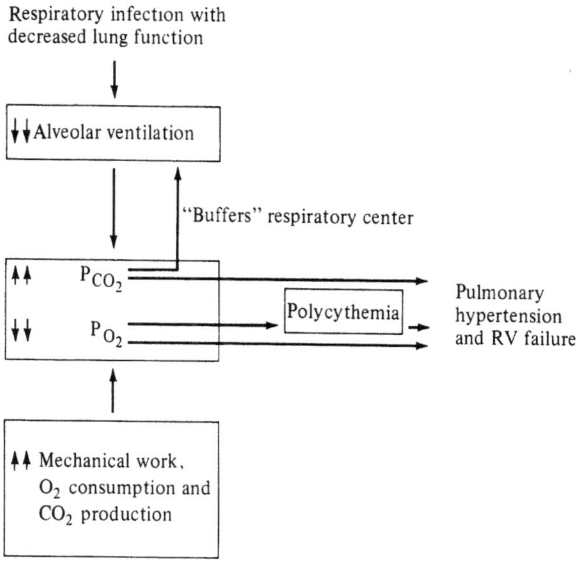

FIGURE 2 Sequence of events leading to syndrome of respiratory acidosis and cor pulmonale in chronic obstructive lung disease. Increased mechanical work increases the carbon dioxide production of the body, while decreased alveolar ventilation interferes with the clearance of carbon dioxide. While respiratory infriction frequently initiates the sequence, decreased respiratory-center activity due to bicarbonate buffering of medullary neurons and injudicious use of both sedation and oxygen lead to further retention of carbon dioxide. From *Care of the Critically Ill*, Second Edition, 1974. Courtesy of Appleton-Century-Crofts.

tension of 80 mm Hg in a patient with a bicarbonate concentration of 30 meq/l leads to a pH of 7.3, whereas the pH declines to 7.0 when the bicarbonate concentration is only 20 meq/l. Chronic elevations of body buffer stores protects the patient against subsequent acute elevations of carbon dioxide.

MINUTE VENTILATION IN RESPIRATORY FAILURE

Hyperventilation is an important defensive response that prevents carbon dioxide tension from rising early in the course of chronic airways obstruction. This defensive response is ultimately lost, however, when carbon dioxide retention leads to chronic bicarbonate accumulation within the central nervous system. Increased bicarbonate concentration buffers intracellular hydrogen ion and renders the respiratory center relatively insensitive to changes in carbon dioxide tension. In Figure 4, this reversible depression of the respiratory center is documented. During acute respiratory failure a low concentration of administered oxygen increased arterial oxygen tension from 44 to 88 mm Hg, and removal of the hypoxic stimulus to ventilation raised carbon dioxide tension from 56 to 77 mm Hg. The patient

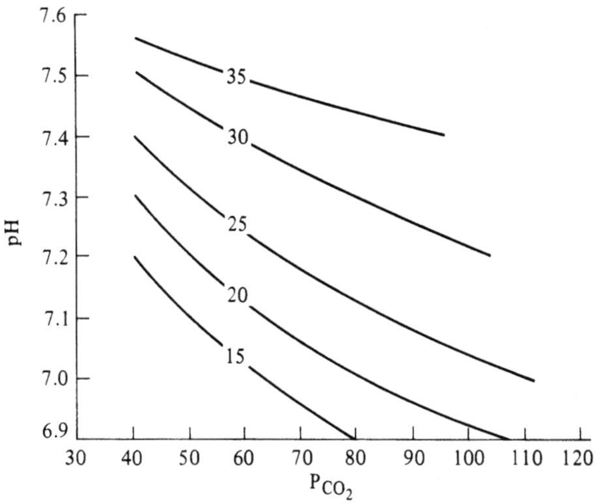

FIGURE 3 Variation in pH response to acute hypercapnia is shown for different plasma bicarbonate concentrations. Each curve represents the total body buffer effect to changes in carbon dioxide tension. Note the progressive flatness of the response curves with increasing plasma bicarbonate. Acute hypercapnia is obviously much more hazardous to a patient with normal or low plasma bicarbonate concentration. From *Care of the Critically Ill,* Second Edition, 1974. Courtesy of Appleton-Century-Crofts.

became comatose. Following vigorous treatment including the administration of diuretics, acetazolamide, corticosteroids, and antibiotics, the response of the respiratory center to oxygen administration was restored to normal. Sedation of any type can also precipitously decrease ventilation and lead to marked rise in carbon dioxide tension. McNicol and Campbell [10] emphasized that severe hypercapnia and acidosis in respiratory failure are almost always due to the injudicious use of oxygen and pH levels below 7.2 are never observed in the untreated patient; as they quoted Peters and Van Slyke, "CO_2 excess . . . is unlikely of itself to be of dangerous or even serious significance."

PRINCIPLES OF TREATMENT

Acute respiratory failure is due to sudden decreases in regional ventilation relative to perfusion; treatment strategy is directed to improving regional ventilation as quickly as possible and, at the same time, preventing severe tissue hypoxia by the controlled administration of oxygen (Table 2). Situations such as inactivity, unnecessarily high concentrations of oxygen, and sedation, which depress minute ventilation, must be avoided.

Low concentrations of oxygen should be administered immediately by either nasal cannulas or Venturi mask. King, Ali, and others [8] reported an oxyhemoglobin saturation increase of 15% following 30–60 min of breathing 24% oxygen, an observation predicted from the theoretic con-

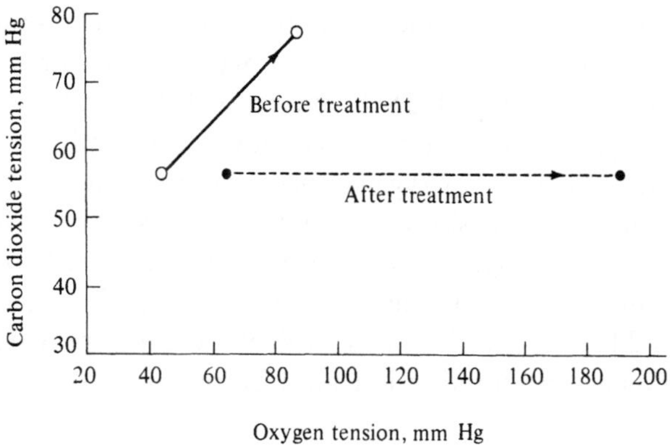

FIGURE 4 Reversible depression of the respiratory center in a patient with chronic obstructive lung disease. Prior to treatment a small increase in oxygen tension led to a decrease in alveolar ventilation and an increase in carbon dioxide tension. Following treatment, high oxygen tensions could be tolerated without changes in ventilation. From *Care of the Critically Ill*, Second Edition, 1974. Courtesy of Appleton-Century-Crofts.

siderations discussed above. Since a rise in arterial oxygen tension (Pa_{O_2}) from 50 to 75 mm Hg results in a mere 25% decrease in carotid-sinus nerve activity, while an increase to 100 mm Hg produces a 50% decrease [10], arterial oxygen tensions of 60–70 mm Hg are relatively safe. Optimal oxygen delivery should be provided in patients with concomitant circulatory collapse by raising oxyhemoglobin saturation to 95%; direct spectrophoto-

TABLE 2 Treatment of Respiratory Failure in Patients with Chronic Obstructive Lung Disease

1. Administration of low concentrations of oxygen (24–35%) by nasal cannula at flow rate of 1–3 l/min or ventimask.
2. Vigorous treatment including:

Bronchodilators	Antibiotics
Physical therapy	Steroids
Diuretics	Phlebotomy
Digitalis	Acetazolamide (Diamox)

No sedation

3. Intubation and controlled ventilation indicated if:
   - P_{O_2} cannot be raised to > 66 mm Hg
   - pH remains below 7.25–7.35
   - P_{CO_2} rises at rapid rate

   There are clinical findings of somnolence, coma, hypotension, or cardiac arrhythmias

metric measurements of saturation may be useful in such situations. The choice between nasal cannula and Venturi mask varies with each patient. The nasal cannula delivers 24–38% oxygen with flow rates of 2-3 l/min but arterial oxygen tension must be monitored frequently to protect the patient from sudden rises in oxygen concentration. A major advantage of the oxygen cannula over masks of all types is that it remains in place during eating, talking, or coughing. The Venturi mask entrains fixed proportions of room air and thus delivers a constant concentration of oxygen. Available for delivery of 24%, 28%, 35%, and 40% oxygen, they provide a precisely controlled oxygen concentration but must be removed for meals or other activities.

A decrease in airways obstruction increases regional ventilation and is the key goal of therapy. Adequate humidification of the inspired air, maintenance of hydration, purposeful and productive coughing, proper positioning in bed, and supervised walking or chair-sitting all assist in clearance of secretions, [9]. Mucolytic agents are useful in some patients, although acetyl cysteine has been reported to produce occasional bronchospasm. Nebulized bronchodilators should be administered at regular intervals; tachycardia may be avoided by using a preparation such as Bronkosol, which contains both α- and β-stimulating sympathomimetic amines. Corticosteroids are indicated if there is evidence of severe unresponsive bronchospasm, although the possibility of gastric irritation and stress ulceration must be considered.

Intermittent positive-pressure breathing (IPPB) is controversial and overutilized [13]. If properly administered by a skilled nurse or therapist, it may be useful in clearing secretions. A dilute solution of sympathomimetic amine in the nebulizer provides both humidification and bronchodilatation. The individual administering IPPB should be prepared to assist the patient in coughing and to perform nasotracheal suctioning if necessary immediately following treatment. An oxygen mixing valve prevents administration of excessively high concentrations of oxygen; under no circumstances should the unit be powered directly from a source which delivers 100% oxygen to the patient.

Infection should be treated by clearing secretions as described above and by administering antibiotics. Probably all patients should receive an antibiotic agent. Our practice is to obtain a sputum sample and begin tetracycline prior to identification of specific bacterial species. While this appears imprecise, there is considerable evidence that the administration of either tetracycline or ampicillin is effective for treatment of bronchopulmonary inflammation in patients with chronic airways obstruction.

Hypervolemia and polycythemia should be corrected by the use of diuretics and phlebotomy. Increased intravascular volume increases the work of the right ventricle, and interstitial accumulation of fluid within the lungs further impairs gas exchange.

Digitalis should be administered cautiously and only if specific indications such as left ventricular failure or supraventricular arrhythmias are identified. Since tissue hypoxia enhances the likelihood of digitalis toxicity, relatively low doses must be used.

Carbonic anhydrase inhibitors such as acetazolamide (Diamox) may be useful since they are believed to improve respiratory-center responsiveness by hastening changes in CNS bicarbonate concentrations. We frequently administer acetazolamide, 500 mg IV for one or two days but carefully monitor arterial bicarbonate concentration to prevent development of uncompensated respiratory acidosis.

Intubation and Artificial Ventilation in Chronic Airways Obstruction

The vigorous attempts to improve regional ventilation outlined above, together with the controlled administration of oxygen to relieve potentially fatal tissue hypoxia, are almost always successful. Campbell [2] reported only eight of 70 patients treated in this manner requiring intubation; Zwillich; Pierson, and others [13] reported 26 of 304 patients with chronic airways obstruction and acute respiratory failure requiring intubation. The clinical indications for intubations are given in Table 2. Inability to raise arterial oxygen tension to 55–65 mm Hg with low concentrations of oxygen suggests the presence of pneumonitis or atelectasis with venoarterial shunting. Since higher concentrations of oxygen almost always lead to hypoventilation and increased acidosis, intubation may be necessary. The conduct of intubation and artificial ventilation in the patient with chronic airways obstruction differs significantly from that in the patient with nonobstructive respiratory failure. Assisted ventilation and intermittent mandatory ventilation is preferable to controlled ventilation to prevent deconditioning of respiratory muscles. During intubation the patient should be allowed to ambulate or at least to sit for many hours each day. Extubation should be attempted early, even if arterial blood gases are quite abnormal, and should be based on the clinical appearance of the patient. A patient with an alert, responsive expression is probably ready for extubation. Tracheostomy should be avoided; the probability of increased tracheobronchial infection and loss of an adequate cough reflex substantially reduces chances of survival following tracheostomy. There should usually be several attempts at extubation prior to tracheostomy. If necessary, nasotracheal intubation may be continued for many days.

The short-term prognosis in acute respiratory failure due to chronic airways obstruction is excellent, whereas the long-term prognosis is dismayingly dismal. Gottlieb and Balchum [6] found a 66% death rate among 30 patients within two years following the first attack of respiratory failure. Perhaps nowhere in medicine today are preventive measures more fruitful than in the patient with chronic airways obstruction. More than 80% of all such patients are cigarette smokers, and the disease would not have developed had the patients been nonsmokers at an early age.

References

1. *Am. Rev. Resp. Dis. 6* (part 2), 1974.
2. **Campbell, E. J. M.** (1967). The J. Burns Amberson Lecture. The management of acute respiratory failure in chronic bronchitis and emphysema. *Am. Rev. Resp. Dis. 96:*626.
3. **Enson, Y., Guintini C.,** and **Lewis, L.** (1964). The influence of hydrogen ion concentration and hypoxemia on the pulmonary circulation. *J. Clin. Invest. 43:*1146.
4. **Filley, G. F., Beckwitt, H. J., Reeves, J. T.,** and **Mitchell, R. S.** (1968). Chronic obstructive bronchopulmonary disease. II. Oxygen transport in two clinical types. *Am. J. Med. 11:*26–38.
5. **Gilbert, R., Keighley, M. B.,** and **Auchincloss, J. H., Jr.** (1965). Mechanisms of chronic carbon dioxide retention in patients with obstructive pulmonary disease. *Am. J. Med. 38:*217–225.
6. **Gottlieb, L. S.,** and **Balchum, O. J.** (1973). Course of chronic obstructive pulmonary disease following first onset of respiratory failure. *Chest 63:* 5–8.
7. **Karpick, R. J., Pratt, P. C., Asmundsson, T.,** and **Kilburn, K. H.** (1970). Pathological findings in respiratory failure. Goblet cell metaplasia, alveolar damage, and myocardial infarction. *Ann. Int. Med. 72:*189–197.
8. **King, T. K. C., Ali, N.,** and **Briscoe, W. A.** (1973). Treatment of hypoxia with 24 per cent oxygen. A new approach to the interpretation of data collected in a pulmonary intensive care unit. *Am. Rev. Resp. Dis. 108:* 19–29.
9. **Lagerson, J. B.** (1973). The cough—its effectiveness depends on you. *Resp. Care 18:*434.
10. **McNicol, M. W.,** and **Campbell, E. J. M.** (1965). Severity of respiratory failure arterial blood-gases in untreated patients. *Lancet* 336–338.
11. **West, B.** (1971). Causes of carbon dioxide retention in lung disease. *New Engl. J. Med.* 1232–1236.
12. **Witzler, E. W.** (1963). The excitation of chemoreceptors by arterial hypoxia and hypercapnia. In: *Regulation of Human Respiration.* Philadelphia: Davis, pp. 173–182.
13. **Zwillich, C. W., Pierson, D. J., Creagh, C. E., Sutton, F. D., Schatz, E.,** and **Petty, T. L.** (1974). Complications of assisted ventilation. A prospective study of 354 consecutive episodes. *Am. J. Med. 57:*161–170.

Humidification, Nebulization, and Bronchodilator Agents

PETER SAFAR, M.D.
Department of Anesthesiology/Critical Care Medicine
University of Pittsburgh School of Medicine
Pittsburgh, Pennsylvania

PULMONARY CLEARING MECHANISMS

These defense mechanisms include: (a) ciliary escalator system—the mucus carpet carrying microorganisms and small foreign particles at a normal rate of about 1 cm/min from bronchioles and bronchi to the larynx entrance, (b) coughing, and (c) phagocytosis—macrophages in alveoli clearing via interstitial spaces (lymphatics) and upward via the ciliary escalator system. Maintaining the soft mucus carpet of the ciliary escalator system requires systemic hydration and tracheal gas with 100% relative humidity (RH) at body temperature. Normally, the nasal mucosa warms even cold dry gas to 37°C and fully humidifies it (100% RH; 44 g H_2O/m^3). The oropharynx is less efficient in this regard. Bypassing the nose with a tracheal tube and inhaling dry gas brings movement of the carpet to a halt. Thus when the nasal air passages are bypassed, inhaled gas should be supplied with at least 100% RH at 37°C.

The "primary humidity deficit" is due to the fact that most ambient air contains less than 100% RH. The "secondary humidity deficit" occurs when the ambient temperature is increased to 37°C. For example, air/O_2 bubbled through water and delivered into the trachea at room temperature with 100% RH will lose about 50% RH when warmed to 37°C. Cold humidification of O_2 is thus adequate only in patients breathing nasally.

To compensate for these humidity deficits, gas inhaled via tracheal or tracheostomy tube must be bypassed via a *heated humidifier,* which adds warm water molecules to the gas, or through a cold or heated *nebulizer,* which adds droplets (i.e., aerosol, mist). If the water is heated—not necessarily above body temperature—nebulizers can deliver gas supersaturated with water vapor.

HEATED HUMIDIFICATION

Gas is passed over a large surface of water by bubbling or cascading. The water is heated above body temperature and the gas is cooled to body temperature in the delivery tube on the way to the trachea. To avoid overheating the patient, inhaled temperature should be kept at about 37–40°C by a nurse or a servocontrol mechanism, readjusting the humidifier temperature based on thermometer readings at the airway.

NEBULIZATION

For *water aerosols* to soften secretions, about 0.45% saline is recommended as water may macerate the mucosa and isotonic saline may become hypertonic.

In order to coat the entire mucosa from the trachea to the terminal bronchioles, droplet sizes of about 1–10 μ in diameter are needed. However, particle sizes change before deposition. On passage into the lungs, some water droplets give off water molecules, and some conglomerate to rain out. Mathematical models on aerosol deposition have been only partially confirmed by experiments with tracer deposits and particles. Most particles greater than 5 μ in diameter will deposit above the epiglottis and in the trachea; most less than 5 μ in the bronchi and alveoli. Most particles of 1 μ or less pass into the alveoli, where most drugs given for bronchial effect are not wanted. One study showed that during nose breathing, 91% of labeled water droplets produced by jet nebulization and 83% produced by ultrasonic nebulization are deposited above the larynx; during normal mouth breathing, 70% of ultrasonic mist is deposited above the larynx. Only when breathing through the wide open mouth (or a tracheal or tracheostomy tube) can one expect about half of the droplets to reach the lower tracheobronchial tree [36].

Nebulization Equipment

Nebulizers are more complicated and thus less reliable than humidifiers. Most aerosol generators (nebulizers) use the gas-jet–capillary junction principle; the Venturi effect at the tip of a gas jet produces a negative pressure, which draws liquid through a thin tube and breaks it up into droplets of various sizes. A ball opposite the jet orifice and the nebulizer's housing and tubings act as baffles to cause rain-out of large droplets.

For aerosol administration of drugs, a metered dose, cartridge-type nebulizer is most popular. *Freon gas,* a propellant in these metered dose nebulizers (particularly flurocarbon 11), can depress myocardial contractility and produce hypotension and arrhythmias [1,16]. For spontaneous inhalation of drug aerosols in critically ill patients, we prefer use of a mainstream small drug-aerosol jet nebulizer (e.g., Bird), with the tail open and the patient breathing to-and-fro through it, with oxygen used for continuous nebulization. For aerosol administration of drugs via mechanical ventilators, sidestream jet nebulizers are usually preferred. Mainstream jet nebulizers are used for water-aerosol administration.

The narrow oxygen delivery tube is commonly used with cold humidifiers or no humidifiers in short-term use of resuscitation equipment. Heated humidification and cold or heated nebulization, however, require a large-bore oxygen/air delivery tube, since the narrow tube would become plugged with condensed water and squirt water into the patient. Ventilator tubings require a water trap to avoid obstructing the tube and drowning the patient with condensed water.

In the ultrasonic nebulizer ultrasonic vibrations of a base plate, transmitted via a coupling liquid, break up the nebulized solution into a dense mist. This ultrasonic mist is capable of thinning thick secretions, but has several drawbacks: (a) absorption of water into the bloodstream may overhydrate the patient, particularly the small child, (b) alveolar flooding may cause hypoxemia, and (c) irritation of the tracheobronchial tree may worsen bronchospasm. In status asthmaticus we use ultrasonic mist only when mucus obstruction is a major factor. After hypoxemia and hypercarbia have been corrected, a bronchodilator is used and administration is intermittent rather than continuing.

CLINICAL SELECTION

The therapeutic superiority of nebulization over heated humidification has not been established, for either the intubated patient with normal lungs or the nonintubated patient with uncomplicated bronchitis, emphysema, or asthma. There is no convincing evidence that the use of mist tents, popular for asthma and mucoviscidosis, is effective in lower respiratory-tract disease. They may even be detrimental, producing iatrogenic infection and bronchospasm [14].

Bacteria can grow in humidifier and nebulizer fluids but are more readily delivered into the patient via droplets. Particularly in hospitals without reliable programs of respiratory-care infection control, which should include regular (12–24 hr) changeovers of sterilized nebulizers and delivery equipment, the routine use of heated humidifiers is safer than that of nebulizers. One heats humidifier pasteurizes water and gas (70°C), and cools and further sterilizes it on the way to the patient through tubing filled with copper wool (Johns Hopkins Hospital, D. Benson).

MUCOLYTICS AND DETERGENTS

Little is known about the quantity and characteristics of bronchial secretions and their therapeutic modifications. The value of mucolytics and detergents is controversial, particularly for chronic obstructive lung disease [5]. There are isolated patient reports [28] that mucus evacuation is promoted by adding detergent, bicarbonate, and glycerin to the aerosolized water. However, small droplets of detergent may harm the surfactant mechanism in the alveoli. In patients with thick tenacious secretions or mucus plugs that cannot be coughed up, acetylcysteine (Mucomyst), which splits the sulfur bonds of mucopolysaccharides, may be of value; but it must be used with a bronchodilator, as it may provoke bronchospasm. Instillation of acetylcysteine via curved-tip bronchial catheter or bronchoscope is preferred over aerosol therapy. The use of alcohol (30–50% via humidifier; 5–10% via nebulizer) to produce an antifoaming effect in pulmonary edema is also controversial.

DRUG AEROSOLS

Drug-aerosol therapy is meant to produce effective concentrations of drugs at the levels of the tracheobronchial mucosa and smooth muscles, producing minimal or no systemic side effects. Limitations of aerosol medication include the fact that aerosols will not be deposited in obstructed airways. Drug aerosol inhalation should be slow, with several seconds of breath-holding to allow optimal distribution and deposition.

The *mechanism of action* of bronchodilators is not clear [26]. Stimulation of beta receptors in the bronchial smooth muscles causes bronchodilation. Whether or not alpha receptors are present in the bronchial smooth muscles is controversial. Alpha-receptor stimulation in the mucosa causes vasoconstriction and decongestion. Sympathetic amines seem to change ATP to cyclic AMP. The xanthines (aminophylline; theophylline) inhibit breakdown of cyclic AMP. Thus, both cause cyclic AMP accumulation in tracheobronchial smooth-muscle cells, binding calcium and thereby promoting relaxation through stabilization of the cell membrane. Secondarily, increased cyclic AMP seems to impede antigen–antibody-mediated release of histamine from leukocytes. Bronchoconstrictors cause accumulation of cyclic GMP (guanosine-3,5-phosphate), which can be blocked by atropine.

Bronchodilator administration should be evaluated objectively by determining improvement in wheezes and maximal expiratory flow rate or timed forced expiratory volume. During mechanical controlled ventilation with fixed tidal volumes, bronchodilation would cause a decrease in airway pressure. Reversible airway obstruction is usually due to some combination of mucosal edema, mucosal congestion, spasm of bronchial smooth muscles, bronchial collapse with air trapping, and viscous secretions. Bronchodilator drugs (Table 1) relax bronchial circumferential smooth muscles (bronchodilation) and relax longitudinal smooth muscle fibers in the alveolar ducts and sacs (pneumodilation). Alpha stimulators also produce mucosal decongestion.

Dosage and duration of aerosol inhalation must be individualized, since the patient's needs vary with age, weight, physical condition, and pulmonary status. Atelectasis and secretions create the need for increased drug dosage. "Pushing" bronchodilator catecholamine aerosols (with ECG monitoring) to slight tachycardia is justified in patients without heart disease. Some of the bronchodilators' aerosol effect seems to be due to systemic absorption of the drug.

Isoproterenol is a beta stimulator that provides bronchodilation without mucosal decongestion. When isoproterenol worsens hypoxemia, it may be causing pulmonary vasodilation and congestion; when it worsens bronchospasm, metabolites may be the cause. Refractoriness to isoproterenol may be due to inspissated secretions or blockage of receptors by a less effective drug, such as ephedrine. *L-epinephrine* and racemic epinephrine are beta–alpha stimulators, causing bronchodilation and mucosal decongestion.

The addition of *atropine* prolongs the actions of catecholamines. Atropine itself has regained some reputation in the treatment of asthma. It seems to offer little risk of thickening bronchial secretions in well-controlled asthmatics.

The addition of *phenylephrine* (Neosynephrine) or *cyclopentamine,* both alpha stimulators, prolongs the action of isoproterenol and aids mucosal decongestion.

The addition of *propylene glycol* and *glycerol* increases particle stability and deposition.

Isoetharine, now the most popular bronchodilator, gives almost as much beta-two receptor stimulation as isoproterenol (bronchodilation and vasodilation), while it produces less than one-tenth of the beta-one activity (cardiac acceleration). Metaproterenol and butylphenylethanol act similarly.

Antihistamine aerosols have not yet been evaluated. Drying of the tracheobronchial mucosa by oral or parenteral antihistamine is given as a contraindication for their use in asthma.

In *status asthmaticus,* the bronchodilator effect of sympathomimetic amines is decreased by acidosis. Catecholamine responsiveness can be restored and tracheal intubation and mechanical ventilation avoided in most cases by rapid normalization of arterial pH with bicarbonate [18]. This

TABLE 1 Bronchodilator Agents

AGENT		APPROXIMATE DOSE[a] (MG)	TIME OF PEAK RESPONSE (MIN)	DURATION OF ACTION (MIN)
TRADE NAME	GENERIC NAME			
Isuprel hydrochloride Aludrine Vapo-N-Iso solution	Isoproterenol hydrochloride 0.5–1%	0.25–1.0	10–15	60–90
Asmolin Asthma meter	L-epinephrine 0.25%	0.25–1.0	<5+90–120[b]	120–180
	L-epinephrine 0.5%	0.2–0.8	<5+90–120[b]	120–180
Vaponefrin Asthmanefrin automatic aerosol mist Micronefrin Solution A	Racemic epinephrine hydrochloride 2.25%	0.2–0.7	<5+90–120[b]	120–180
Dylephrin	Racemic epinephrine 2.25% Atropine 0.5%	0.2–0.7	5–10	180–240
Nebuprel	Isoproterenol 0.4% Phenylephrine 2% Propylene glycol 10%	0.2–0.8	10–15	180–240
Aerolone compound	Isoproterenol hydrochloride 0.25% Cyclopentamine hydrochloride 0.50% Propylene glycol 80%	0.5–1.5	10–15	180–240

TABLE 1 (*Continued*)

AGENT		APPROXIMATE DOSE[a] (MG)	TIME OF PEAK RESPONSE (MIN)	DURATION OF ACTION (MIN)
TRADE NAME	GENERIC NAME			
Bronkospray	Isoetharine hydrochloride 1% Phenylephrine hydrochloride 0.25% Thenyldiamine hydrochloride 0.1%	0.25–1	10–15	90–150

[a] Dose is always diluted with water or saline to 1:2 or 1:4 initial concentration (Aerolone always 1:4).
[b] Exhibit a double peak response; transient initial effect lasting less than 60 min.

should be accompanied by reoxygenation (e.g., by bag-mask 100% O_2 and bronchodilator-aerosol administration from a drug nebulizer interposed between valve and mask). Tracheal intubation is indicated in coma and when the patient cannot clear secretions spontaneously. Titrated intravenous administration of epinephrine [32], isoproterenol [10], or aminophylline (not effective via tracheobronchial tree) has "turned the tide" in some cases of status asthmaticus when obstruction by secretions render aerosol therapy ineffective.

Steroids by aerosol have been tried for asthma and other pulmonary-insufficiency states. In status asthmaticus, short-term intravenous steroid therapy is indicated, but is effective only after several hours. For chronic asthma therapy, the new drugs, *beclomethasone* and *triamcinalone* by aerosol, are said to be minimally absorbed and to have no systemic effects.

Cromolyn (Intal) is not a bronchodilator, but merely blocks histamine release of antigen–antibody reactions in the mast cells. When given by dust inhalation (it is not soluble), it sometimes permits weaning from steroid in young asthmatics. It has no place in critical care.

Aerosol administration of *antibiotics* seems to have little advantage in the prevention or treatment of pulmonary infection over systemic administration. There are several exceptions: (a) severe bronchopulmonary infections that fail to respond to bronchial clearing and oral parenteral antibiotics, (b) amphotericin B aerosol, which can sometimes cause remissions in fungal infections, and (c) prophylactic polymixin B nebulization, which seems to decrease the incidence of pseudomonas pneumonia in intensive care units, although it did not improve mortality from pseudomonas pneumonia [19]. Antibiotic aerosols should be used with a bronchodilator, as they are irritating.

Adjunctive Physical Measures

Aerosol inhalation should be reinforced with chest percussion, vibration, and deep breathing. Intermittent positive-pressure breathing has been overutilized; it probably can improve distributions of aerosols, break up secretions, and help deliver gas via collateral respiration channels into alveoli obstructed by thick secretions. Routine IPPB treatments have no proven value in chronic obstructive lung disease[1] or in preventing postoperative atelectasis but may be of assistance in acute atelectasis (via deep lung inflations), bronchospasm (with bronchodilator), and pulmonary congestion.

SUMMARY

In critically ill patients with nasal air passages bypassed, respiratory gases must be delivered with at least 100% RH at body temperature, in order to protect mucociliary clearing and other pulmonary defense mechanisms. The use of heated humidification (molecular water) versus cold and heated nebulization (water droplets) is discussed. Heated humidification offers less risk of iatrogenic infection. Nebulization (aerosol therapy) with water or mucolytics should be used for specific indications. Chest physiotherapy and adjustment of respiratory-care patterns are important adjuncts to clearing. New knowledge has been gained on deposition and persistence of inhaled aerosols and concepts of pulmonary clearing mechanisms. Aerosols have topical effects on the mucosa and a reflex and pharmacologic effect on smooth muscles. Very small droplets are favored for bronchodilator agents ($< 3\ \mu$), larger ones for other drugs, and large ones (5–40 μ) for humidification.

Choice and dose of bronchodilator and the route of administration should be according to specific indications (e.g., bronchodilation and/or decongestion of mucosa). Bronchodilator aerosols discussed include isoproterenol (Isuprel and Aludrine), racemic epinephrine (Vaponefrin, Asthmanefrin, Micronefrin, and Dylephrin), phenylephrine (Neosynephrine), isoproterenol/phenylephrine/propylene glycol (Nebuprel), isoproterenol/cyclopentamine/propylene glycol (Aerolone), metaproterenol (Alupent), isotharine (Dilabron), and isoetharine/phenylephrine/thenyldiamine (Bronkospray). Acidosis decreases the bronchodilator effect of catecholamines. A therapy protocol for status asthmaticus is presented.

[1] Objective data on aerosol therapy in chronic lung disease are scarce, and are almost lacking in critical care. Evaluation techniques have weaknesses. What is known remains to be synthesized and appraised as to its relevance in critical care.

"Bronchodilators" can produce bronchospasm. Bronchodilators and propellants can be "cardiotoxic." The value of and indications for other drug aerosols are controversial. Cromolyn dust inhalation is sometimes useful prophylactically in allergic asthma, but is not effective for treating bronchospasm.

References and Selected Readings

1. **Aviado, D. M.** (1975). Regulation of bronchomotor tone during anesthesia. *Anesthesiol. 42:*68–80.
2. **Aviado, D. M.** (1975). Toxicity of aerosols. *J. Clin. Pharmacol. 15* (part 2): 86–104.
3. **Barach, A. L.** (1948). *Physiologic Therapy in Respiratory Diseases.* Second Edition, Philadelphia: Lippincott, chapter 25.
4. **Barrett, J. P.** (1975). Clinical epilog on bronchomotor tone. *Anesthesiology 42:*1–2.
5. **Barton, A. D.** (1974). Aerosolized detergents and mucolytic agents in the treatment of stable chronic obstructive pulmonary disease. *Rev. Resp. Dis. 110:*104–110.
6. **Birnbaum, M. L., Cree, E. M., Rasmussen, H., Lewis, P.,** and **Curtis, J. K.** (1966). Effects of intermittent positive pressure breathing on emphysematous patients. *Am. J. Med 41:*552–561.
7. **Cheney, F. W.,** and **Butler, J.** (1970). The effects of ultrasonic aerosols on the total respiratory resistance of intubated patients. *Anesthesiology 32:*456–458.
8. **Cushing, I. E.,** and **Miller, W. F.** (1965). Nebulization threapy. In: Safar, P. (ed.), *Respiratory Therapy,* Philadelphia: Davis.
9. **Dalhamn, T.** (1966). Mucous flow and ciliary activity in the trachea of healthy rats and rats exposed to respiratory irritant gases. *Acta Physiol. Scand. 36:* Suppl. 123.
10. **Downes, J. J., Wood, D. W., Harwood, I., Sheinkopf, H. N.,** and **Raphaely, R. C.** (1973). Intravenous isoproterenol infusion in children with severe hypercapnia due to status asthmaticus. *Crit. Care Med.* 1/2:63–68.
11. **Dautrebande, L.** (1962). *Microaerosols.* New York: Academic.
12. **Finley, T. N.** (1963). Pulmonary surface activity and the problems of atelectasis, wetting, foaming, and detergency in the lungs. *Anesth. Analg. 42:*35.
13. **Forbes, A. R.** (1973). Humidification and mucus flow in the intubated trachea. *Brit. J. Anaesth. 45:*874–878.
14. **Gibson, L. E.** (1974). Use of water vapor in the treatment of lower respiratory disease. *Rev. Resp. Dis. 110:*100–103.
15. **Graff, T. D.,** and **Benson, D. W.** (1969). Systemic and pulmonary changes with inhaled humid atmosphere. *Anesthesiol. 30:*199–207.
16. **Harris, S. W.** (1973). Toxic effects of aerosol propellants on the heart. *Arch. Int. Med. 131:*162–166.
17. **Hatch, T. F.,** and **Gross, P.** (1964). *Pulmonary Deposition and Retention of Inhaled Aerosols.* New York: Academic.
18. **Kampschulte, S., Marcy, J.,** and **Safar, P.** (1973). Simplified physiologic management of status asthmaticus in children. *Crit. Care Med. 1*:69–74.

19. **Glick, J. M., DuMoulin, G. C., Hedley-Whyte, J., Teres, D., Feeley, T. W., Bushnell, L. S.,** and **Finegold, D. S.** (1975). Prevention of gram-negative bacillary pneumonia with polimyxin B aerosol (Abstr.). *Crit. Care Med. 3*:38.
20. **Luisada, A. A., Goldman, M. A.,** and **Weyl, R.** (1952). Alcohol vapor by inhalation in the treatment of acute pulmonary edema. *Circulation 5*:363.
21. **Mercer, T. T.** (1973). Production and characterization of aerosols. *Arch. Int. Med. 131*:39–50.
22. **Milai, A. S., Davis, G.,** and **Safar, P.** (1965). Simplified apparatus for IPPB/aerosol therapy. *Anesthesiology* 26:362.
23. **Miller, W. F.** (1973). Aerosol therapy in acute and chronic respiratory disease. *Arch. Int. Med. 131*:148–155.
24. **Modell, J. H., Giammonas, T.,** and **Alvarez, L. A.** (1966). Effective ultrasonic nebulized suspensions on pulmonary surfactant. *Dis. Chest 50*:627–629.
25. **Morrow, P. E.** (1974). Aerosol characterization and deposition. *Rev. Resp. Dis. 110*:88–99.
26. **Murad, F.** (1974). Mechanisms of action of some bronchodilators: cyclic nucleotide metabolism in tracheal preparations. *Rev. Resp. Dis. 110*:111–121.
27. **Nadel, J. A.** (1973). Aerosol effects on smooth muscle and airway visualization techniques. *Arch. Int. Med. 131*:83–91.
28. **Paez, P. N.,** and **Miller, W. F.** (1971). Surface-active agents in sputum evacuation. *Chest 60*:312 317.
29. **Parks, C. R., Alden, E. R., Stadaert, T. A., Woodrum, D. E., Graham, C. B.,** and **Hodson, W. A.** (1973). The effect of water nebulization on cough transport of pulmonary mucus in the mouth-breathing dog. *Am. Rev. Resp. Dis. 108*:513–519.
30. **Pierce, A. K.,** and **Saltzman, H. A.** (eds.) (1974). Conference on the scientific basis of respiratory therapy. *Rev. Resp. Dis. 110*:1–202.
31. **Proctor, D. F., Andersen, I.,** and **Lundsuist, G.** (1973). Clearance of inhaled particles from the human nose. *Arch. Int. Med. 131*:132.
32. **Safar, P.** (1973). IPPB: indications and complications. In: Caldwell, T. B., and Moya, F. (eds.), *Advances in Respiratory Care and Physiology.* Springfield, Illinois: Thomas, pp. 96–108.
33. **Sheldon, G. P.** (1963). Pressure breathing in chronic obstructive lung disease. *Med. 42*:197.
34. **Stuart, B. O.** (1973). Deposition of inhaled aerosols. *Arch. Int. Med. 131*:60–73.
35. **Williams, M. H.** (1974). Steroid and antibiotic aerosols. *Rev. Resp. Dis. 110*:122–127.
36. **Wolfsdorf, J., Swift, D. L.,** and **Avery, M. E.** (1969). Mist therapy considered; an evaluation of the respiratory deposition of labelled water aerosols produced by jet and ultrasonic nebulizers. *Pediatr. 43*:799–808.

Acute Respiratory Failure in the Critically Ill: "Shock Lung"

RICHARD W. CARLSON, M.D., PH.D., RICHARD C. SCHAEFFER, PH.D., URI FREUND, M.D., and WILLIAM FRENCH, M.D.
Shock Research Unit and the Department of Medicine, University of Southern California, School of Medicine, Los Angeles County/USC Medical Center, and the Center for the Critically Ill, Hollywood Presbyterian Medical Center, Los Angeles, California

Pulmonary failure has emerged as the single most lethal complication in the practice of critical care medicine. "Shock lung" or "adult respiratory distress syndrome" (ARDS) represents a clinical constellation often referred to as "shock lung." The purpose of this chapter is to review some of the current concepts of the pathophysiology and principles of management of acute respiratory failure (ARF) following shock or complicating a critical medical or surgical illness. Our own studies have been with special emphasis on fluid accumulation in the lung.

DESCRIPTION AND HISTORICAL PERSPECTIVE

The ARF syndrome is characterized by hypoxia—a marked decrease in arterial oxygen tension in the critically ill patient in the absence of acute pneumonia or chronic cardiac or pulmonary disease. Other causes of pulmonary failure must therefore be excluded.

[1] This study was supported by United States Public Health Service Research Grants HL-05570 from the National Heart, Lung and Blood Institute, GM-16462 from the National Institute of General Medical Sciences, RO1 HS 01474 from Health Resources Administration, and the Parker B. Francis Foundation.

Prior to and during World War I, pulmonary complications of injuries or shock were believed to be due to infection or atelectasis. However, some investigators recognized that patients often developed a delayed form of pulmonary pathology termed "secondary shock." In World War II, with vastly improved techniques for resuscitation and volume repletion, cases of "congestive atelectasis" or "wet lung" were observed more frequently. Pulmonary failure following resuscitation was even more common during the Korean conflict. During the Vietnam conflict it evolved as a major clinical problem (Table 1). Comparable disturbances of lung function were also encountered in civilian practice. Similarities between the adult form and hyaline membrane disease of the newborn were recognized. The increasing incidence of the syndrome was attributed in a large part to more effective resuscitation of critically ill patients who in former years may not have survived long enough to present with ARF. After resuscitation from a variety of shock states, including volume depletion, sepsis, traumatic shock, and myocardial infarction, ARF was observed. Aspiration, fat embolization, extracorporeal circulation, and the use of ventilators with high inspired oxygen tensions were also implicated. Multiple transfusions and the administration of large volumes of resuscitation fluids were suspect.

In the past five years investigators have sought a more precise description of the clinical syndrome to help clarify its mechanism and to improve its management. Moore and his colleagues [1] viewed the process as "posttraumatic pulmonary insufficiency" and regarded traumatic and hypovolemic shock as etiologic factors. He divided the clinical syndrome into four phases: (a) shock and resuscitation, (b) hypoxia, congestion, and hyperventilation, (c) progressive pulmonary failure, and (d) terminal cardiopulmonary failure. Although Moore's emphasis was on traumatic shock, more recent studies have directed attention to sepsis, aspiration,

TABLE 1 Historical Perspective of Acute Respiratory Failure in the Critically Ill

DATE	INVESTIGATOR	TERMINOLOGY
1927	Surgeon General	Secondary shock
1932–1945	Moon, Eaton	Edema, atelectasis
1945	Burford	Wet lung
1950	Jenkins	Congestive atelectasis
1961	Capers	Hyaline membrane
1962	Chu	Hypoperfusion
1967	Henry	Surfactant
1970	Thomas	Oxygen toxicity
1972	Ashbaugh	Sepsis
1972	Pontoppidan	Acute respiratory failure

TABLE 2 Acute Respiratory Failure. *Clinical Settings*

1. Perfusion failure
    - Septic shock
    - Trauma
    - Cardiogenic shock
    - Hypovolemic shock
2. Infection
    - Sepsis
    - Pneumonia—especially viral
3. Chemical injury
    - Aspiration
    - Inhaled toxins—O_2, smoke
4. Coagulation and/or embolization
    - Fat
    - Thrombin
    - Particles—platelets, white blood cells, etc.
5. Central nervous system injury and/or hypoxia
6. Toxins—autopharmacologic
    - Histamine, kinins, serotonin
    - Prostaglandins, catecholamines
    - Endotoxin

microembolization, disturbances of coagulation, and both autopharmacological and neurogenic reflex mechanisms as factors. The clinical settings in which this form of respiratory failure is likely to develop are summarized in Table 2.

Two major defects of lung structure and function are shown. Pulmonary extravascular fluid is increased. This may be regarded as a type of pulmonary edema. Abnormal distribution lung volume represents the other major defect (Table 3).

TABLE 3 Acute Respiratory Failure Pathophysiology

1. Increased pulmonary extravascular fluid
    - "Pulmonary edema"
2. Abnormal gas volume and distribution
    - Airway closure
    - Decreased functional residual capacity
    - Ventilation–perfusion defects

TABLE 4 Acute Respiratory Failure "Pulmonary Edema"

MECHANISMS
1. Vascular integrity
Permeability
Anatomic defects
2. Hydrostatic–oncotic
3. Insufficient lymphatic clearance

A hallmark of the syndrome is the accumulation of pulmonary extravascular fluid. Many investigators regard this as one of the earliest lesions. Fluid first appears in the pulmonary interstitium and subsequently enters the alveoli. The accumulation of fluid may be due to decreased ability of the lymphatics to clear the interstitium. An increase in the escape of fluid into the interstitium may be due to a defect in the endothelial integrity of the microvasculature. The balance of hydrostatic and oncotic forces between plasma and interstitial fluid may also be implicated. There may be either functional (permeability) or anatomic ("breaks") defects in the vascular integrity of the pulmonary arterioles, capillaries, and venules. The extent to which the bronchial circulation participates in this process in man remains unresolved. If vascular permeability increases, fluid resembling plasma escapes into the interstitium. Conversely, if structural alterations in the endothelium or its basement membrane develop, plasma as well as formed elements and cells are deposited in the interstitium. If lymphatic clearance is inadequate, the accumulation of interstitial protein may favor fluid egress from the circulation by its effect on the hydrostatic–oncotic forces between the vasculature and interstitium (Table 4). Several agents and conditions have been implicated in the genesis of pulmonary edema by affecting vascular permeability (Table 5).

TABLE 5 Pulmonary Edema Due to Alterations in Vascular Integrity

ETIOLOGIES
1. Perfusion failure (shock)
2. Sepsis
3. Embolization–coagulation
4. Chemical–autopharmacologic
Histamine
Serotinin
Kinins
Oxygen toxicity

An increase in microvascular pressure or interstitial oncotic pressure (COP), a decrease in plasma COP or interstitial or a combination of these effects, may also lead to edema. Pulmonary capillary pressure can be assessed by measurement of the pulmonary-artery wedge pressure (PAWP). Plasma COP can be measured directly or estimated from the plasma protein concentration. Interstitial hydrostatic pressure cannot be measured directly, and estimates of values for this factor vary widely. Pulmonary interstitial fluid has not been sampled in man, although in experimental studies pulmonary lymph has been collected and its protein content measured. The albumin content and COP of this fluid have been found to be relatively high, indicating that even under normal conditions a modest but not insignificant leakage of protein enters the interstitium.

For clinical purposes the risk of edema may be judged by measurements of the capillary wedge pressure and the plasma COP. If the gradient between these two factors is calculated (COP–PAWP gradient), one may predict with greater precision the risk of pulmonary edema. Decreases in this gradient to < 3 torr are predictably associated with pulmonary edema, whereas increases in the gradient may favor a decrease in the leakage of fluid into the interstitium. Sequential calculations of the COP–PAWP gradient are thus helpful in the management of critically ill patients. Several factors may be operative in the development of edema by affecting the hydrostatic–oncotic forces in the lung. These are listed in Table 6.

Major disturbances in the distribution and volume of gas in the lung develop in this syndrome. Airway closure, atelectasis, a decrease in the functional residual capacity (FRC) and compliance, with a corresponding increase in the work of breathing, develop in concert with the increase in lung water. Disturbances in the mucous transport, a loss of surfactant, producing further airway closure and a decrease in lung volume, secondary infection, as well as changes in Types 1 and 2 alveolar lining cells and macrophages, complicate the picture. Effective gas exchange is further compromised by ventilation–perfusion mismatching and diffusion blocks.

TABLE 6 Pulmonary Edema Related to Hydrostatic–Oncotic Forces

FACTORS
1. Shock and transcapillary refill
2. Overhydration–congestive failure
3. Oncotic dilution
4. Pulmonary capillary hypertension
Humoral, toxins, neurogenic
Autopharmacologic
Embolization–vascular obstruction
5. Interstitial colloid osmotic pressure (COP)

TABLE 7 Prevention and Management: Pulmonary Edema

1. Identify high-risk patients
2. Hemodynamic monitoring during treatment of shock
3. Avoid overhydration and oncotic dilution
4. Corticosteroids
    - Aspiration, fat emboli, sepsis, shock
5. Blood filtration systems
6. Adjust COP–PAWP gradient.
    - Restrict fluids
    - Diuretics
    - Oncotic agents
    - ? Digitalis
    - ? Dialysis

MANAGEMENT OF PULMONARY EDEMA IN ARF

The options for prevention, detection and management of pulmonary edema associated with ARF are shown in Table 7. The high-risk patient must be identified. Hypoxemia and the accumulation of edema fluid can be detected early in the course of the syndrome by sequential examinations of the patient, as well as frequent arterial blood-gas determinations. The chest x-ray will provide further documentation of interstitial and alveolar fluid.

Vigorous treatment of perfusion failure may decrease the incidence of subsequent pulmonary complications. Although the controversy centering on the choice of crystalloid or colloid resuscitation fluids has not been resolved, overhydration with either fluid may lead to edema. This may be partially avoided with the early use of pulmonary-artery pressure monitoring during resuscitation and calculation of the COP–PAWP gradient. Decreases in this gradient may be managed by restriction of fluids, diuretics, the administration of oncotic fluids (albumin), and, occasionally, dialysis and digitalis.

Ultrafiltration systems should be employed for administration of blood to prevent exogenous microembolization. Endogenous microembolization and disturbances of coagulation are treated primarily by correction of perfusion defects and infection. Pharmacologic doses of corticosteroid analogs may be of value in aspiration, fat embolization, and sepsis. Antibiotics should be employed for documented invasive infections and sepsis, but prophylactic broad-spectrum antibiotics may lead to the development of superinfections.

Table 8 lists steps in prevention and treatment of abnormal gas volume and distribution. Prolonged use of high inspired oxygen tensions ($FI_{O_2} > 0.5$) and lack of adequate humidification of gases is further injurious to the lining cells. Chemical injury to the airways may also be pro-

TABLE 8 Prevention and Management of Abnormal Gas Volume and Distribution

1. Identify high-risk patients
2. Prevent aspiration
3. Avoid prolonged $FI_{O_2} > 0.5$
4. Monitor Pa_{O_2} and A–a D_{O_2}
5. Physical measures
   - Position and drainage
   - Suction
   - Physiotherapy
6. Humidification
7. Corticosteroids (aspiration, chemical injury)
8. Antibiotics
9. Intubation, volume ventilator, high tidal volumes, positive end-expiratory pressure.
10. Extracorporeal oxygenation in fulminant cases

duced by aspiration of intestinal contents or inhaled toxins such as smoke. If the patient presents with tachypnea, dyspnea, cyanosis, and congestion, hypoxia is present, usually with a decrease in the Pa_{CO_2}, an increase in dead space to tidal volume ratio (V_D/V_T), and a sharp reduction in the FRC.

Physical measures, including frequent changes in the position of the patient, suctioning, humidification of inspired gases, and physiotherapy, constitute vital elements in the management of ARF. Corticosteroids are of value in cases with aspiration. When hypoxia, atelectasis, and the work of breathing persist or worsen, endotracheal intubation and mechanical ventilation with generous tidal volumes are indicated.

The use of positive end-expiratory pressure (PEEP) has revolutionized the management of this form of respiratory failure. With careful monitoring of the hemodynamic effects of PEEP, this modality can facilitate improvement in oxygenation, help prevent airway closure and atelectasis, and allow for a reduction in the FI_{O_2}.

A trial of extracorporeal membrane oxygenation may be selected in certain cases when this method of therapy is available and the course has not been reversed by conventional measures. Effectiveness of extracorporeal techniques, however, is not proven.

Reference

1. **Moore, F. D., Lyons, J. H., Pierce, E. C., Jr., Morgan, A. P., Jr., Drinker, P. A., MacArthur, J. D.,** and **Dammin, G. J.** (1969). *Post Traumatic Pulmonary Insuffiency*. Philadelphia: Saunders.

Selected Readings

Pontoppidan, H., Geffin, B., and **Lowenstein, E.** (1972). Acute respiratory failure in the adult. *New Engl. J. Med. 287:*690,743,799.

Robin, E. D., Cross, C. E., and **Zelis, R.** (1973). Pulmonary edema. *New Engl. J. Med. 288:*239,292.

Staub, N. C. (1974). Pulmonary edema. *Physiol. Rev. 54:*678.

Mechanical Ventilators: Critical Assessment and Methods of Use

B. W. KIRK, M.D. and W. L. MACKEEN, R.R.T.
Department of Medicine, University of Manitoba, Department of Respiratory Technology and Intensive Care Unit,
Health Sciences Centre, Winnipeg, Manitoba, Canada

INTRODUCTION

We use a "consumer-report" format in this chapter to present information on a variety of ventilators. Given a limitless budget, we would buy the most versatile, reliable, and powerful ventilator available. Where funds are limited, however, the physician may have great difficulty deciding what is best in terms of his needs and the funds available. Furthermore, there has as yet been no attempt to critically evaluate each new ventilator by an unbiased central agency, and comparisons based on manufacturers' claims can be misleading.

The evaluations in this chapter reflect the experience of an intensive care unit in a teaching hospital. Because of our teaching role, we try to have all ventilators available for use by our trainees. Unfortunately, two newer ventilators (Searle and Gill) are not yet available for evaluation in Canada. Hence we are only able to give the specifications provided by the manufacturer (see Table 1).

TABLE 1 Manufacturers' Specifications. *Adult Ventilators*

CHARACTERISTICS	BIRD MARK 7	BEN-NETT PR II	MONA-GHAN 225	GILL I	EMER-SON POST-OP	OHIO M560	SEARLE VVA	BEN-NETT MA I	ENG-STROM ER312/322	PHILIPS AV 3
Canadian price	$1,000	$1,295	$3,500	$4,025	$4,111	$4,500	$4,945	$5,680	$6,570	$6,905
Price code	1–3	1–4	1–6	1–6	1–4, 6	1–6	1–6	1–6	1–6	1–6
Electric	–	–	–	+	+	+	+	+	+	+
Pneumatic	+	+	+	–	–	–	–	–	–	–
Pressure cycle	+	+	+	–	–	–	–	–	–	–
Time cycle	–	+	+	+	+	–	–	–	–	–
Volume cycle	–	–	+	+	–	+	+	+	+	–
Assistor	+	+	+	+	–	+	+	+	–	+
Controller	–	–	+	+	+	+	–	–	+	–
Assistor–controller	+	+	+	+	–	+	+	+	–	+
Rate range	6–60	6–45	4–60	6–60	5–55	4–60	5–60	6–60	12–35	6–60
Volume range (ml)	Pressure dependent	100/2200	100/3300	150/2100	0/2000	0/2200	300/2200	0/2200	N.A.	50/1800
Big breaths	–	–	–	+	+	+	+	+	–	+
Maximum pressure (cm/H_2O)	40	45–50	80	100	100	100	100	80	90	100
Maximum flow rate (l/min)	110[A]	110[A]	100[C]	120[N.A.]	N.A.	140[B]	200[N.A.]	100[A]	N.A.	150[A]

Sensitivity control	+	+	+	+	—	+	+	+	—	+
Nebulizer	+	+	+	+	—	—	—	+	—	+
FI_{O_2} range	40 & 100	60 & 100	21–100	21–100	21–100	21–100	21–100	21–100	21–100	21–100
FI_{O_2} accuracy	Venturi	Venturi	±5%	N.A.	±2%	±3%	±3%	±2%	±2%	N.A.
PEEP	—	—	+	+	—	+	+	+*	+	+*
Inflation hold	—	—	—	+	—	+	—	—	+	+
Disconnect alarm	—	—	—	+	—	+	+	—	+	+
Volume alarm	—	+*	+	+	—	—	+*	+*	—	+
Rate alarm	—	—	+	—	—	—	—	—	—	+
Failure to cycle	—	—	—	+	—	+	+	—	+	—
Pressure alarm	—	—	—	+	—	+	+	+	+	+

Legend:

PRICE CODE
(1) Basic unit
(2) Humidifier
(3) Patient circuit
(4) Spirometer
(5) PEEP attachment
(6) Alarm-system component

FLOW RATE
(A) Unrestricted flow
(B) 40 cm H_2O back pressure
(C) 100 cm H_2O back pressure

OTHER CODES
+ Feature present
— Feature absent
N.A. Not advertised
* Available as attachment

CHOOSING A VENTILATOR

Volume- or Pressure-cycled

For the adult we believe that a lower-priced time- or volume-cycled ventilator is usually superior to a pressure-cycled machine. To maintain a constant minute ventilation, too much nursing time may be spent adjusting a pressure-cycled ventilator; this is valuable time better spent looking after the patient. A combination of volume- and pressure-cycled ventilators can also lead to confusion in monitoring, alarm settings, and adjustments. For these reasons and because of many restrictions due to their relatively simple design, there is a steady trend away from pressure cycled ventilators in the intensive care unit despite their lower cost.

Electric or Pneumatic

The choice will often depend on the funds available. The low cost Bird and PR II are good transport ventilators because of their small size. The newer fluidic pneumatic ventilators (Monaghan 225) may have a high gas consumption even on standby but have greater power. This would be a poor ventilator in any location relying on tanks of oxygen unless shut off at the tank when not running. The electric ventilators, although more expensive initially, do not need compressed air, are generally more reliable, and their use throughout an intensive care unit could negate the need for a large air compressor.

Assistor Controller or Controller

Beginning with the Bird and Engstrom, opinions in Europe and North America have varied regarding this choice. The European attitude is that the doctor should determine the minute ventilation. The North American attitude favors letting the patient set his own rate under most circumstances. A controller will work optimally postoperatively, with sedation or spontaneous deep coma, and minimally in head injuries and lung injury where there is a high central or peripherally mediated respiratory drive. Emerson, the North American manufacturer of a strict controller, remains popular because of its simplicity, reliability, and low noise level, but our own bias is to let the patient assist where possible and thus we do not consider the controller a good investment.

Oyxgen Concentration (FI_{O_2})

Venturi operated air-mix controls tend to decrease air entrainment as the mouth pressure rises. The Bird, although nominally delivering 40% O_2, shows a rapidly rising FI_{O_2} as pressure rises in the patient circuit. The PR II is less back-pressure dependent but only 60% or 100% O_2 is available. It is necessary to use an air–oxygen blender to achieve a range of accurate

FI_{O_2} on these ventilators, adding to their cost. The Emerson and Engstrom both use a proportioning system and the added oxygen must be calculated from the minute ventilation; however, this is somewhat awkward.

The newer bellows-driven ventilators supply FI_{O_2} with an accuracy of ±5% or better over the entire range of 21–100%. This is extremely useful in the management of patients with hypoxemic respiratory failure, where a gradual decrease in FI_{O_2} is part of the management. In our experience the accuracy and reliability of FI_{O_2} on the Bennett MA I has been above average.

Maximum Flow Rate and Pressure

The ability of a ventilator to continue to deliver a high minute ventilation in the face of a high resistance is determined by the output power. The engineering concepts involved are beyond the scope of this chapter but are reviewed in another publication [2]. Most volume ventilators have adequate power to ventilate a severe asthmatic or a patient with rigid lungs. However, neither the PR II nor the Bird will provide a high minute ventilation at high pressures, because of control pressure and rate limitations in the PR II and low flows and low cutoff pressure in the Bird Mark 7. High flow rates are important in shortening inspired time in patients with severe airway obstruction; thus the use of these low cost ventilators must be restricted to patients with relatively normal lungs and chest wall.

ADVANTAGES AND DISADVANTAGES OF SPECIFIC VENTILATORS

Gas Powered, Pressure-cycled Ventilators

BIRD MARK 7 AND BIRD MARK 8

Advantages. These models are of lowest cost and small size and can double as IPPB machines. They are easy to repair and have high sensitivity and a wide range of tidal volumes. They can be used as transport ventilators and are safe and effective for use with infants.

Disadvantages. Tidal volumes vary with resistance, these models have less power and lower flow rates than most ventilators, and FI_{O_2} can reach toxic levels in some situations. There are neither PEEP attachments, disconnect alarms, nor spirometer accessories on these units.

BENNETT PR II

Advantages. This model is of lower cost than most ventilators and small size. It can double as an IPPB machine and be time-cycled, and FI_{O_2} on air mix is relatively stable at 60%. This unit can be used upright as a transport ventilator, and its accessories include an effective spirometer and humidifier.

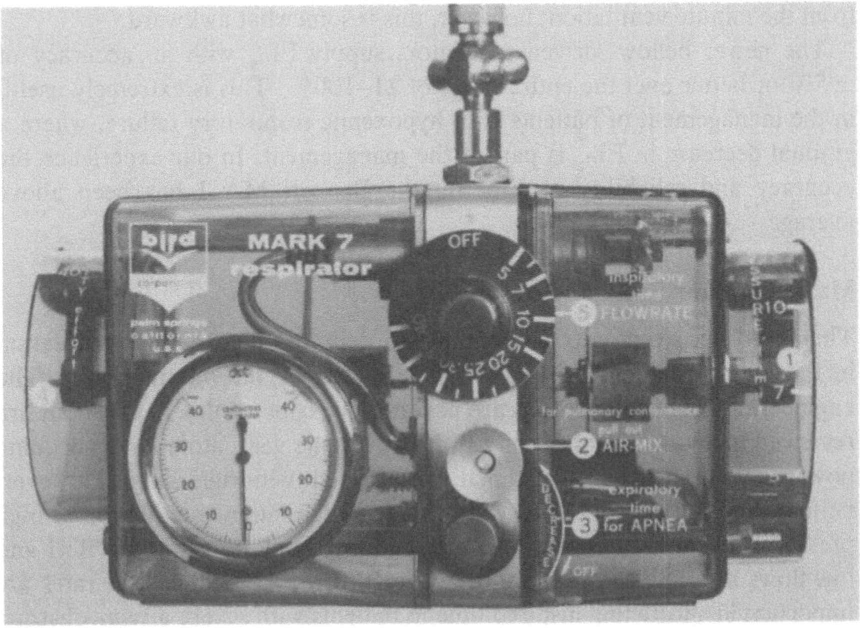

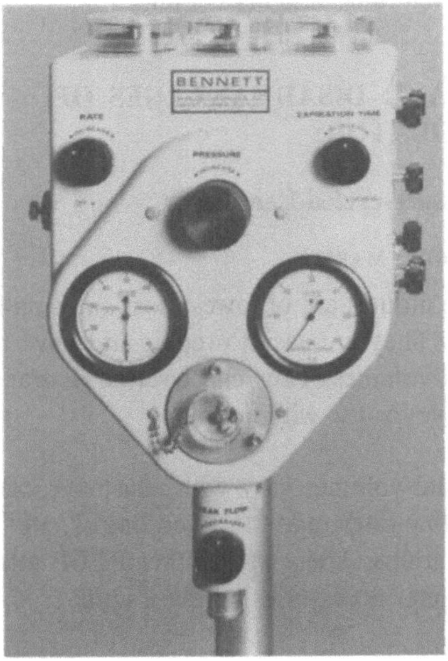

FIGURE 1 Top: Bird Mark 7 ventilator: useful all-purpose ventilator–IPPB machine for the small hospital. A good transport ventilator but not recommended for routine use in intensive care units. Bottom: Bennett PR II Ventilator: Can double as IPPB and ventilator in small hospital. May be used as intensive care unit ventilator in time cycled mode (see text).

Disadvantages. This model requires frequent maintenance, and its tidal volume can vary somewhat with resistance in time-cycled mode. It will not function above rate of 30/min on most adults, and FI_{O_2} is not variable (60% and 100% only). There are neither attachment nor disconnect alarms on this unit.

Electrically Operated Strict Controllers

EMERSON 3 PV

Advantages. This model is very quiet, needs fewer repairs than most, and has good power. It has an optional disconnect alarm, spirometer, a good PEEP attachment, and an IMV accessory.

Disadvantages. This model functions only as a controller, and the FI_{O_2} is difficult to set. There is no oxygen alarm, and the spirometer does not have low-volume alarm.

ENGSTROM ER 312/322

Advantages. This model is well constructed, very quiet, its major parts are autoclaveable, and it has good power and maximum flows. It has a spirometer, a disconnect alarm, and "inflation hold." This unit requires fewer repairs than most.

Disadvantages. This model functions only as a controller, is more expensive than most, and FI_{O_2} is difficult to set. There is neither low-volume alarm nor low-oxygen alarm.

Gas-powered, Volume-cycled

MONAGHAN 225

Advantages. This model is of lower cost than other volume ventilators and medium size. It has good power and flows and variable FI_{O_2} (21–100%). Accessories include humidifier, electronic spirometer, and PEEP attachment.

Disadvantages. The tidal volume of this model is somewhat awkward to adjust, and there is high gas consumption due to fluidic circuits (8–10 l/min in off position). Also, the electronic spirometer adds significantly to cost. The frequency of repairs is not established.

GILL AND SEARLE

There is no information available in Canada from users of these ventilators at this time.

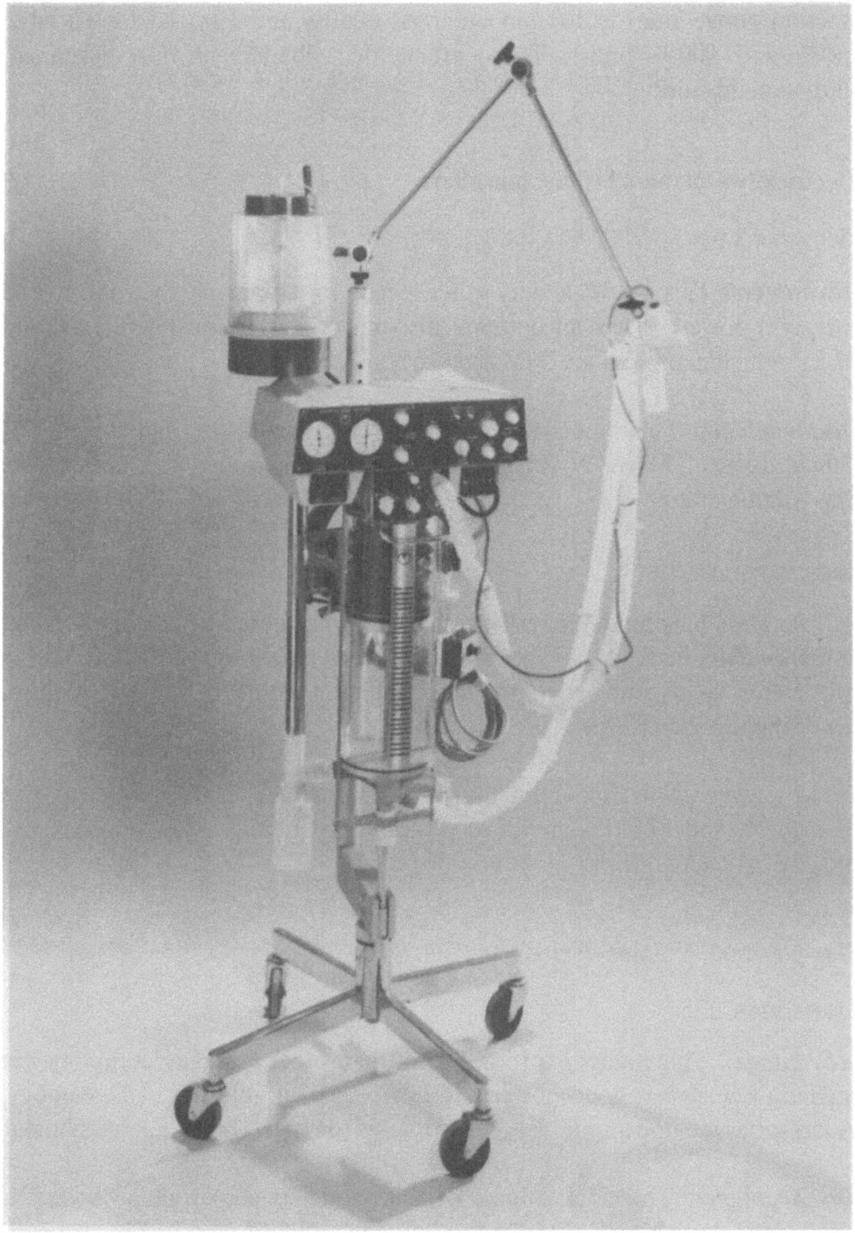

FIGURE 2 Monaghan 225 ventilator equipped with bellows spirometer: A "best-buy" general-purpose volume ventilator.

BENNETT MA I

Advantages. It has an easily adjustable tidal volume, good power, and maximum flows. There are alarms for overpressure, I/E ratio, and low-oxygen gauge. This model requires fewer repairs than most. It has a nebulizer outlet, PEEP attachment, and sigh. The accuracy is excellent. The spirometer accessory has a low-volume alarm, and the humidifier is the heated-water type.

Disadvantages. This model is somewhat noisy, has no rate meter, and is of relatively large size. Rate will not go below 6/min and therefore limits IMV (an IMV card is available from the manufacturer). Also, there is no low-pressure disconnect alarm.

FIGURE 3 Bennett MA I ventilator: A reliable volume ventilator for the seriously ill patient.

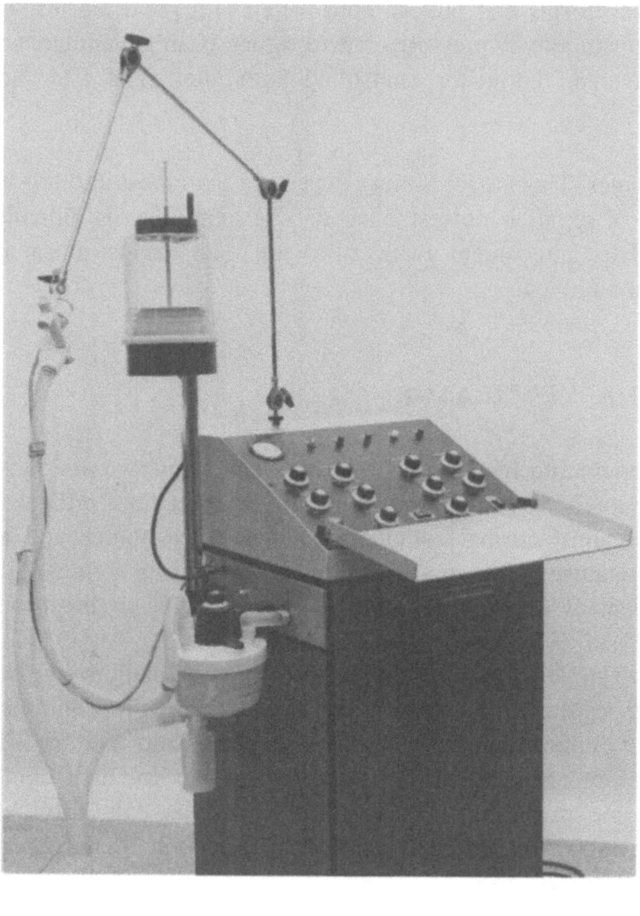

OHIO M560

Advantages. This model has an easily adjustable tidal volume, high sensitivity, and is very powerful, with high flows. It has a low-pressure disconnect alarm, electrical disconnect, high-pressure alarms, PEEP control, and inflation hold. The FI_{O_2} accuracy is good. This model has a rate meter, which is an advantage.

Disadvantages. This model is noisy, of large size, and requires more frequent repairs than most. Also, the manufacturer has discontinued North American production (available in Europe as M250). The flow rates are difficult to adjust, the ultrasonic humidifier is difficult to clean, and there is no nebulizer outlet. Rate will not go below 6/min and therefore limits IMV and the oxygen-line pressure alarm is only visual (i.e., not audible).

PHILLIPS AV_3

Advantages. This model is very quiet. It has good power, maximum flows, variable waveforms and built-in spirometer with good alarms. It also has peak and mean airway pressure control, which is an advantage, and a built-in autoclavable, thermistor controlled humidifier. The FI_{O_2} accuracy is acceptable.

Disadvantages. This model is more expensive than most and top heavy. The frequency of repair is not established. The humidifier is difficult to clean and the PEEP attachment awkward to use. The oxygen alarm lights only (i.e., is not audible).

TESTING A VENTILATOR

Ideally a pneumotachograph, with flow, volume, and two pressure channels, along with an O_2 sensor, should be used to evaluate the ventilator. It should be tested against normal compliance and flow resistance and at the abnormal resistance and compliance likely to be seen in seriously ill patients. A great deal of information on testing is available in the proposed ISO standard [1,3].

A much simpler but still useful test setup can be made with a set of metal drums and resistances and a sampling port as shown in Figure 4. This will give tidal volume, minute ventilation, pressure, and average FI_{O_2}. When ventilators are compared in this way, the reasons for their clinical limitations become much more clear. This apparatus can also be used for demonstrating the effect of equipment malfunction to nurses, respiratory technicians, and doctors.

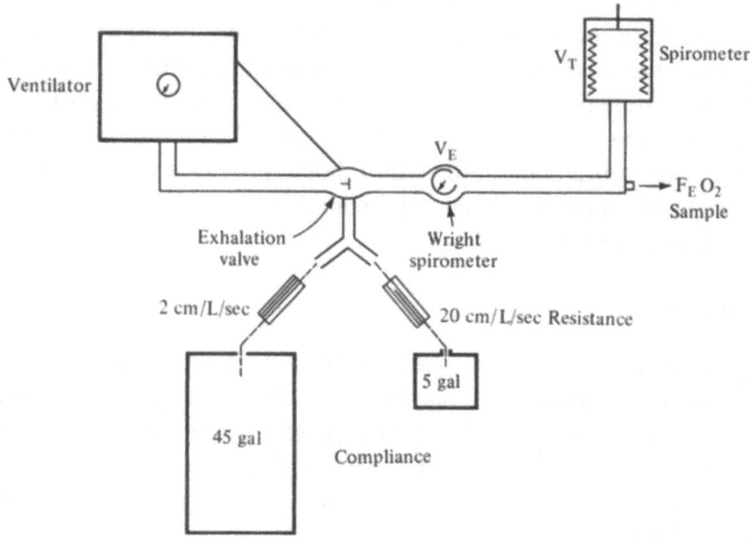

FIGURE 4 Simple test system for evaluation of a ventilator. V_T = tidal volume, V_E = minute volume, F_EO_2 = average expired oxygen concentration. A more comprehensive system is described in the proposed LSO standard.

GUIDELINES IN PURCHASING VENTILATORS

Never buy equipment without evaluation. A month is minimum. Keep careful records of criticisms from respiratory technicians, nurses, and other staff. Where possible, test the ventilator against a set of resistances and compliance at a variety of rates. Measure the minute ventilation and FI_{O_2} accuracy. Find out about service. Obtain a written service contract if possible. Be wary of new products unless guarantees of service are provided. For the small hospital a ventilator that can double as an IPPB machine and transport ventilator is ideal since long-term ventilation will not usually be attempted. Either a Bird or Bennett PR II would be a good choice in this situation. For the medium-sized hospital (50 + beds) with blood-gas facilities, a ventilator may be required for postoperative and trauma patients and patients with airway obstruction. The best buy for this situation at present is the Monaghan 225, which has most of the important features of the more expensive ventilators at half the cost. To keep the cost down, a Bennett spirometer should be substituted for the electronic spirometer which is sold along with this unit. The medium-sized hospital may also require one or more of neonatal ventilator, an anesthesia ventilator, and will have several IPPB machines. The larger community hospital will require at least one ventilator that can handle their most seriously ill patients. Most currently available electric controllers or assistor–controllers will handle most patients with decreased compliance and increased airway resistance. At the present time the Bennett MA I remains justifiably popular for the seriously ill patient because of its reliability, simplicity, and excellent service. To economize, the hospital may have in addition a number of low-cost machines for routine postoperative care and patients with drug overdose.

Generally, the physician "gets what he pays for" in terms of performance. However, the information in the tables should provide some basis for selection, keeping in mind that local requirements and local service may become major criteria in the final choice.

SUMMARY

The routine use of volume-cycled ventilators in preference to pressure-cycled units for mechanical ventilation of the adult provides substantial advantages of operation. Electrically powered ventilators are generally preferred over pneumatic units. The option of assisting ventilation rather than strictly controlling ventilation should be preserved. Newer bellows-driven ventilators provide greater accuracy in establishing inspired oxygen concentrations. The maximum flow rate must be adequate for delivery of high minute volumes in patients with markedly increased airway resistance. Guidelines for testing ventilators, preparatory to purchase are detailed.

References

1. **Mills, M.** (1973). Problems with mechanical ventilators. *Anesth. Analg. Curr. Res. 52:*747–752.
2. **Mushin, W. W., Rendell-Baker, L., Thompson, P.,** and **Mapleson, W. W.** (1969). *Automatic Ventilation of the Lungs.* Second Edition, Oxford: Blackwells Scientific Publications.
3. **Saklad, M.** (Chairman, ISO Sectional Committee ISO/TC 121/WG3). Proposed ISO standard specifications for breathing machines for medical use. To be published by American National Standards Institute, New York.

Weaning from Mechanical Ventilation

HENNING PONTOPPIDAN, M.D. and
DOREEN R. G. BROWNE, M.B., B.S.
Department of Anesthesia, Harvard Medical School,
Massachusetts General Hospital, Boston, Massachusetts

Weaning from mechanical ventilation is a poorly understood and often frustrating phase of management of acute respiratory failure (ARF) [6]. With the exception of diseases known to require prolonged, uninterrupted, mechanical ventilation (MV)—i.e., severe tetanus, polyneuritis, and massive chest trauma with severe flailing—consideration should be given to weaning from MV as soon as certain simple criteria are met. These criteria are as follows: (a) vital capacity > 4–5 ml/kg, (b) inspiratory force > 10 cm H_2O, (c) A–a P_{O_2} < 350 torr, (d) positive end-expiratory pressure requirement < 10 cm H_2O, (e) stable cardiovascular system, (f) chest-wall flailing not severe, and (g) close supervision by experienced physicians.

GENERAL PRINCIPLES OF WEANING

If the patient has been hyperventilated and is acclimatized to a low a P_{CO_2}, hypocapnia should be gradually corrected prior to weaning by reducing minute ventilation (reduced respiratory rate and/or tidal volume) or by increasing inspired CO_2 concentration by insertion of mechanical dead space [10] or use of a CO_2 blender [2]. If major problems are anticipated in weaning, or if chronic hypercapnia has been a feature of the patient's history, induced hypercapnia to a P_{CO_2} level of 50–60 torr may facilitate weaning and minimize cardiovascular complications.

Regardless of weaning technique employed, the daily program of the patient should be planned with weaning as first priority. Before weaning is initiated, the procedure and weaning plan should be explained in detail to the patient, who must be informed that dyspnea can be expected, but will not be harmful. The patient's confidence must be obtained by starting weaning slowly without exceeding his tolerance limit (sec; min) and inducing panic. Each weaning episode should end with a sense of accomplishment, not on a note of failure. Consequently, weaning by the clock

TABLE 1

	10 MIN		
	START	END	P
Vital capacity, ml/kg	10.72[1] ±5.33	11.20 ±5.09	
V_T, ml/kg	4.74[1] ±2.48	5.33 ±2.65	
Inspiratory force, cm H_2O	22.63[1] ±10.63	24.50 ±11.60	
Respiratory rate/min	25.60 ±9.69	26.56 ±7.57	
A–a D_{O_2}, mm Hg ($FI_{O_2} = 1$)	225.40 ±82.87		
a P_{CO_2}, mm Hg	39.40 ±8.89	47.35 ±10.19	<0.001
Heart rate	91.28 ±17.12	98.16 ±16.83	0.004
Static compliance, ml/cm H_2O	51.59 ±11.48		
V_D/V_T	0.46 ±0.15		
FRC%, predicted	88.25 ±29.86		

Legend: Mean values and standard deviation of selected parameters measured in 25 patients during weaning from mechanical ventilation; P values refer to significance of changes recorded within the respective weaning period. Where significant changes in a parameter occurred as weaning time progressed, numbers are marked by [1]($p < 0.001$) or [2]($p < 0.05$).

according to tolerance is preferred rather than pushing the patient to the point of exhaustion.

"CONVENTIONAL" WEANING: TECHNIQUES AND PRINCIPLES

Use a T piece, high flow, and high-humidity gas. For initial weaning and until oxygen requirements have been established, adjust FI_{O_2} to 10–20% above maintenance. Most patients benefit from use of continuous positive airway pressure of 3–10 cm H_2O and with the trunk elevated 20–40°.

1 HR			24 HR		
START	END	*P*	START	END	*P*
13.86[2]	13.93		16.18[1]	16.30	
±1.70	±5.26		±7.52	±7.78	
5.12[2]	5.75	0.05	5.77[1]	5.15	
±2.58	±2.30		±2.79	±2.19	
24.79	26.17		28.48[1]	33.68	0.004
±9.74	±10.20		±13.79	±14.16	
24.00	28.71	<0.001	25.38	27.44	
±7.73	±8.45		±7.82	±9.38	
211.40			205.20		
±78.86			±73.47		
40.64	46.63	<0.001	42.44	45.22	
±9.26	±9.91		±10.39	±12.48	
88.12	95.57	<0.001	90.38	91.81	
±16.12	±18.47		±15.67	±17.35	
52.19			52.53		
±13.85			±15.50		
0.47			0.50		
±0.11			±0.13		
			86.67		
			±43.07		

It is of interest that no statistical significance in physiologic values were found among three groups of patients studied, namely, muscular disease, acute respiratory failure without COPD, and those with acute respiratory failure superimposed on COPD. In this group of patients hypoxemia was never a problem which limited weaning.

Wean every 30 min according to tolerance for a specified period of time, no more no less. Delay nightly weaning until weaning is essentially complete during the day. When nightly weaning is initiated, many patients fear they will "stop breathing" and may initially remain awake when disconnected from the ventilator despite assurance and reinforcement. Patience and a thorough explanation of the physiological considerations will usually resolve this problem rapidly.

The time to complete weaning is not predictable from duration of MV or type of illness. In a recent study of blood-gas exchange and pulmonary mechanics in a group of patients being weaned from mechanical ventilation, physiologic data were obtained at a time when the patient could breathe spontaneously for 10 min, 1 hr and 24 hr, respectively (see Table 1). Complete independence from the ventilator cannot be expected until vital capacity exceeds 16–18 ml/kg ideal body weight.

PHYSIOLOGIC EFFECTS OF WEANING

Changeover from mechanical to spontaneous ventilation, as well as abrupt withdrawal of high PEEP levels, may be associated with several acute and subacute changes in hemodynamic function and pulmonary mechanics, such as redistribution of blood volume to the chest, arrhythmias, and fall in cardiac output. "Circulatory weaning" may be required.

Hemodynamic changes. These result from abrupt changes in intrathoracic pressure, presumably causing an acute rise in cardiac filling pressures (preload). They include cardiac output changes and arrythmias. As a rule, a reduction in mean intrathoracic pressure causes an increase in cardiac output; however, under certain circumstances the opposite response may take place [1]. The most likely explanation for such a "paradoxical" fall in cardiac output is a move toward the descending part of the ventricular-function curve caused by the acute rise in right or left ventricular preload [11]. Continuous positive airway pressure presumably will reduce the cardiovascular effects of sudden "autotransfusion" following disconnection from the ventilator or PEEP. Cardiac arrythmias are seldom serious and rarely necessitate treatment. However, hypoxemia or acute hypercapnia must be ruled out.

Changes in lung mechanics. These are secondary to changes in breathing pattern and lung volume and include small airway closure, increase in small airway resistance, gas trapping, and progressive, diffuse atelectasis. These in turn increase ventilation–perfusion inequality, and cause a fall in lung compliance and an increase in the work of breathing. The most effective prevention is careful monitoring and use of continuous positive airway pressure.

Impairment of ventilation–perfusion inequality secondary to airway closure and atelectasis may to some extent be offset by increased ventilation of dependent lung regions during spontaneous ventilation, as compared to controlled ventilation [4].

Work of Breathing and Weaning. The best correlate of ability to breathe spontaneously appears to be the work (*W*) of breathing [7]. Unfortunately, this measurement requires insertion of an esophageal balloon and access to sophisticated computer technology, and is presently not technically applicable.

INTERMITTENT MANDATORY VENTILATION

Intermittent mandatory ventilation (IMV) [9] as an alternate approach to weaning is gaining increasing acceptance and is a superior approach in many patients. As the frequency of ventilator-provided breaths is progressively reduced, the patient gradually assumes a greater fraction of the alveolar ventilation. Intermittent mandatory ventilation permits earlier start of weaning than does "conventional weaning," requiring less time and attention from nurses and physicians than frequent weaning by respirator disconnect. This method presumably also facilitates gradual circulatory adaptation to a change in intrathoracic pressure, and each ventilator breath may reverse progressive atelectasis and airway closure occurring with shallow, spontaneous breathing (ultrafrequent sighing). Finally, intermittent mandatory ventilation may cause an improvement in the ventilation–perfusion distribution in the lungs by favoring ventilation to dependent lung regions during spontaneous ventilation, and may reduce the tendency to systemic and pulmonary edema to the extent that spontaneous ventilation favors lymphatic drainage from the lung and thoracic duct [8].

DIFFICULTIES IN WEANING

In many cases weaning progresses poorly, frequently for unexplained and unclear reasons. Whenever difficulties in weaning are encountered, the following two possibilities should be considered: (a) an increased work of breathing due to low compliance, increased airway resistance, or reduced chest-wall compliance (i.e., abdominal distention) and (b) unexplained reduction in ventilatory reserve, due to either prolonged negative nitrogen balance and muscle wasting or disuse atrophy of respiratory muscles following prolonged mechanical ventilation. Condition (b) is unproven. Finally, chronic low cardiac output syndrome and impaired respiratory muscle perfusion may lead to a decreased ventilatory reserve.

Respiratory muscle discoordination, manifested by a lack of synchrony of chest wall and diaphragmatic muscle activity, is common in patients following acute respiratory insufficiency [9]. Simultaneous on-line measurement of AP diameter of chest wall and upper abdomen, using magnetometers [5], is the most reliable method of documenting this condition.

SUMMARY

Weaning must start early and follow a planned, systematic approach. It is the most important facet of the patient's daily program.

A major advantage of "intermittent mandatory ventilation" (IMV) circuit is that spontaneous respiratory effort can be maintained without the problems associated with having a patient breathing out of phase with the ventilator. This is particularly useful when PEEP is used, an essential feature of weaning in many patients with tendency to progressive airway closure, atelectasis, or pulmonary edema.

Ventilatory dyscoordination is common in patients with acute and chronic respiratory insufficiency.

References

1. **Beach, T., Millen, E.,** and **Grenvik, A.** (1973). Hemodynamic response to discontinuance of mechanical ventilation. *Crit. Care Med. 1:*85–90.
2. **Breivik, H., Grenvik, A., Millen, E.,** and **Safar, P.** (1973). Normalizing low arterial CO_2 tension during mechanical ventilation. *Chest 63:*525–531.
3. **Downs, J. B., Klein, E. F.,** and **Desautels, D. A.** (1973). Intermittent mandatory ventilation: A new approach to weaning patients from mechanical ventilation. *Chest 64:*331–335.
4. **Froese, A. B.,** and **Bryan, A. C.** (1974). Effects of anesthesia and paralysis on diaphragmatic mechanics in man. *Anesthesiology 41:*242–255.
5. **Goldman, M. D.,** and **Mead, J.** (1973). Mechanical interaction between the diaphragm and rib cage. *J. Appl. Physiol. 35:*197–204.
6. **Hodgkin, J. E., Bowser, M. A.,** and **Burton, G. G.** (1974). Respirator weaning. *Crit. Care Med. 2:*96–102.
7. **Peters, R. M., Hilberman, M.,** and **Hogan, J. S.** (1972). Objective indications for respiratory therapy in post-trauma and post-operative patients. *Am. J. Surg. 124:*262–269.
8. **Pilon, R. N.,** and **Bittar, D. A.** (1973). The effect of positive end-expiratory pressure on thoracic-duct lymph flow during controlled ventilation in anesthetized dogs. *Anesthesiology 39:*607–612.
9. **Pontoppidan, H., Geffin, B.,** and **Lowenstein, E.** (1973). *Acute Respiratory Failure in the Adult.* Boston: Little, Brown.
10. **Suwa, K., Geffin, B., Pontoppidan, H.,** and **Bendixen, H. H.** (1968). A nomogram for deadspace requirement during prolonged artificial ventilation. *Anesthesiology 29:*1206–1210.
11. **Trichet, B., Falke, K.,** and **Togut, A.** (1975). The effect of preexisting pulmonary vascular disease on the response to mechanical ventilation with PEEP following open-heart surgery. *Anesthesiology 42:*46–57.

Management of Flail Chest

B. W. KIRK, M.D. and J. ALI, M.D.
Departments of Medicine and Surgery, University of Manitoba and the Adult Intensive Care Unit, Health Sciences Centre, Winnipeg, Canada

It has been estimated that thoracic injuries account for 25% of deaths from motor-vehicle accidents. Although many injuries to the heart and great vessels are immediately fatal, analysis of delayed deaths provides strong evidence that early skilled first aid, rapid transport, and expert resuscitation would improve the mortality rate from such accidents by as much as 20%. A significant number of these would be patients with chest injuries.

EMERGENCY MEASURES

At the Scene of Injury. Endotracheal intubation and/or insertion of a chest tube may be life-saving early measures. Unfortunately, few ambulance systems in North America are adequately equipped for these procedures. Efforts must be made to improve this aspect of health-care delivery. Even with the present ambulance systems an alert well-trained attendant could improve patient salvage by performing such simple maneuvers as clearing the upper airway, occluding a sucking chest wound, needle aspiration of a tension pneumothorax, or temporarily stabilizing a flail segment by the use of sandbags.

At the Hospital. The casualties must be classified according to priorities of treatment. Generally, the chest injury must be sorted out from other injuries during resuscitation measures. Bruising of the chest or an obvious flail segment will usually be recognized early. Yet, the flail may not be immediately obvious because of muscle splinting so that serial examination of the chest is necessary. In children, however, even extremely forceful trauma is much less likely to break ribs and the underlying injury may be missed.

Endotracheal Intubation

An adequate airway and oxygenation have top priority in any injured patient. Endotracheal intubation secures the airway and should be carried out early in the cyanosed patient. Clinical skills assuring that both endotracheal intubation and insertion of chest tubes may be accomplished competently and rapidly are mandatory for physicians serving in emergency and critical care services.

Pneumothorax and hemothorax, if clinically detectable, usually requires prompt intervention with tube thoracostomy. Chest x-rays are essential since physical signs are often extremely unreliable. A lateral decubitus chest x-ray with the injured side superior makes it possible to detect pneumothorax of less than 30% intrathoracic volume in the patient who cannot be placed in sitting position. Any patient who requires mechanical ventilation, even though the pneumothorax may be small, should have a chest tube inserted as a safety measure when positive pressure ventilation is begun because sudden tension pneumothorax is a relatively common and fatal complication. A small hemothorax need not be aspirated but larger hemothorax requires drainage in order to ensure lung expansion and quantification of continued bleeding. Continued massive hemorrhage usually represents bleeding from a systemic rather than pulmonary vessel and warrants surgical evaluation with open thoracotomy. Similarly, massive pneumothorax that is uncontrolled by adequately functioning chest tubes requires bronchoscopy in order to determine the site of a suspected tracheobronchial tear, with the expectation that surgical repair may be required.

CATEGORIZATION OF CHEST INJURIES

It is useful to classify patients into four groups on the basis of management and outcome. In examining the patient we pay particular attention to his ability to cooperate and to cough effectively to clear secretions. Vital capacity should be measured frequently as it provides objective information about the factors limiting chest expansion. Blood-gas determinations at intervals of four to six hours, with the patient breathing room air, provide essential information on gas exchange. Finally, the natural history of the other injuries must be taken into account. The final assessment also takes into account the patient's age and his clinical course.

Group I. These are patients who, despite a chest injury, do well and do not require ventilation but only physiotherapy and analgesia. In adults, there are usually only one to five broken ribs, no flail segment, and no major head or abdominal injury or multiple extremity fractures. Such patients may not show bruising of the chest but always complain of pain. Cough, although painful, is effective. Chest x ray may show a small pneumothorax and/or hemothorax. Blood gases show moderate hypoxemia on room air but the Pa_{O_2} is usually $\geqq$ 50 torr and vital capacity is $>$ 12 ml/kg body weight.

Group II. These are patients who struggle to maintain ventilation at bed rest. Either the chest injury is more extensive and a small flail segment may be present, or there are extensive injuries to the head with altered state of consciousness, abdominal injuries requiring laparotomy, and pelvic or lower-limb fractures requiring immobilization with the high risk of fat embolization. Alternatively, chronic bronchitis or other obstructive lung disease may have preceded the injury. In patients in whom the primary injury involves the chest wall, breathing and coughing are inadequate. Atelectasis and secondary pneumonia are likely to appear as complications between 48 and 72 hr after injury. Pa_{O_2} while breathing air may be 40 torr and vital capacity $<$ 12 ml/kg after 72 hr.

Group III. These are patients who require mechanical ventilation from early in their course but who generally survive. This group includes patients with extensive, often bilateral, rib fractures, four or more rib-flail segments, often pneumothorax and hemothorax, and evidence of traumatic injury to underlying lung within 24–48 hr. Alternatively, there may be patients in whom the chest trauma is less severe, but major head, abdominal, or bony injuries necessitate postinjury or postoperative ventilation. Vital capacity is usually less than 10 ml/kg and Pa_{O_2} is generally less than 40 torr within 24 hr following injury.

Group IV. These are patients with injuries to lung resulting from forces during the accident that often diffusely damage both lungs, the patient somehow having escaped death from cerebral or major vessel injury. Alternatively, a usually nonfatal traumatic injury to lung may become fatal if complicated by head injury, aspiration, prolonged shock, chronic lung disease, coronary artery disease, fat emboli, and other secondary causes of lung injury. The Pa_{O_2} is usually less than 300 torr on a ventilator on 100% oxygen.

Mechanical Factors versus Gas Exchange in Chest Injury

Our modern concept of chest injury places greater emphasis on hypoxemia than the mechanical effects of obvious flail as the ultimate cause of death in many patients. Pa_{O_2} is of the greatest value in following these patients, but for the Pa_{O_2} to be meaningful the patient must breathe a gas of known oxygen concentration. Room-air blood gases ($FI_{O_2} = 0.2093$) should be assessed at frequent intervals and can be useful in categorizing patients, as shown in Table 1.

MANAGEMENT

In Groups I and II the major problem is painful fractured ribs, poor cough, and low vital capacity. Skilled nursing care is vital. The response to narcotics is variable and thus the orders must be written in a way that will allow the nurse to find the optimal dose of morphine on the basis of comfort, cough and vital capacity. Either excessive or insufficient analgesia can lead to clinical and laboratory deterioration. Intercostal nerve block may be of value in these patients, but we have observed thoracic epidural anesthesia to be superior with prompt pain relief and resumption of effective cough, increased vital capacity, and rising Pa_{O_2}.

In the unconscious or immobilized patient turning is most important but is frequently done improperly. Dependent atelectasis may be the complication which later requires mechanical ventilation.

In Groups III and IV the initial tidal volume (V_T) is generally set at $\geqq$ 10–12 ml/kg. The use of this basic volume plus sighs of $>$ 15 ml/kg or a larger V_T without sighs appears to be a matter of local preference. We do not now believe that ventilation must be strictly "controlled" as long as inspiratory efforts do not result in major flail. Sensitivity of the ventilator must be adjusted to minimal. Following head injury, it is often important to avoid both morphine and curare in the early period. The basic respiratory frequency should result in slight hyperventilation ($Pa_{CO_2} = 30$–35) to minimize the drive to breathe. High inspiratory flow rates of 80–120/min are usually required in order to settle the patient.

The alveolar–arterial oxygen partial-pressure gradient (A–a D_{O_2}) becomes the most important pulmonary laboratory parameter to follow. The A–a D_{O_2} is easily calculated from samples of expired gas and arterial blood.

Worsening Gas Exchange—Group IV. Large ($>$20–30%) right-to-left shunts are associated with a high mortality rate. Patients with an A–a D_{O_2} in excess of $>$350–400 torr fall into this category. The large shunt reflects major pulmonary edema and/or collapse of large segments of lung. Adequate arterial oxygen tensions cannot be maintained on less than 70% (toxic) concentrations of oxygen. A careful search must be made to identify

TABLE 1 Patient Categories

	EXAMINATION OF CHEST	CHEST X RAY	ASSOCIATED INJURIES	BLOOD GAS AND VITAL CAPACITY
Group I	Bruising, rib fractures, but no flail. Pain on cough or deep breath. Usually minimal or no hemothorax or pneumothorax	Initially clear. May show discoid atelectasis	No associated major injuries or surgery required	Pa_{O_2} on air greater than 50 torr. Vital capacity >12 ml/kg
Group II	May have small flail. Marked pain from fractured ribs. Pneumothorax or hemothorax	May show early local traumatic infiltrate. May show segmental or lobar atelectasis	Head injury with stupor or uncooperative. Laparotomy, extremity fractures, minor aspiration	Pa_{O_2}, 40–50 on room air. Vital capacity 10–12 ml/kg
Group III	Major flail or other major injury to chest. Bronchial BS, pneumothorax, and often hemothorax	May show lung contusion involving both lungs and/or segmental or lobar collapse	Often serious injuries in head, abdomen, or pelvis, and aspiration	Pa_{O_2}, <40 torr on room air. A–a $D_{O_2} >300$ torr on 100% oxygen. Vital capacity <10 ml/kg
Group IV	Bilateral flail. Major consolidation. Bloody tracheal secretion	Bilateral diffuse pulmonary infiltrates plus local trauma. May also have local collapse	Often serious aspiration, sepsis, fat emboli, or head injury in very elderly	Pa_{O_2} <30 torr on air. A–a D_{O_2} >400 torr on 100% oxygen

TABLE 2 Causes of Severe Hypoxemia Following Chest Injury

ALVEOLAR EDEMA AND MICROATELECTASIS	COMPRESSION OR COLLAPSE
Lung injury and contusion	Misplaced endotracheal tube
Pulmonary fat emboli	Pneumothorax
Liquid aspiration	Hemothorax
Bacterial pneumonitis	Secretions
Crystalloid overload[a]	
Myocardial failure and infarction[b]	
Colloid overload[b]	

[a] Positive fluid balance and low colloid osmotic pressure.
[b] Elevated pulmonary capillary wedge pressure.

the possible causes of the severe hypoxemia and steps taken to correct them (Table 2). A Swan–Ganz catheter should be inserted to allow a measurement of pulmonary wedge pressure and for subsequent calculations of shunt, since A–a D_{O_2} is affected by cardiac output. Measurements of plasma-protein oncotic pressure are useful but a simple intake–output following admission will often identify crystalloid overinfusion. There should be repeat examinations for pneumothorax, retained secretions, or segmental atelectasis.

Positive-end Expired Pressure (PEEP)

Criteria for PEEP are worsening gas exchange with arterial desaturation in the face of maximal safe inspired oxygen concentrations (A–a-$D_{O_2} > 300$–350). Gas exchange should be assessed as increments of 5 cm H_2O PEEP are added every 2–3 hr until improvement occurs or a level of 15–20 cm is reached. Excessive alveolar pressure can further damage the lung, thus the minimum PEEP allowing adequate oxygenation should be used. The patient must be carefully observed for signs of falling cardiac output and tension pneumothorax during PEEP, especially following chest trauma.

Failed PEEP means that at 15–20 cm H_2O PEEP, arterial saturation is less than 80%. Attention should be directed to the causes of edema and alveolar collapse and measures to correct them. The hemoglobin should be kept near 15 g%. Arterial saturation can be improved by producing mild alkalosis, shifting the oxyhemoglobin dissociation curve to the left. The arteriovenous oxygen content difference should be followed carefully since too much alkalosis can impair unloading at the tissues. Optimally cardiac output determinations may be useful for assessing oxygen delivery to tissues.

Crystalloid Overinfusion

Despite the controversy currently surrounding the use of crystalloid infusions in shock and trauma, we still firmly oppose massive crystalloid infusions in patients with lung injury, particularly when blood or fresh frozen plasma are available. Lung trauma leads to an increase in pulmonary extravascular fluid and this appears to be aggravated by a lowering of plasma oncotic pressure. In Group IV patients, crystalloid should be kept to a minimum and diuresis or dialysis may be required to remove fluid. The circulation should be supported with blood, packed cells, plasma, or albumin as required.

Tracheostomy

There appear to be few indications for tracheostomy without mechanical ventilation. We usually perform elective tracheostomy at 24–72 hr where prolonged mechanical ventilation is anticipated. Removal of secretions is accomplished far more readily through a tracheostomy than an endotracheal tube.

CONTINUING CARE

The usual time between injury and successful weaning from the ventilator is 10 days to 3 weeks. During this period the psychological needs of the patient should be met with visitors, music, television, and conversation from the bedside nurse. Cardiovascular deconditioning can be avoided using a stationary bicycle provided there are no lower-extremity or pelvic fractures. Nutrition needs must be met in order to prevent excessive muscle wasting, a common cause of difficulty weaning. Oral nourishment, tube feedings, or intravenous alimentation may be required.

Weaning from the Ventilator

First, the patient must satisfy a set of weaning parameters. These include the ability to cooperate and cough, a vital capacity of $\geqq$ 12 ml/kg, an inspiratory "force" of greater than —30 cm H_2O, and an A–a D_{O_2} of <250 torr on 100% oxygen. During weaning, alveolar collapse is detected by an increase in A–a D_{O_2} during spontaneous ventilation of gradually increasing duration. If the A–a D_{O_2} does not increase during weaning, the period off the ventilator is gradually increased until a level of 5 min on and 55 min off is reached. Decannulation is usually preceded by a 1–3 day period utilizing a tracheostomy dummy, button, or fenestrated tube. Fiberoptic bronchoscopy and tracheal x-rays allow detection of tracheal and laryngeal injury and should be an integral part of the follow-up of these patients.

Although the mechanical ventilation aspect of the treatment of chest injuries has remained the focus of popular attention, patients requiring mechanical ventilation represented 50 out of 160 patients with primary thoracic injuries seen in our Health Sciences Centre over a 2-year period. In a number of cases we believe mechanical ventilation might have been avoided by more vigorous early assessment and treatment. It is obviously better to avoid mechanical ventilation if this course of management is consistent with patient safety. With meticulous care ventilatory support can result in the recovery of patients with severe thoracic injuries. Out of the 15 patients who died, nine had been transferred from outside, and all but two died of nonthoracic causes. This highlights the favorable prognosis of the chest injury alone.

SUMMARY

Immediate care of the patient with traumatic injury of the chest cage includes maneuvers by which the airway is cleared and tension pneumothorax is relieved by needle aspiration. Initial management may require endotrachial intubation and insertion of a chest tube for management of pneumothorax and hemothorax, together with mechanical ventilation.

A method for categorization of severest of chest injuries is detailed. Methods of management are related to severity of injurity. Selective use of positive and expiratory pressure (PEEP), caution in the use of crystalloid solution, and elective tracheotomy in patients who may require prolonged mechanical ventilation are advised.

Selected Readings

1. **Ballinger, W. F., Rutherford, R. B.,** and **Zuidema, G. D.** (1968). *The Management of Trauma.* Philadelphia: Saunders.
2. **Moore, F. D.,** and **Lyons, J. H.** (1969). *Post Traumatic Respiratory Insufficiency.* Philadelphia: Saunders.
3. **Pontoppidan, H., Geffin, B.,** and **Lowenstein, E.** (1973). Acute respiratory failure in the adult. *New Engl. J. Med. 287:*14–16.

Diagnosis and Treatment of Acute Pulmonary Thromboembolism and Fat Emboli

FRANCIS Y. K. LAU, M.D.
Department of Medicine and Radiology
The Los Angeles County/University of Southern California Medical Center
Los Angeles, California

Pulmonary embolism and infarction are often associated phenomena, but the terms should not be used synonymously. Although pulmonary infarction may follow embolism, many emboli are not followed by infarction. The probability of infarction is increased in the presence of elevated pressures in the pulmonary circulation, such as is seen with left ventricular failure or mitral stenosis. Thrombi may originate in the venous channels of the lower extremities, pelvis, right atrial appendage, or a malignant organ. The venous disease and/or stasis as seen with congestive failure, infectious diseases, malignancies, blood dyscrasias, toxic agents, and convalescent periods for surgical procedures, childbirth, or fracture, may predispose to venous thrombi and potential pulmonary emboli.

The diagnosis of pulmonary embolism is frequently missed, since there may be a primary disease fostering secondary venous thrombosis, and the clinician may be misled by the symptoms and signs of the primary disease, either simulating or overshadowing the signs and symptoms of pulmonary emboli. Postmortem studies report as many as 50% of the adult population having evidence of pulmonary thromboembolism [4,6] it is the most common cause of sudden, unexpected hospital deaths [10]. Many emboli are never detected because they are asymptomatic and, for the most part, resolve spontaneously without known ill effects.

SYMPTOMS

Pulmonary Embolism

The classical symptoms of clinically-evident pulmonary embolism are: (a) sudden onset of dyspnea, (b) chest pain, and (c) collapse. Death frequently occurs within 15 minutes in nearly 50% of patients suffering from a massive pulmonary embolus.

Pulmonary Infarction

The symptoms of pulmonary infarction are pleuritic chest pain and bloody sputa, which may accompany any of the symptoms of pulmonary emboli.

The symptoms of pumonary embolism—shortness of breath, syncope, and chest pain—are frequently confused with an acute myocardial infarction. It is not unusual that the substernal precordial chest pain cannot be distinguished from that experienced with an acute myocardial infarction or pericarditis. Chills with fever greater than 102° may suggest a pneumonia, rather than pulmonary embolism.

PHYSICAL SIGNS

Pulmonary Embolism

In the presence of significant pulmonary hypertension, the following signs may be present: (a) accentuated P_2, (b) right ventricular lift, (c) third and fourth heart sounds, (d) distended and prominent systemic venous channels, and (e) enlarged liver. Partial occlusion of the pulmonary vascular channels by thromboemboli may give rise to systolic and diastolic murmurs located centrally, but they may radiate peripherally. The pulmonary examination may be normal; however, unilateral expansion lag and diminished breath sounds may suggest areas of atelectasis.

Pulmonary Infarction

The following signs may be present over an area of pulmonary consolidation: (a) increased fremitus, (b) dullness to percussion, (c) accentuated bronchial breath sounds and diminished vesicular breath sounds, and (d) rales. If there is involvement of the pleural surfaces, a pleural and/or pericardial friction rub may be present. The signs of pleural effusion should be searched for, such as (a) absence of fremitus, (b) flatness to percussion, and (c) loss of breath sounds. With the breakdown of infarcted lung, there may be icteric sclera, skin, and urine.

A low-grade fever is often present, and increases in heart and respiratory rates are out of proportion to the minimal rise in temperature. Atrial arrhythmias are not unusual in pulmonary thromboemboli and infarction.

LABORATORY STUDIES

I. Hematologic and Enzyme Changes
   A. Mild to moderate leukocytosis
   B. Anemia
   C. Increased sedimentation rate
   D. Elevated serum bilirubin, serum lactic dehydrogenase, alkaline phosphatase, with a usually normal SGOT.

II. Electrocardiographic Findings
   A. Rhythm changes: Sinus tachycardia, atrial arrhythmias, ventricular ectopy, ventricular fibrillation, sinus bradycardia and arrest, and conduction defects.
   B. Depolarization changes: Right axis shift or deviation; Q waves in leads II, III, and aVF; S waves in leads I, aVL, V_5, and V_6; prominent R waves in $V_{1,2,3}$ representing right ventricular hypertrophy may be seen with chronic recurrent pulmonary thromboembolism.
   C. Repolarization changes: Inverted T waves in leads II, III, aVF, V_1-V_3.
   D. Right atrial hypertrophy: P waves in leads II, III, aVF, and/or V_1, with voltages greater than 0.25 millivolt.

Since electrocardiographic changes occur in less than 30% of patients with thromboembolic disease, it is a poor screening test.

III. Arterial Blood Gases
   A. Arterial desaturation ($P_aO_2 < 80$ mmHg). These values may not correlate with the degree of vascular obstruction.
   B. A difference (at least 5 mmHg) between the arterial and end tidal (alveolar) CO_2 tension.

IV. Radiologic Findings
   A. Chest x-ray. About 80% of patients with positive angiographic evidence of pulmonary emboli show abnormal x-ray findings [12]. These findings are: Unilateral elevation of the diaphragm (80%); consolidation (60%); prominent pulmonary artery (50%); pleural effusions (35%); unilateral hypoperfusion (Westermark's sign); contralateral overperfusion; enlarged pulmonary artery, right-sided cardiac chambers, and great veins.
   B. Lung scans. Perfusion scans utilize radioactive-tagged microscopic

particles injected intravenously. Albumin particles (about 15 micra) act as microemboli temporarily obstructing less than 0.1% of the vasculature delineating areas in which pulmonary arterial circulation may be deficient. Perfusion scans do not detect pulmonary emboli, but show the distribution of the pulmonary arterial blood flow. Although perfusion scans cannot pick up areas of less than 2–3 cm, one would expect evidence of 30–50% of the capillary bed involved in patients with signs of tachycardia, tachypnea, and systemic hypotension. A normal radioactive perfusion scan in the presence of these physical signs would infer that some other serious pathologic condition might be present. The use of the chest x-ray and radioactive ventilation scans may assist in differentiating bronchopulmonary disease from thromboembolism.

C. Pulmonary arteriography. This is the most specific diagnostic test for pulmonary embolism and is mandatory prior to embolectomy or any operative intervention. It is also the gold standard used to evaluate medical or surgical therapy. The prime requisite for the angiographic diagnosis is the presence of intravascular filling defects. However, vessel cut-offs may be the only finding in thromboembolic disease.

V. Cardiopulmonary Hemodynamics [11,12]

A. In patients free of prior cardiopulmonary disease

1. Pulmonary artery mean pressures (normal 7–15 mmHg) may elevate after 20–30% of the circulation is obstructed. Mean pressures of 30–40 mmHg usually indicate severe obstruction. In acute pulmonary thromboembolism, mean pulmonary artery pressures rarely exceed 40 mmHg because the right ventricle is unable to cope with the obstructive load.
2. Cardiac index is usually normal or increased in thromboembolism, and decreases only when the obstruction is greater than 50%.

B. In patients with prior cardiopulmonary disease

1. Mean pulmonary artery pressures are higher and may relate more to the cardiopulmonary disease. It is not unusual to have systemic levels of pressures even with minor pulmonary emboli.
2. Cardiac outputs are generally low in patients with prior cardiopulmonary disease.

Of all laboratory studies, radioactive pulmonary perfusion scans, correlated with the chest x-ray, remain the best combination of screening tests for pulmonary thromboembolism. The gold standard for diagnosis remains the pulmonary angiographic study. Arterial blood gases, blood enzymes, and electrocardiograms may be useful in monitoring patients with pulmonary thromboembolism.

TREATMENT

Patients clinically suspected of having significant pulmonary emboli should be in a critical care area for diagnosis and treatment.

I. Monitoring
   A. ECG.
   B. Intake and output.
   C. Pressures.
      1. Venous. Preferably with a Swan-Ganz balloon catheter for pressures and cardiac output (thermodilution).
      2. Arterial. These pressures may be obtained by cuff in a normotensive patient or by catheter in a hypotensive individual.
   D. Arterial blood gases.

II. Medical Management
   A. Supplemental oxygen therapy to maintain arterial PO_2 80–100 mmHg by the use of nasal catheter, mask, tent, or endotracheal tube with pressure assistance if necessary.
   B. Heparin therapy. Initial doses of 10–15,000 units and maintenance doses of 5–10,000 units every 4 to 6 hours to keep the clotting times (Lee-White) 2–3 times greater than the initial clotting time, or the use of a continuous pump infusion to maintain the PTT (partial thromboplastin time) 1.5–2 times that of the starting value.
   C. Medication for shock and pain.
   D. Long-term anticoagulants. Coumadin or Dicumarol to be started on the third to the tenth day and to be continued for at least 3 to 6 months at 20–30% of normal prothrombin time.
   E. Thrombolytic agents [18,19]
      1. Clot resolution with intravenous urokinase or streptokinase (12-hour infusion) may be more rapid than with heparin alone, and may lessen the convalescent period. The mortality at the end of two weeks of therapy did not seem to be significantly different with thrombolytic agents.
      2. Malayan pit viper (Arvin) limited trials [8] showed no significant difference between heparin, streptokinase, or Arvin on resolution of deep vein thrombi.

III. Surgical Measures
   A. Embolectomy. Indications are controversial and are reserved for angiographically-proved massive central pulmonary emboli with refractory hypotension and persistent hypoxia. Mortality rates are still 50–90%.
   B. Inferior vena caval obstruction.
      1. Plication or ligation
      2. Catheter-placed umbrella [13]

Indications for these procedures are in patients where anticoagulant therapy has been unsuccessful or contraindicated when fatal pulmonary emboli are imminent.

The primary disease associated with the pulmonary emboli should be treated. Active and passive exercise programs should be instituted with all postoperative and bedrest patients as soon as possible. Anticoagulant therapy with heparin [1,9,14] has shown a decline in mortality rate in pulmonary embolism from 25% to 5% or less. Spontaneous recovery and recanalization of obstructed pulmonary artery passages may be expected even in nontreated individuals [3].

FAT EMBOLISM SYNDROME

Fat emboli can be demonstrated at necropsy in 90 to 100% of patients with recent fractures [16], and occurs in association with diabetes, osteomyelitis, steroid therapy, burns, pancreatitis, cardiopulmonary bypass, metastatic tumors, and other unrelated diseases. The clinical syndrome of fat embolism primarily occurs with multiple fractures of the long bones and depends on the amount of embolic fat in the circulation [7]. Only 1–2% of patients with fractures of the long bones may develop the syndrome [2].

I. Signs, Symptoms, and Clinical Findings
  A. The following symptoms are present after a 2- to 12-hour lucid interval:
    1. Pulmonary distress
      (a) shortness of breath
      (b) labored breathing
      (c) rapid respiration
      (d) expectoration of blood
    2. Cerebral distress
      (a) anxiety
      (b) restlessness
      (c) confusion
      (d) convulsions
      (e) partial paralysis
      (f) coma
    3. Systemic complaints
      (a) dizziness or fainting
      (b) fever
  B. The following signs are present:
    1. Vital signs
      (a) elevated temperature
      (b) tachycardia
      (c) tachypnea
      (d) low blood pressure

2. Skin
   (a) cyanosis
   (b) petechial hemorrhages in the axillary folds and lower eyelids
3. Respiratory findings
   (a) rapid, labored breathing
   (b) wheezing
   (c) rales
4. Neurologic findings
   (a) mental confusion
   (b) abnormal nonlocalizing neurologic signs which may include paresis, changes in sensory modalities, abnormal reflexes of a transient nature.

C. Laboratory data
1. Hematologic changes
   (a) mild anemia
   (b) mild leukocytosis
   (c) decreased platelet count due to intravascular clotting
2. Electrolytes. The serum calcium level may drop as the fat emboli hydrolyze and free fatty acids are released to combine with calcium.
3. Enzymes. The lipase levels may elevate in both the blood and the urine in massive fat embolization.
4. Arterial blood gases.
   (a) hypoxia with Pa_{O_2} values of less than 80 mmHg
   (b) hypocarbia with Pa_{CO_2} values less than 40 mmHg
5. Electrocardiographic changes consistent with acute cor pulmonale similar to that seen with pulmonary thromboembolic disease.
6. Chest x-ray. "Snowstorm" appearance of pulmonary edema.
7. Urine and sputum analyses for lipids may be positive, but are not always found in the fat embolism syndrome.

The pathophysiology of pulmonary fat emboli is unknown. The fat emboli particles are usually microscopic and do not cause mechanical obstruction as seen with pulmonary thromboembolism. Some of the suggested mechanisms are: (1) biochemical injury by the fat or byproducts to the endothelial lining of the pulmonary capillary, with resultant deposition of platelets and platelet release factors which may cause alveolar edema and hemorrhage [5]; (2) neuro pulmonary edema due to neurogenic cause with alterations in the pulmonary capillary endothelial permeability [4].

The primary cause of symptoms and progressive pulmonary distress is the marked pulmonary edema that develops with loss of compliance of the lungs and the severe hypoxia.

II. Treatment

Close attention for signs of pulmonary edema and neurologic disorders should be given to any patient with multiple fractures. Close observance of the skin folds of the axillary area and eyelids for petechial hemorrhages may be helpful in anticipating the more serious pulmonary and neurologic problems.

A. Monitoring
   1. Blood gases
   2. Intake and output
   3. Venous and arterial pressures
   4. Cerebral symptoms
   5. Skin manifestations
B. Therapy
   1. Oxygen therapy is indicated for any patient with respiratory distress and an arterial oxygen less than 80 mmHg. Early endotracheal intubation should be used if the oxygen therapy by nasal catheter, mask, or tent does not provide normal levels of monitored arterial oxygen.
   2. Limitation of fluid to 1000 cc/day should be instituted unless the patient is suffering from a depleted circulating volume. Diuretics may be of temporary help.
   3. Measures of controversial usage. These include administration of the following: (a) hydrocortisone 250 mg intravenously four times daily for a period of two days, then rapidly reduced over a period of five to seven days; (b) Dextran 40, 250–500 ml per day for two to three days, then 250 ml for three to four days; (c) ethyl alcohol 10 cc of 5% solution per kilogram weight every four hours intravenously; and (d) heparin therapy as given for pulmonary thromboembolism.

Usually there is no residual pulmonary or cerebral damage in those patients who recover. Definitive surgical or orthopedic procedures can be performed within a week after recovery.

SUMMARY

Pulmonary thromboembolism is usually heralded by the sudden onset of dyspnea, chest pain, and collapse. Physical signs of pulmonary hypertension may be present. Pulmonary infarction may be associated with signs of pleural involvement, increases in serum bilirubin, LDH, and chest x-ray findings of consolidation and/or pleural effusion. Radioactive pulmonary perfusion scans are excellent screening tests, but the pulmonary angiographic changes of emboli remain the gold standard for diagnosis. Guidelines for treatment include oxygen therapy, anticoagulation with heparin followed by coumadin, and supportive measures for shock and pain. Thrombolytic agents may effect an earlier clearing of thromboemboli, but with the expense of added complications of bleeding. Surgical treatment includes embolectomy and inferior vena caval obstructive devices and may be indicated in those individuals not responding to medical management.

References

1. **Barritt, D. W.,** and **Jordan, S. C.** (1960). Anticoagulant drugs in the treatment of pulmonary embolism. *Lancet 1:*1309.
2. **Benatar, S. R.,** *et al.* (1972). Some clinical observations and a review of controversial aspects of fat embolism. *Quart. J. Med. 51:*85.
3. **Chait, A.,** *et al.* (1967). Observations in the fate of large pulmonary emboli. *Am. J. Roentgen. 100:*364.
4. Editorial (1972). Fat embolism. *Lancet 1:*672 (March 25).
5. **Fleischner, F. G.** (1962). Pulmonary embolism. *Clin. Radiol. 13:*169.
6. **Freiman, D. G.** (1965). *Pathological Observations on Experimental and Human Thromboembolism, Pulmonary Embolic Disease.* New York: Grune and Stratton.
7. **Ishida, O.,** and **Taji, Y.** (1964). Fat emboli syndrome. *Med. J. Osaka Univ. 14:*275.
8. **Kakhar, V. V.,** *et al.* (1969). Treatment of deep vein thrombosis. *Brit. Med. J. 1:*806.
9. **Kernohan, R. J.,** and **Todd, C.** (1966). Heparin therapy in thromboembolic disease. *Lancet 1:*621.
10. **McIntyre, K. M.,** and **Levine, H. J.** (1965). *Cardiac Arrest and Resuscitation, Emergency Medical Management.* New York: Grune and Stratton.
11. **McIntyre, K. M.,** and **Sasahara, A. A.** (1971). The hemodynamic response to pulmonary embolism in patients free of prior cardiopulmonary disease. *Am. J. Cardiol. 28:*288.
12. **McIntyre, K. M.,** *et al.* (1972). Pulmonary thromboembolism, current concepts. *Adv. Int. Med. 18:*199.
13. **Mobin-Uddin, K.,** *et al.* (1969). A new catheter technique of interruption of inferior vena cava for prevention of pulmonary embolism. *Am. Surgeon 35:*889.
14. **O'Sullivan, E. F.,** *et al.* (1968). Heparin in the treatment of thromboembolic disease: Administration, control, results. *Med. J. Australia 2:*153.
15. **Sevitt, S.** (1962). *Fat Embolism.* London: Appleton-Century-Crofts.
16. **Sevitt, S.** (1966). Fat emboli.*Lancet 2:*1203.
17. **Szues, M. M.,** *et al.* (1971). Diagnostic sensitivity of laboratory findings in acute pulmonary embolism. *Ann. Int. Med. 74:*161.
18. Urokinase-streptokinase embolism trial, cooperative study. (1974). *J. Am. Med. Assoc. 229:*1606.

Selected Readings

1. **Sabiston, D. C., Jr.,** and **Wagner, H. N.** (1965). Pathophysiology of pulmonary embolism. *J. Thorac. Cardiovasc. Surg. 50:*339–356.
2. **Saldeen, T.** (1970). Fat embolism. *J. Trauma 10:*287.
3. **Soloff, L. A.,** and **Rodman, T.** (1967). Acute pulmonary embolism (clinical). *Am. Heart J. 74:*829.
4. **Soloff, L.,** *et al.* (1967). Acute pulmonary embolism. *Am. Heart J. 74:*710–847.
5. **Thomas, D. P.** (1970). The management of pulmonary embolic disease. *Am. J. Med. Sci. 259:*157–163.
6. Urokinase pulmonary embolism trial, cooperative study. (1974). *J. Am. Med. Assoc. 214:*2163.
7. **Wertzberger, J. J.,** and **Peltier, L. F.** (1968). Fat embolism. *Surg. 63:*626.

II

SHOCK AND TRAUMA

Treatment of Shock and Trauma States: Use of Cardiorespiratory Patterns to Define Therapeutic Goals, Predict Survival, and Titrate Therapy

Department of Surgery, Harbor General Hospital, Torrance, California, and the University of California at Los Angeles School of Medicine, Los Angeles, California

For maximal effectiveness, therapy should be directed against the basic underlying pathophysiologic mechanisms and toward optimal physiologic values. Therapy should be given vigorously in the early stages where it is most effective, as no amount of belated therapy can be expected to compensate for previous failure to recognize the insidious onset of shock. The major problems are to define with precision the pathophysiologic mechanisms and the therapeutic goals so that the therapy may be given in the optimal order and be titrated to ensure maximal survival.

PATHOPHYSIOLOGIC MECHANISMS

Understanding of the essential nature of shock states must be predicated upon adequate descriptions of the sequential cardiorespiratory patterns obtained during periods remote from therapy. Physiologic mechanisms underlying the *early* cardiorespiratory events may have pathogenic significance in the subsequent development of shock syndromes, whereas those of the late stage probably reflect only terminal mechanisms. Clinically, shock is usually recognized after hypotension develops. However, the major pathophysiologic reactions are initiated in the early period immediately after the etiologic event but before the initial hypotensive episode; hence this is before the patient is recognized as being in shock.

In several studies various etiologically defined shock states were described by sequential cardiorespiratory observations in 180 patients with over 10,000 sets of physiologic measurements [3,4,7,10]. The physiologic data were divided into early, middle, and late periods by criteria of time and arterial pressure. Objective criteria for staging were devised to analyze the data at comparable periods since some patients go through their course of shock more rapidly than others. The control period (Stage A) was defined as the preillness or preoperative period. Stage B was the initial period of declining arterial pressure immediately after the etiologic event. The lowest recorded arterial pressure (Stage Low) separated Stage B from Stage C, the middle period. The latter was divided into Stages C_1 and C_2 by the point in time when arterial pressure returned halfway to control values. Stage D was the late or recovery period for surviving patients; it started when arterial pressures had returned to normal or nearly normal values. Stage E was the preterminal period in patients who subsequently died; it covered the time from Stage C to the terminal stage, Stage F, about 1–2 hr prior to death.

In this system, the "early" period extends from the time of etiologic event until the initial hypotensive episode, which usually is the time when it is first recognized that the patient is in serious difficulty and requires vigorous therapy. This, in contrast to most other temporal systems in which "early" designates the period early after shock is recognized, is comparable to our "middle" period.

The major common denominator in the early period of shock states was not low flow, but normal and high flow (unless limited by blood-volume deficit or myocardial function), which was maldistributed at the microcirculatory level to a degree that compromised oxygen transport.

Hemorrhagic shock. In the early period immediately after onset of hemorrhage, there are decreases in arterial pressure, cardiac output, central venous pressure (CVP), central blood volume, stroke volume, stroke work, and oxygen consumption (V_{O_2}), as well as increases in heart rate, systemic (peripheral) vascular resistance, a-vD_{O_2}, and O_2 extraction (see Table 1 and Figs. 1–3). The compensations to hemorrhage are tachycardia, systemic and pulmonary metrateriolar vasoconstriction, and increased myocardial contractility. Vasomotor changes are produced by increased sympathetic neural activity, which unevenly redistributes blood volume and flow in hypovolemia and low blood-flow states [3,4,7,10].

The redistribution of blood volume and cardiac output produces relatively greater perfusion to the liver, heart, and brain and lesser perfusion to the kidney, gut, and skin. Neural regulatory mechanisms also redistribute blood flow at the microcirculatory level. Initially, the tissues extract oxygen more completely because less blood is flowing through them and at a slower

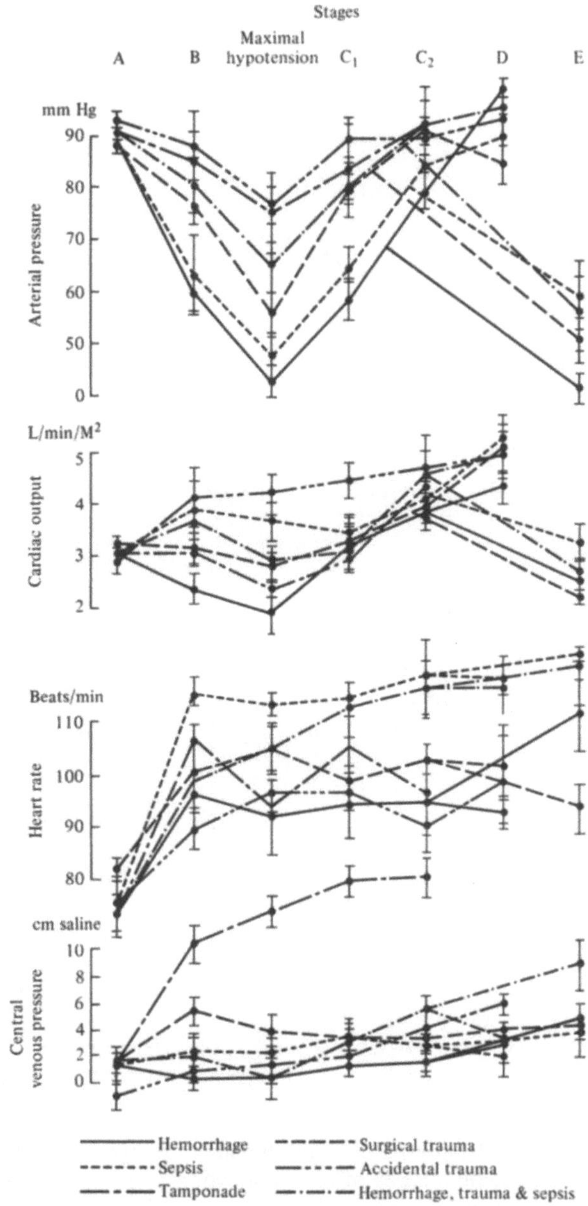

FIGURE 1 Serial hemodynamic changes at each temporal stage after various etiologic types of shock illustrating the sequential patterns. Means (dots) and S.E. of the mean (vertical bars) are shown for mean arterial pressure, cardiac index, heart rate, and CVP. Note the fall in cardiac index in Stages B and Low after hemorrhagic shock and to a lesser extent after cardiac tamponade, while the cardiac index values of the other groups were normal or increased. Heart rates increased in all etiologic groups but were greatest in the two groups with sepsis. The venous pressures were within the normal range except in the tamponade patients. From Shoemaker [7].

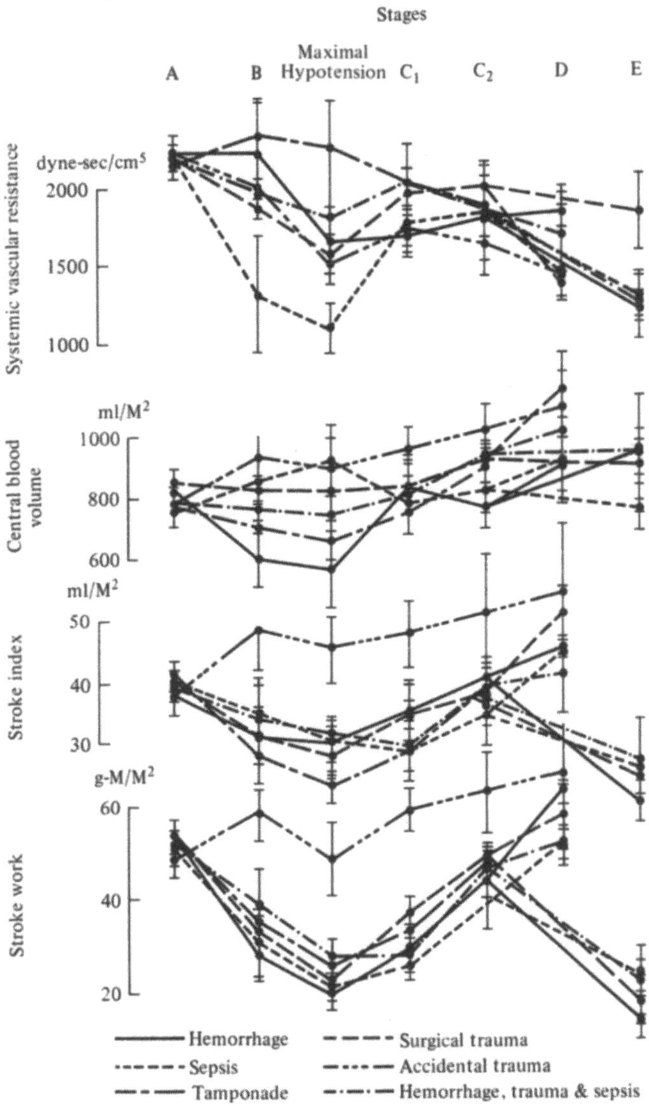

FIGURE 2 Sequential patterns of hemodynamic changes at each temporal stage for various etiologic types of shock showing systemic (peripheral) vascular resistance, central blood volume, stroke index, and left-ventricular stroke work. Note the slight transient rise in peripheral resistance in Stage B after hemorrhage and tamponade and the subsequent progressive decrease with time in all categories. Also in Stages B and Low of hemorrhage and tamponade patients central blood-volume values tended to be low, but the values of the other stages were normal or high. The stroke volume and stroke work increased progressively in accidental trauma, but these variables decreased in the Stages B, Low, and C_1 in the other groups. From Shoemaker [7].

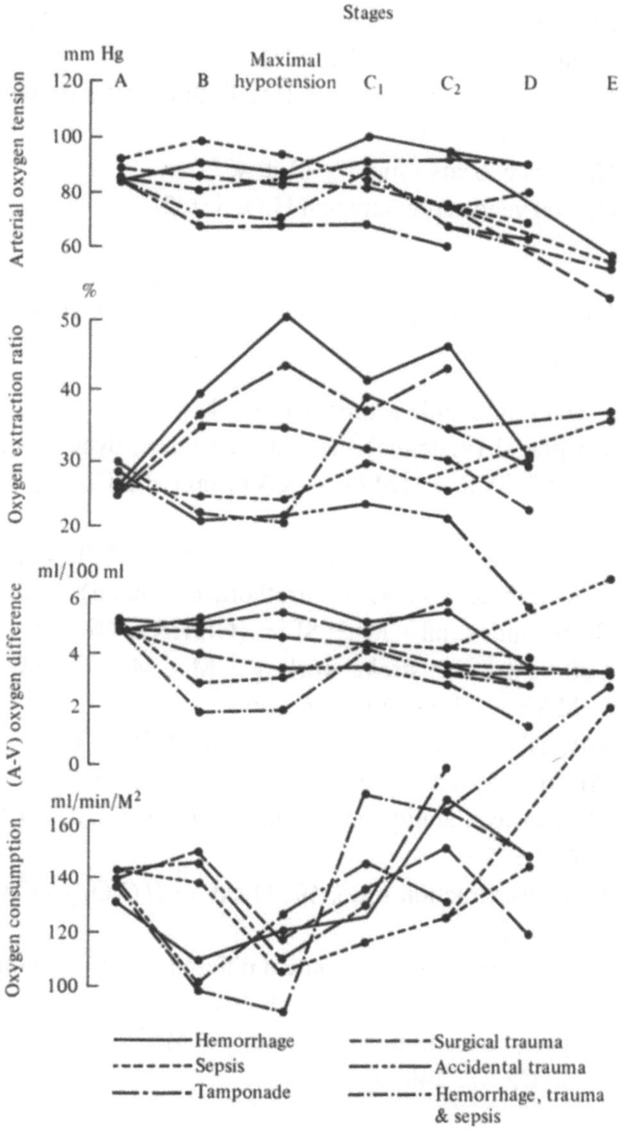

FIGURE 3 Sequential patterns in oxygen metabolism including P_aO_2, oxygen-extraction ratio, a-vD_{02} (arteriovenous oxygen-content differences) and oxygen consumption after various etiologic types of shock. Note that P_aO_2 values, although somewhat low, did not fall alarmingly until the late stages. The oxygen-extraction ratios and to a lesser extent the a-vD_{02} rose in the hemorrhage and tamponade patients. The a-vD_{02} fell in the accidental trauma, sepsis, and hemorrhage-trauma-sepsis groups. Oxygen consumption fell in the early (Stages B or Low) period and rose in the middle periods in all groups. From Shoemaker [7].

TABLE 1 Abbreviations, Units, Formulas, Definitions, Normal Values

CI	Cardiac index, $1 \cdot min^{-1} \cdot m^{-2}$; cardiac output per m^2 body surface area, 3.2 ± 0.2 (SD)
MAP	Mean arterial pressure, mm Hg, diastolic pressure plus ⅓ pulse pressure, 90 ± 5
HR	Heart rate, beats $\cdot min^{-1}$, 72 ± 4
CVP	Central venous pressure, cm H_2O, 5 ± 2
MTT	Mean transit time, sec; $MTT = \dfrac{\int_0^\infty tc(t)\,dt}{\int_0^\infty c(t)\,dt}$; where c is dye concentration and t is time, 15 ± 1.4
SVR	Peripheral (systemic) vascular resistance, dyne $\cdot$ cm $\cdot\ sec^{-5} \cdot M^{-2}$, SVR = (MAP − CVP, mm Hg/CI) × 79.96, 2180 ± 210
CBV	Central blood volume, ml $\cdot\ m^{-2}$; CVB = MTT × CI (catheter-to-catheter volume or intrathoracic volume), 830 ± 86
SI	Stroke index, ml $\cdot\ M^{-2}$; SI = (CI/HR), 46 ± 5
LVSW	Left-ventricular stroke work, g $\cdot$ M $\cdot\ M^{-2}$; LVSW = (SI × MAP × 13.6/1000), 56 ± 6
C_aO_2	Arterial oxygen content, ml $\cdot$ 100 ml^{-1}, 19 ± 1
P_aO_2	Arterial oxygen tension, torr $\cdot$ 100 ml^{-1}, 86 ± 8
O_{2av}	Oxygen availability, ml $\cdot\ min^{-1} \cdot m^{-2}$; $O_{2av} = CI \times C_aO_2$, 600 ± 50
O_2ext	Oxygen-extraction ratio, %; $O_2ext = [(C_aO_2 - C_vO_2)/C_aO_2]$, 26 ± 2
a-v D_{O_2}	Arteriovenous oxygen-content difference, ml $\cdot$ 100 ml^{-1}; a-vD_{O_2} = $(C_aO_2 - C_vO_2)$, 4.6 ± 0.4
V_{O_2}	Oxygen consumption, ml $\cdot\ min^{-1} \cdot M^{-2}$; $V_{O_2} = CI \times (C_aO_2 - C_vO_2)$, 140 ± 25.

rate, but despite this compensation, the uneven flow results in inadequate tissue oxygenation. With prolonged, intense vasoconstriction, the redistribution of flow eventually leads to maldistributed flow. Metabolic acidosis occurs with hypovolemia and maldistributed blood flow; under these conditions, respiratory alkalosis arises as a compensatory mechanism.

Traumatic shock. In trauma, the early cardiorespiratory pattern consists of increase in cardiac output, heart rate, central blood volume, stroke volume, stroke work, and O_2 availability and decrease in arterial pressure, peripheral resistance, oxygen extraction, a-vD_{O_2}, and V_{O_2} [3,4,7,10]. In essence, acute injury increases autonomic neural activity, which in turn stimulates the central cardiac and respiratory centers to increase heart rate, myocardial contractility, and alveolar ventilation (Figs. 1–3). When hypovolemia is not present, the stroke volume increases because of enhanced myocardial contractility and cardiac output increases as a result of increased stroke volume and heart rate. Increased ventilation in the absence of hypovolemia leads to hypocarbia and respiratory alkalosis.

The initial physiologic responses to trauma and hemorrhage are primarily mediated by generalized increases in autonomic neural activity, which may stimulate central cardiac and respiratory centers. The duration and magnitude of these effects depend on many factors. For instance, the stimulation of cardiac function increases cardiac output after trauma and sepsis, but this response may be limited by hypovolemia and impaired myocardial function. Furthermore, metabolic influences and the cellular breakdown products of direct tissue injury tend to intensify both the increase and redistribution of flow.

Septic shock. The early cardiorespiratory pattern in sepsis consists of hypotension, tachycardia, normal or high cardiac output, and decreases in peripheral resistance, stroke volume, stroke work, a-vD_{O_2}, and V_{O_2}. Compensatory response to sepsis includes neural mechanisms that stimulate heart rate, myocardial contractility, and alveolar ventilation [2,11,12]. This leads to increased cardiac output when blood volume is not reduced by dehydration or other factors. Hyperpnea, tachypnea, and respiratory alkalosis result from increased respiratory drive.

Cardiogenic shock. The early cardiorespiratory pattern in cardiogenic shock consists of hypotension, tachycardia, high CVP, and decreases in cardiac output, stroke work, O_2 extraction, and V_{O_2}. In the early period of cardiogenic shock, increased neural activity accounts for tachycardia and transiently vascular resistance; increased CVP may result from failure of the heart to keep up with the venous return, as well as increased venomotor tone from neural mechanisms. Later, the tendency to increase myocardial contractility in cardiac tamponade, for example, may be transient and succumb to rapid deterioration from progression of the underlying disease and the failure of compensatory responses [5,11].

Physiologic Common Denominator in Various Types of Shock

In essence, the striking initial physiologic response to each of the various etiologic events is the stimulus to increased cardiorespiratory function manifest by: (a) increased heart rate and myocardial contractility, which produce increased cardiac output unless limited by reduced blood volume or myocardial function and (b) increased alveolar ventilation, which produces respiratory alkalosis unless balanced by metabolic acidosis from anaerobic metabolism. Thus, the common physiologic denominator of the various states is not *low flow,* but *uneven flow* with inadequate oxygen transport at the microcirculatory level that occurs in the early period prior to the initial hypotension and often before the patient is recognized as being in shock.

The stimulus for increased cardiorespiratory function arises from: (a) stimulation of cardiac centers of the brain stem by the stress response, which produces a generalized increase in autonomic nervous-system activity; (b) cellular breakdown products, hyperthermia, vasoactive peptides, metabolic end-products, and endotoxins, and (c) increased metabolic needs of the peripheral tissues. The latter are reflected in the augmented oxygen transport of the middle period, Stages C_1 and C_2 (Fig. 3) [2,9].

THERAPY

Therapeutic Goals

Normal hemodynamic values are not appropriate goals of therapy, since compensatory physiologic reactions produce abnormal values and these protective compensations have survival value. Moreover, it is not apparent whether a given physiologic alteration is compensatory or decompensatory, advantageous or disadvantageous. Therefore, therapeutic goals must be defined in terms of optimal physiologic interactions in order to develop an integrated plan that will reduce mortality.

Cardiorespiratory variables were described in a retrospective series of critically ill patients who had major surgical procedures for life-threatening conditions [1,6,9]. The results were confirmed by a prospective series [8]. The data remote from therapy were analyzed by the conventional statistics [9] and by a nonparametric statistical analysis [1,6] using the differences in the ranges of cardiorespiratory variables in the survivors and nonsurvivors as predictors (Figs. 4–7 and Table 1). This was done to define therapeutic goals from the physiologic patterns of the survivors, to identify for each cardiorespiratory variable the probable limits compatible with survival, and to identify which variables associated with the early appearance of circulatory deterioration may serve as an early warning of impending death.

Table 2 shows the values for 21 cardiorespiratory parameters of nonsurvivors and survivors during the early period (Stages B and Low), the "cutoff" points that divide the region shared by both groups from the region unique to only one group, and a tentative list of "optimal" therapeutic goals.

The differences in the patterns of mean values and the ranges between

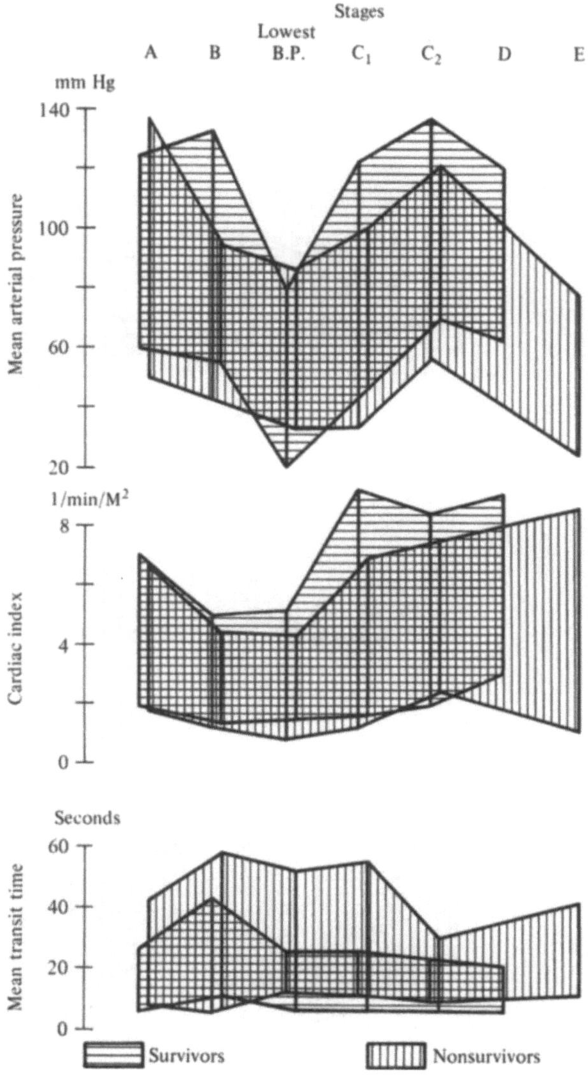

FIGURE 4 The sequential patterns in the ranges of values of mean aterial pressure, cardiac output, and mean transit-time values in surviving and nonsurviving patients. The ranges of the survivors are indicated by the horizontal lines and the ranges of nonsurvivors by the vertical lines. In general, the ranges of arterial pressure and flow were higher in survivors, while the ranges of mean transit time were higher in the nonsurvivors. From Shoemaker [6].

these two groups were more pronounced in the early period (Stages B and Low) and in the late period (Figs. 4–7). Nevertheless, the values of the two groups were widely overlapping.

With respect to the mean hemodynamic values in this small series, arterial

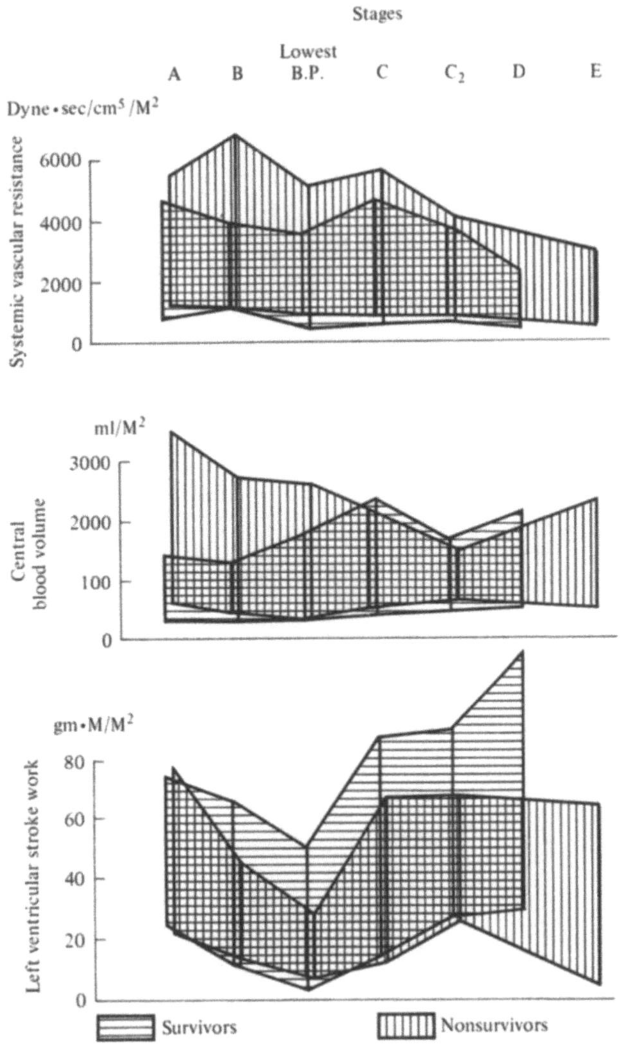

FIGURE 5 The sequential patterns in the ranges of systemic vascular resistance, central blood volume, and left-ventricular stroke work in surviving and nonsurviving patients. The resistance ranges of nonsurvivors were higher throughout all stages; the ranges of stroke were higher in the survivors. From Shoemaker [6].

pressure was not a good index of survival in the early period (Stages B and Low). Cardiac index, stroke index, left-ventricular stroke work, and heart rates were somewhat greater in the survivors; the average mean transit time, peripheral resistance, and central blood volume of survivors were lower

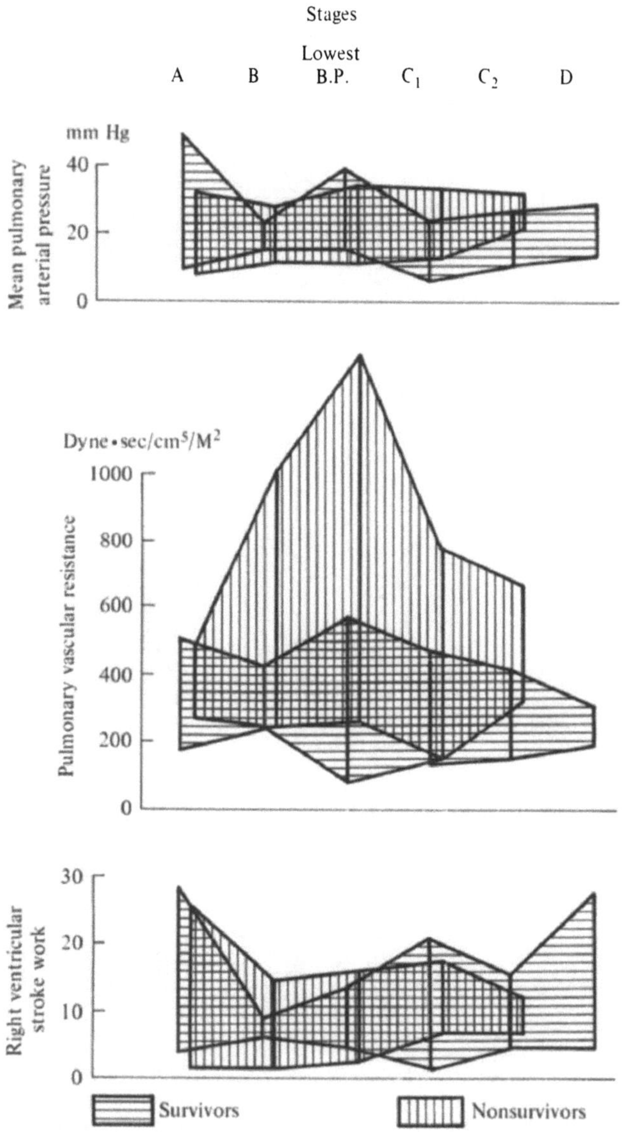

FIGURE 6 The sequential patterns of mean pulmonary arterial pressure, pulmonary vascular resistance, and right-stroke-work ranges of surviving and nonsurviving patients. Note the pronounced early increase in pulmonary vascular resistance of nonsurvivors. From Shoemaker [6].

than those of the patients who died in the early period. There was no significant discrepancy in the mean CVP values of the two groups in this period. In the middle period (Stages C_1 and C_2), the differences between survivors and nonsurvivors generally decreased, but the mean values and ranges for arterial pressure, cardiac index, stroke index, and left-ventricular

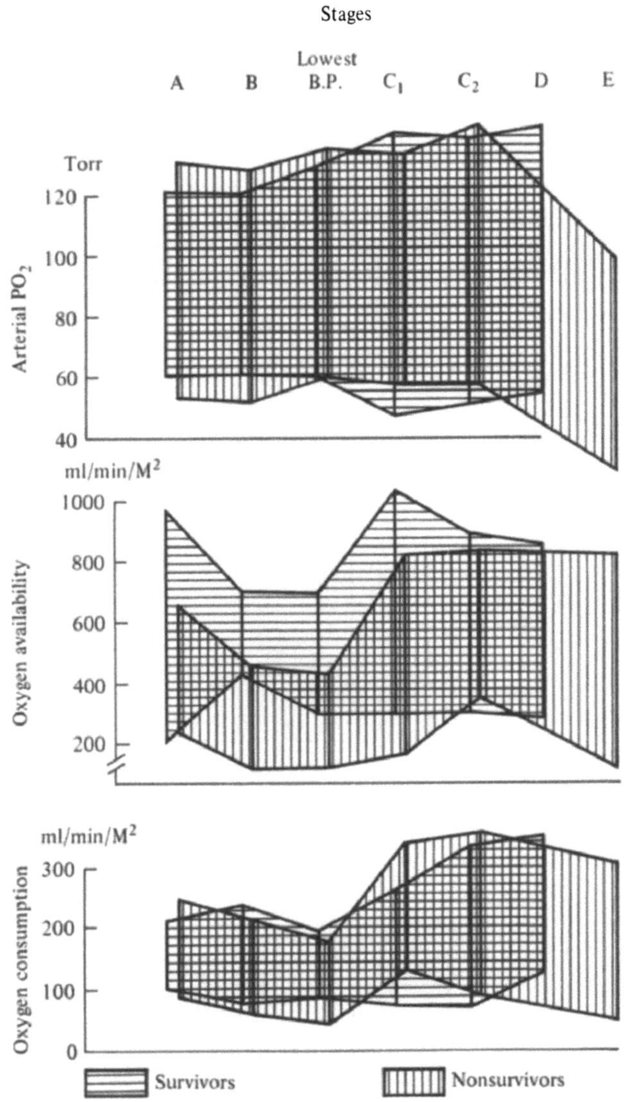

FIGURE 7 The sequential patterns of ranges in oxygen-transport variables of surviving and nonsurviving patients. Note the pronounced lowering of the oxygen availability range in the nonsurvivors, especially in the early period; similar changes, but to a lesser degree, occurred in oxygen consumption. From Shoemaker [6].

stroke index were slightly higher in survivors [9]. In the late period, there were again appreciable differences in both mean values and ranges; arterial pressure, cardiac index, central blood volume, stroke index, and stroke work were higher in survivors than nonsurvivors (Figs. 4–5).

The sequential patterns of the mean pulmonary hemodynamic values and the ranges of the survivors were significantly different from those of the nonsurvivors (Fig. 6). In the early period, nonsurvivors had slightly higher pulmonary arterial pressures and markedly higher pulmonary vascular resistance than did survivors.

In the early period, the mean arterial oxygen tensions and saturations were relatively well maintained in both groups. The ranges of the two groups were quite similar in the early and middle periods. Pronounced desaturation occurred in the late period of the nonsurvivors. In the early period, oxygen availability and rate of oxygen consumption were greater in survivors, but in the middle period, the oxygen consumption was greater in patients who died (Fig. 7). The mean arterial pH values in all postoperative periods were slightly higher in survivors. The pH fell markedly in the late period of nonsurvivors.

In the early period, hemoglobin and hematocrit values were higher in survivors; there were minimal differences between the two groups in the middle and late periods. Blood-volume measurements of survivors were close to the normal predicted values throughout the postoperative periods. In contrast, the average blood-volume deficit of the nonsurvivors postoperatively was 780 ml less than their predicted norms.

Wide differences in the ranges of pulmonary vascular resistance, oxygen availability, oxygen consumption, left and right ventricular stroke work, P_{CO_2}, pH, and mean transit time rendered these parameters useful as classifiers, but no one variable was capable of separating the two groups. However, various sets of variables that predominantly reflected blood flow, blood volume, neurohumeral influences, oxygen transport, and acid–base-related influences considered aggregately furnished information on the relative frequency with which each of the sets of variables was related to survival or death.

In the early period (Stages B and Low), nonsurvivors were identified by the following values, which fell outside the ranges of the survivors.

1. Cardiac-related variables: (a) cardiac index below 1.8 $l \cdot min^{-1} \cdot m^{-2}$, (b) mean transit time >35 sec, (c) systolic ejection rate <80 $ml \cdot min^{-1} \cdot m^{-2}$, (d) tension-time index <700, and (e) right-ventricular stroke work <4 $g \cdot M \cdot m^{-2}$.
2. Volume-related variables: (a) blood-volume deficit >1500 ml, (b) red-cell mass deficit >600 ml, (c) central blood volume >1700 $ml \cdot m^{-2}$, (d) CVP $>18H_2O$, and (e) stroke index <12 $ml \cdot m^{-2}$.
3. Neurohumeral-related variables: systemic vascular resistance >3500 $dyne \cdot sec \cdot cm^{-5} \cdot m^{-2}$.
4. Oxygen-transport–related variables: (a) arterial P_{O_2} <60 torr, (b) oxygen-extraction ratio $>40\%$, (c) hemoglobin concentration <9.0 $g \cdot 100\ ml^{-1}$, (d) a-vD_{O_2} >5.5 $ml \cdot 100\ ml^{-1}$, (e) oxygen availability <400 $ml \cdot min^{-1} \cdot m^{-2}$, and (f) V_{O_2} <80 $ml \cdot min{-1} \cdot m^{-2}$.

TABLE 2 Cardiorespiratory Values of Survivors and Nonsurvivors in the Early Period (Stages B and Low)

		NONSURVIVORS		SURVIVORS		
	NORMAL VALUES ±1 STANDARD ERROR	MEAN VALUES ±1 STANDARD ERROR	CUTOFF POINT[1]	MEAN VALUES ±1 STANDARD ERROR	CUTOFF POINT	"OPTIMAL" VALUES[2]
Cardiac-related variables						
Cardiac index ($l \cdot min^{-1} \cdot M^{-2}$)	3.2 ± 0.2	2.2 ± 0.4	<1.8	2.8 ± 0.4	>4.4	4 – 4.5
Mean transit time (sec)	14 ± 1	27 ± 6	>40	20 ± 3	<12	10 – 15
Mean systolic ejection rate ($ml \cdot min^{-1} \cdot M^{2}$)	230 ± 36	190 ± 50	<50	240 ± 53	>350	150 – 300
Tension-time index		620 ± 190	<600	940 ± 180	>1350	800 –1500
Left-ventricular stroke work ($g \cdot M \cdot M^{-2}$)	50 ± 5	23 ± 4	>10	28 ± 4	>42	35 – 50
Volume-related variables						
Blood volume ($l \cdot M^{-2}$)	2.7 ± 0.1	2.3 ± 0.2	<1.8	2.6 ± 0.1	—	3 – 3.5
Hemoglobin ($g \cdot 100\ ml^{-1}$)	14 ± 1	9.3 ± 0.5	<8.8	11.1 ± 0.4	>13.2	10 – 12
Mean arterial pressure (mm Hg)	86 ± 3	56 ± 8	—	59 ± 4.5	>80	80 – 100
Central venous pressure (cm H_2O)	4 ± 1	6 ± 2.5	>19	7 ± 2	<0	2 – 10
Central blood volume ($ml \cdot M^{-2}$)	770 ± 72	950 ± 106	>1400	830 ± 100	—	700 – 900
Stroke volume ($ml \cdot M^{-2}$)	43 ± 36	27 ± 4.5	<15	30 ± 4	>40	30 – 45

Neurohumeral-related variables						
Systemic vascular resistance ($dyne \cdot sec \cdot cm^{-5} \cdot M^{-2}$)	2090 ± 112	2360 ± 700	>4000	1950 ± 270	<1000	900 –2400
Pulmonary vascular resistance ($dyne \cdot sec \cdot cm^{-5} \cdot M^{-2}$)	270 ± 43	720 ± 130	>500	320 ± 48	<250	200 – 350
Heart rate ($beat \cdot min^{-1}$)	75 ± 5	96 ± 8	<70	106 ± 7	>145	90 – 110
Oxygen-transport-related variables						
Arterial hemoglobin saturation (%)	96 ± 0.3	96 ± 2	—	97 ± 2	>93	96 – 99
O_2 extraction ratio (%)	26 ± 1	36 ± 6	>40	25 ± 6	<25	20 – 30
a-vD_{O_2} ($ml \cdot 100 \cdot ml^{-1}$)	4.4 ± 0.4	5.2 ± 1.2	>5.6	4 ± 1.7	—	3 – 5
O_2 availability ($ml \cdot min^{-1} \cdot M^{-2}$)	560 ± 43	290 ± 37	<350	506 ± 24	>460	500 – 650
O_2 consumption ($ml \cdot min^{-1} \cdot M^{-2}$)	142 ± 8	105 ± 18	<75	140 ± 25	>200	150 – 200
pH-related variables						
pH_a	7.40 ± 0.02	7.37 ± 0.02	<7.3	7.46 ± 0.01	>7.48	7.4– 7.45
P_aCO_2 (torr)	40 ± 2	33 ± 3	>35	25 ± 4	—	25 – 40

[1] Cutoff point is the point beyond which the values of only one group lie.
[2] "Optimal" values are tentatively regarded as the values most crucial for therapy of the critically ill postoperative patient.

5. Acid–base-related variables: (a) pH_a <7.34 and (b) arterial P_{CO_2} <25 torr (Table 2).

Survivors were identified in the early period by the following sets of values, which fell outside the ranges of the nonsurvivors:

1. Cardiac-related variables: (a) cardiac index > 4.5 $1 \cdot min^{-1} \cdot m^{-2}$, (b) mean transit time <11 sec, (c) tension-time index >1300, (d) left-ventricular stroke work >44 $g \cdot M \cdot m^{-2}$, (e) and left cardiac work >5 $kg \cdot M \cdot m^{-2}$.
2. Volume-related variables: (a) maintenance of blood volume at or near preoperative values, (b) central blood volume <500 $ml \cdot m^{-2}$, and (c) stroke index >40 $ml \cdot m^{-2}$.
3. Neurohumeral–related variables: systemic vascular resistance <1000 $dyne \cdot sec \cdot cm^{-5} \cdot m^{-2}$.
4. Oxygen-transport-related variables: (a) oxygen-extraction ratio <25%, (b) a-vD_{O_2} <3.0 $ml \cdot 100\ ml^{-1}$, (c) oxygen availability >450 $ml \cdot min^{-1} \cdot m^{-2}$, and (d) oxygen consumption >200 $ml \cdot min^{-1} \cdot m^{-2}$.
5. Acid–base-related variables: pH_a >7.45 (Table 2) [1,6].

Over 90% of the patients studied in the early period and all of those who died in shock in that period were correctly classified by the range criteria [6]. However, there was more overlap in the ranges of the physiologic variables during the middle period (Stages C_1 and C_2) and, therefore, differentiation between survivors and nonsurvivors was not as marked in this period as in the early and late periods.

Since most of the patients were observed at several stages, the cumulative number observed and the cumulative number of positive identifications rose gradually at each successive stage. Ninety-four percent of the survivors and 87% of the entire series were ultimately identified with one or more variables; 87% of the survivors and 65% of the nonsurvivors were identifiable by two or more variables [1,6].

Data of the prospective series were used to test the validity of the methods as well as the results. The patients of the second or prospective series were classified according to criteria developed by the initial retrospective study. These results were also comparable to the initial series; specifically 94% of the survivors and 89% of the entire series were predicted by one or more variables, and 89% of the survivors and 86% of the entire series were correctly predicted by two or more variables in the prospective series [8]. As in the retrospective series, the highest percentage of correct predictions was in the early period at or before the initial hypotensive episode. Variables reflecting oxygen and CO_2 transport, cardiac performance, pH, and pulmonary vascular resistance were the most frequently positive predictors [6].

Priorities of Therapy

Ultimately, therapy should be directed to the common underlying physiologic problem of shock, which is inadequate oxygen transport from maldistribution of flow at the organ and microcirculatory levels. The rate of oxygen consumption, which is low in the early period and normal or high in the middle or late period, is inadequate to meet the increased metabolic needs of the shock state. Moreover, the shock patient who is resuscitated by correction of the hypotension and hypovolemia becomes critically ill with multiple vital-organ failures.

Since compensatory physiologic reactions represent departures from the normal, the therapeutic goals are not to maintain the normal values. If this were done, it would eliminate the beneficial compensations. After therapeutic goals are well defined according to "optimal" values such as those seen in survivors of similar conditions, treatment may be arranged by priorities according to the life-threatening capability of the functional derangement of each vital organ. Therapy under these circumstances should be not proscribed by a definitive or standardized dose but titrated to an optimal physiologic end-point.

Hemorrhage, fluid loss, airway obstruction, and hypoxia from any origin are all life threatening and must be corrected immediately and simultaneously. With this reservation, the following is a list of the most common problems and their therapy in rough order of priorities.

1. Control hemorrhage and restore blood volumes, and maintain arterial pressures and volume load to about 500–1000 ml in excess of predicted norms, unless there are contraindications.
2. Prevent or correct fluid maldistributions (i.e., excess interstitial water with deficient plasma volume) during resuscitation by adequate plasma expansion with oncotically active agents and by avoidance of salt and water overload from excessive volumes of Ringer's lactate solution.
3. Maintain open upper airway and provide adequate ventilation.
4. Provide respiratory care, including: (a) frequent coughing by patient, (b) tracheobronchial toilet with endotracheal suction as needed, (c) side-to-side repositioning every two hours, (d) postural drainage, (e) humidification of inspired air, (f) avoidance of water overload, (g) tracheal intubation, (h) chest physical therapy, (i) enriched oxygen in inspired air via mask or nasopharyngeal catheter, (j) mechanical ventilation when P_aO_2 falls below 50–60 torr or P_aCO_2 rises above 60 torr, (k) enriched concentrations of oxygen as needed to maintain P_aO_2 above 70 torr, (1) avoidance of overadministration of oxygen therapy, which produces P_aO_2 values over 120 torr.
5. Correct acid–base alterations: (a) metabolic acidosis with sodium bicarbonate administration, fluids, and improvement of blood flow,

(b) respiratory acidosis with endotracheal suction and mechanical ventilation, (c) respiratory alkalosis by sedation, proper adjustment of mechanical ventilatory volume, increase in dead space, and addition of CO_2 to the inspired air, and (d) metabolic alkalosis (when appreciable) with ammonium chloride.

6. Use cardiotonic agents for cardiac failure with pulmonary edema: (a) inotropic agents (digitalis, isoproterenol, and dopamine), (b) fluid and salt restriction, (c) diuretics, (d) glucagon and glucose, (e) antiarrhythmic agents, (f) blocking agents such as phentolamine, nitroprusside, and chlorpromazine when fluid overloads occur, and (g) phlebotomy or dialysis with large fluid overloads unresponsive to other therapy. Resort to vasopressors if all other measures have been tried and found ineffective.
7. Correct extracellular fluid (ECF) overload by restriction of salt and water, provision of normal plasma volume and albumin concentration, and diuretics such as furosemide, ethacrynic acid, mannitol, or 50% glucose. If these are ineffective, resort to dialysis.
8. Provide for nutritional needs: (a) 2000–3000 cal/day with hypertonic (50%) glucose, (b) amino-acid solutions, and (c) albumin, 250–750 ml/day.
9. For semiconsciousness, which may be associated with cerebral edema, give high doses of steroids, urea, fluid and salt restriction, diuretics, and adequate parenteral alimentation.
10. Control infections: (a) culture all potentially infected body fluids, (b) drain abscesses or fluid collections, (c) provide wound care, and (d) give appropriate antibiotics.

Summary

Our concept of the underlying pathophysiology of shock and trauma states is based on a description of the natural physiologic history of the various shock syndromes. This was obtained from sequential cardiorespiratory measurements during periods remote from therapeutic interventions. The common physiologic response to stress is increased cardiorespiratory drive that results in increased cardiac output unless limited by hypovolemia or functional myocardial impairment and increased minute ventilation. The common physiologic denominator of the various etiologic types of shock is inadequate oxygen transport from uneven flow at the organ and microcirculatory level. Oxygen consumption may be low, normal, or high, but it is inadequate to meet the increased metabolic needs associated with the shock state, tissue repair, and concomitant complications including pyrexia.

Normal values are not appropriate goals of therapy, because compensatory physiologic reactions which have survival value also represent changes from the normal values. In survivors, the cardiorespiratory patterns remote from therapy reflect the physiologic effects of the etiologic events and the patient's own compensations; as such, these patterns represent a first approximation to therapeutic goals. By contrast, cardiorespiratory patterns of nonsurvivors reflect the physiologic effects of the etiologic events and the effects of inadequate compensations or decompensations; early warning criteria of impending disaster and death were developed from these patterns.

Predictors of death and survival were defined by the ranges of each variable; a high percentage of patients were classified in the early period. The frequency that changes in each of the variables identify survivors or nonsurvivors reflects their relevance to pathophysiology and therapy.

When the therapeutic goals are defined appropriately, treatment can be arranged by priorities according to the life threatening capability of each cardiorespiratory derangement. Then a therapeutic program may be developed with each therapy titrated to the optimal goals with due consideration for the unique aspects of each individual patient.

References

1. **Shoemaker, W. C.** (1972). Cardiorespiratory patterns in clinical shock as physiologic criteria for therapy and early warning of death. In: *Advances in Automated Analysis.* Vol. 2: 15–22. Tarrytown, New York: Medical Inst.
2. **Shoemaker, W. C.** (1971). Cardiorespiratory patterns in complicated and uncomplicated septic shock. *Ann. Surg. 174:*119.
3. **Shoemaker, W. C.** (1973). Pathophysiologic basis of therapy for shock and trauma syndromes. *Semin. Drug Treat. 3:*211.
4. **Shoemaker, W. C., Boyd, D. M., Kim, S. I., Brown, R. S., Dreiling, D. A.,** and **Kark, A. E.** (1971). Sequential oxygen transport and acid–base changes after trauma to the unanesthetized patient. *Surg. Gynec. Obstet. 132:*1023.
5. **Shoemaker, W. C., Carey, J. S., Yao, S. T., Mohr, P. A., Amato, J. J., Printen, K. J., Corley, R. D.,** and **Monson, D. O.** (1970). Hemodynamic alterations in acute cardiac tamponade after penetrating injuries of the heart. *Surg. 67:*754.
6. **Shoemaker, W. C., Elwyn, D., Levin, H.,** and **Rosen, A. L.** (1974). Use of nonparametric analysis of cardiorespiratory variables as early predictors of death and survival in postoperative patients. *J. Surg. Res. 17:*301.
7. **Shoemaker, W. C., Lim, L., Boyd, D. M., Corley, R. S., Reinhard, J. M., Dreiling, D. A.,** and **Kark, A. E.** (1971). Sequential hemodynamic events after trauma to the unanesthetized patient. *Surg. Gynec. Obstet. 132:*651.
8. **Shoemaker, W. C., Montgomery, E. S., Elwyn, D. H., Levin, H.,** and **Rosen, A. L.** Early prediction of death and survival by prospective analysis of cardiorespiratory variables in postoperative shock patients. *Curr. Topics Crit. Care Med. 2:*44–59, 1977.
9. **Shoemaker, W. C., Montgomery, E. S., Kaplan, E.,** and **Elwyn, D. H.** (1973). Physiologic patterns in surviving and nonsurviving shock patients. *Arch. Surg. 106:*630.

10. **Shoemaker, W. C., Printen, K. J.,** and **Amato, J. J.** (1967). Hemodynamic patterns after acute anesthetized and unanesthetized trauma. *Arch. Surg. 951:*492.
11. **Weil, M. H.,** and **Shubin, H.** (1966). *Diagnosis and Treatment of Shock.* Baltimore, Williams and Wilkins.
12. **Wilson, R. F., Jablonski, D. V.,** and **Thal, A. P.** (1964). The usage of dibenzyline in clinical shock. *Surgery 56:*172.

Prognostic Indices as a Basis for Assessing Severity of Shock

HERBERT SHUBIN, M.D.,[2] MAX HARRY WEIL, M.D.,
LAWRENCE PORTIGAL, M.S., and POTTER CHANG, PH.D.
Shock Research Unit and the Department of Medicine,
University of Southern California School of Medicine,
the Los Angeles County/University of Southern
California Medical Center,
and the Center for the Critically Ill, Hollywood Presbyterian
Medical Center, Los Angeles, California

In the management of patients in shock, objective measurements facilitate the physician's understanding of the mechanisms underlying circulatory and respiratory failure. In turn, the indications for therapy are clarified. With the availability of large numbers of parameters and measurements, however, it is apparent that the available data on the various variables may appear contradictory with respect to the patient's status. For example, the administration of a vasopressor drug to a patient in shock may increase arterial pressure, but this may be accompanied by an undesirable reduction in cardiac output and elevation in blood lactate. The evaluation of the patient's status becomes increasingly complex as three or more simultaneous measurements are taken into account.

In view of the variety of variables available on patients in shock, a number of questions arise: (a) is there a single individual variable or a single set of variables which is most reliable for assessing the condition of the

[1] This study was supported by U.S.P.H.S. Research Grants HL-05570 from the National Heart, Lung and Blood Institute, GM-16462 from the National Institute of General Medical Sciences, and RO1 HS 01474 from the Health Resources Administration.

[2] Deceased June 29, 1975.

patient in shock, (b) if a number of variables are available, what is their order of reliability for evaluating the severity of the patient's condition, and (c) does the same order of variables or the same subset of variables apply to all patients regardless of the etiology of shock?

Prognostic indices, derived for patients with acute myocardial infarction [2], drug overdose [3], gram-negative bacteremia [5], and hypovolemia [12] were investigated in an effort to answer these questions.

PATIENT MATERIAL

Group I—myocardial infarction complicated by shock. Twenty-nine patients who had sustained an acute myocardial infarction were included in this group [2]. All of the patients developed unequivocal manifestations of shock. The patients' ages ranged from 47 to 84 years (mean, 63 years). Seven of the patients recovered from shock. In all except one the ECG findings included Q waves and ST–T wave changes characteristic of acute transmural myocardial infarction. Serum transaminase and lactate dehydrogenase values were significantly increased in each patient. The heart was examined at autopsy in 13 patients, including the patient who had equivocal ECG changes, and acute transmural myocardial infarction with extensive muscle necrosis was confirmed in each instance.

Group II—drug overdose complicated by shock. Fifty-two patients who had attempted suicide by ingestion of large doses of barbiturate, glutethimide, or meprobamate were investigated [3]. Intoxication in each was documented by measurement of toxic levels of the drugs in serum. Included were 39 women and 13 men ranging in age from 16 to 79 years (mean, 37 years). The patients were observed and treated in the Shock Research Unit for an average period of 53 hr. Cardiorespiratory arrest occurred in 11 patients before admission to the Unit, and seven of these died. Among the 18 deceased, all but three had significant underlying diseases or injuries not directly related to drug intoxication.

Group III—gram-negative bacteremia and shock. This group included 32 patients in whom shock was associated with bacteremia caused by gram-negative bacilli [5]. The source of infection was in the intestinal tract in nine patients. This was most often related to peritonitis following perforation of a viscus or infarction of bowel. Twenty-three patients had nonenteric foci of infection, with the urinary tract as the most common site. Gram-negative bacteria were recovered on blood culture and there was evidence of perfusion failure with an increase in lactate concentration to levels exceeding 2 mM/l in each instance. The patients ranged from 34 to 85 years (mean, 64 years) in age. Twelve patients survived. Cirrhosis was found in four patients at autopsy; nine other patients had a history of heavy alcohol intake without evidence of cirrhosis. There was evidence of heart disease in 10 patients including cardiomegaly, left-ventricular hypertrophy, and/or atrial fibrillation.

Group IV—hypovolemic shock. This group included twenty-nine patients in circulatory shock following depletion of intravascular volume [12]. There were 17 men and 12 women, ranging from 18 to 87 years (mean, 54.8 years) in age. Each had unequivocal clinical signs of circulatory shock. Hypovolemia was related to hemorrhage in 17 patients, to loss of extracellular fluid other than blood in 11 patients, and to a combination of fluid losses in one patient. Multisystemic trauma was the cause of volume depletion in 16 of the patients. Fourteen patients were mechanically ventilated. All had a systolic arterial pressure of less than 90 mm Hg, cloudy sensorium, clammy skin, and a decrease in urine output to levels of <20 ml/hour. Blood lactate was increased in all except three patients (mean, 5.5 ± 3.6 mM/l).

Initial treatment included infusion of crystalloid and/or colloid fluids, and in some instances, whole blood immediately after hypovolemic shock had been identified. Seven patients died during the acute episode. Three of the 22 patients who survived the acute periods died after an interval of more than two weeks because of sepsis, pulmonary embolism, or ruptured aortic aneurysm. These three are considered "survivors" since death was from causes not directly attributable to initial volume depletion.

METHODS

Measurements

Hemodynamic, metabolic, and respiratory variables were measured at intervals ranging from every 5 min to every 4 hr. The individual parameters are shown in Table 1, which also serves as a glossary of abbreviations for these parameters as employed in this report. For each patient, the last measurement before death or discharge, excluding the agonal period, comprised the data for this study. Values of intraarterial systolic, diastolic, and mean pressures, mean CVP (right atrial), and heart rate were obtained by methods previously described [14]. Cardiac index, stroke index, cardiac work, stroke work, mean circulation time, appearance time, and central blood volume were obtained with dye-dilution methods and digital-computer techniques [13]. Respiratory rate was obtained from the central venous pressure. Hourly urine outputs were measured with an indwelling urethral catheter and an automated urinometer. Rectal and toe temperatures were measured by means of thermistor probes. Hematocrit and hemoglobin were measured on an IL Co-oximeter. These methods have been previously described [15]. Plasma volume was determined with ^{125}I-tagged iodinated

TABLE 1 Abbreviations

AT (sec)	Appearance time
C_{O_2} (%)	Blood oxygen content
CBV (l)	Central blood volume
CI (l/min/m^2)	Cardiac index
CW (g m)	Cardiac work
DP (mmHg)	Diastolic blood pressure
Hct (%)	Hematocrit
Hgb (g/dl)	Hemoglobin
HR (b/min)	Heart rate
LAC (mM/l)	Lactate
LDF	Linear discriminant function
MAP (mmHg)	Mean arterial pressure
MCT (sec)	Mean circulation time
MVP (mmHg)	Mean central venous pressure
P_aCO_2 (mmHg)	Arterial carbon dioxide tension
P_aO_2 (mmHg)	Arterial oxygen tension
pH_a (units)	Arterial pH
PVI (ml/kg)	Plasma-volume index
RCI (ml/kg)	Red-cell index
RES (dynes sec cm^{-5})	Peripheral vascular resistance
RT (C)	Rectal temperature
S_aO_2 (%)	Arterial oxygen saturation
SI (ml/beat/m^2)	Stroke index
SP (mmHg)	Systolic blood pressure
SW (g m/beat)	Stroke work
T_{O_2} (cc)	Oxygen transport
TT (C)	Toe temperature
TUO	Transformed urine output
UO (ml)	Urine output
$\dot{V}O_2$ (cc)	Oxygen consumption

serum albumin and red cell mass with ^{51}Cr-tagged red blood cells, and both of these values were than standardized by weight to obtain plasma volume index and red-cell index [11]. Laboratory procedures used for measurement of lactate and of arterial pH, partial pressures of carbon dioxide and oxygen, and oxygen saturation are described in previous publications [16,17].

For the calculation of oxygen consumption, blood was sampled simultaneously from the pulmonary artery or right-atrial catheter within an interval of <15 min following inscription of the indicator dilution curve. Oxygen concentration (c) was calculated by the standard formula:

$$C_aO_2 = \text{Hgb} \times S_aO_2 \times 1.39 + (P_aO_2 \times 0.0031)$$

Oxygen transport was computed as the product of the arterial oxygen concentration and cardiac output. Oxygen consumption was calculated from measured values of cardiac output (CO) according to the formula:

$$V_{O_2} = \text{CO}\,[C_aO_2 - C_{\bar{v}}O_2]$$

which represents the difference between arterial and mixed venous oxygen contents.

Statistical Analysis

The final values of the four groups of patients were analyzed separately. For each group, the data were divided into subgroups of survivors and nonsurvivors. Each variable was first examined to evaluate its reliability for the assessment of severity of illness. For each group of patients, the statistical technique of linear discriminant analysis was used to establish a reference value for each variable by which a patient would be classified as a survivor or nonsurvivor. The probability of correct classification, as a survivor or nonsurvivor, with respect to the reference value was then determined. The reliability was expressed as 100 times the probability of correct classification. The variables were then ranked according to the magnitude of their reliabilities.

Since the estimate of the probability of correct classification requires that the frequency distributions of the variables follow Gaussian distributions, the frequency distribution of each variable was examined separately. Appropriate transformations were applied to the variables when distributions deviated significantly from the normal distribution.

The statistical technique of linear discriminant function (LDF) analysis also offers a method for combining the values of several variables to predict survival in an optimal way [1]. A stepwise linear discriminant analysis program was used to determine the smallest number of variables (k), which provided a degree of reliability such that inclusion of additional variables did not significantly improve the reliability of indices [7]. The reliabilities of the LDF analysis, based on all possible combinations of K variables, were compared in order to select an LDF that combined maximal reliability and clinical availability to serve the best interest of patient management.

RESULTS

The reliabilities and the reference values for individual variables are shown in Table 2, together with a sign indication of the direction of change in which survival is predicted. The most reliable combinations of variables are summarized in Table 3.

TABLE 2 Reference Values and Reliabilities for Final Values of Survivors for Each Shock Group

MYOCARDIAL INFARCTION			DRUG OVERDOSE			BACTERIAL SHOCK			HYPOVOLEMIA		
VARIABLE	REFERENCE VALUE	RELIABILITY (%)	VARIABLE	REFERENCE VALUE	RELIABILITY (%)	VARIABLE	REFERENCE VALUE	RELIABILITY (%)	VARIABLE	REFERENCE VALUE	RELIABILITY (%)
LAC	<2.99	85	SP	>105	80	V_{O_2}	>172	91	TUO	>1.3	93
SW	>41	82	MAP	>74	77	DP	>48	90	MAP	>72	86
UO	>56	78	RT	>36.3	76	MAP	>64	89	DP	>53	85
CW	>3123	77	pH_a	>7.39	76	CW	>4899	88	LAC	<4.7	84
SI	>25	73	LAC	<3.17	76	SP	>97	83	pH_a	>7.36	77
AT	<12	72	S_aO_2	>92	74	LAC	<5.76	77	SP	>116	76
DP	>53	71	DP	>58	73	T_{O_2}	>73	75	Hgb	>9.8	75
MAP	>66	71	UO	>78	69	pH_a	>7.40	73	CW	>5679	74
MCT	<26.8	71	CW	>5137	68	CBV	>1.61	72	HCT	>28.9	72
CI	>1.8	70	MVP	<7.2	66	CI	>3.0	70	T_{O_2}	>7554	70
PVI	>48	70	CI	>2.95	66	SI	>33	65	RT	>36.3	70
SP	>91	68	SI	>31	64	RT	>36.6	64	MVP	<9.9	67
pH_a	>7.40	64	MCT	<15.7	64	TT	>27.8	64	S_aO_2	>94	63
P_aCO_2	>41	62	P_aO_2	<40	62	RES	>926	60	P_aO_2	>36	62

TABLE 3 Most Reliable Combinations of Two Variables

GROUP	VARIABLES	RELIABILITY (%)
Myocardial infarction and shock (I)		
LAC included	LAC, P_aCO_2	89
	LAC, SI	88
	LAC, MVP	87
LAC excluded	SI, DP	84
	SI, MAP	81
	SI, SP	78
Drug overdose (II)		
LAC included	SP, S_aO_2	92
	SP, pH	90
	SP, LAC	87
LAC excluded	SP, S_aO_2	86
	SP, pH	86
Bacterial shock (III)		
LAC included	MAP, V_{O_2}	94
	DP, CBV	92
	Log LAC, V_{O_2}	91
Hypovolemia (IV)		
LAC included	UO, MAP	97
	UO, log RES	97
	TUO, T_{O_2}	93

Group I—myocardial infarction and shock. In the analysis of individual variables, the lactate (LAC) was the best single predictor. The only other variable that contributed to the reliability of LAC was P_aO_2, but this was of borderline significance ($p<0.07$). Exclusion of patients whose LAC values were not available rendered the stroke index (SI) the most reliable single variable. Diastolic blood pressure (DP) contributed most significantly ($p<0.01$) to SI. Inclusion of additional variables did not significantly improve the reliability of prediction. Analysis of the data in the 24 patients whose LAC were available revealed the combination of systolic blood pressure (SP) and S_aO_2 was most reliable. It was followed by the combinations of SP with pH, and SP with LAC.

Group II—drug overdose. When LAC was excluded from the analysis (it was measured in only 44 patients), SP was the most reliable single variable.

When other single variables were combined with SP, pH_a contributed most ($p<0.01$). Inclusion of additional variables did not significantly improve the reliability of the prediction. Other highly reliable combinations of two variables were SP and S_aO_2, mean arterial pressure (MAP) and S_aO_2, MAP and pH, and CVP. Systolic blood pressure, individually or combined with other variables, emerged as the single most useful measurement for predicting survival (Table 3).

Group III—bacterial shock. The most reliable single variable, was V_{O_2} followed by DP, MAP, and CW. Among all variables, the final values of MAP contributed most to V_{O_2} ($p<0.005$), giving a combined reliability of 94%. Inclusion of any other single variable did not significantly improve the reliability of the prediction nor did it increase the number of patients classified correctly. Among hemodynamic variables, the best combination was DP and central blood volume (CBV). Among all variables, the best combination was V_{O_2} and log LAC.

Group IV—hypovolemic shock. When the value of urine output (UO) was transformed to urine output (TUO), by adding 5 ml to each value and then taking its logarithm, its final values yielded a reliability of 93%. The MAP, DP, and LAC variables were more reliable than others (Table 2).

The best combinations of two variables was TUO with the logarithm of cardiac work (CW) (93% reliability). The addition of the third and fourth best variables did not increase reliabilities. For this reason, only two variables were employed for the computation of the F index. The results of all combinations of two variables were then examined. The following pairs: (a) MAP with UO, (b) log RES (peripheral vascular resistance) with UO, and (c) T_{O_2} with TUO, proved to be more reliable than other combinations (Table 3).

DISCUSSION

Attempts to estimate the severity of circulatory, respiratory and metabolic abnormalities in patients in shock have been based largely on the physician's clinical judgment supplemented by a limited number of quantitative physiologic measurements. The availability of techniques and instrumentation suitable for bedside monitoring of the critically ill patient has made it possible to rapidly measure changes in physiologic status. The final measurements of the hemodynamic, respiratory, and metabolic variables, obtained before the patient was discharged as a survivor or during the late stages prior to death, excluding the agonal period which reflects terminal events, may be used to objectively assess the severity of the patient's illness and his response to treatment.

This study failed to expose a consistent group of variables which would be applicable to all patients in shock regardless of cause. For patients with acute myocardial infarction a metabolic deficit reflecting reduced tissue blood flow, arterial blood lactate was the most valuable single measurement with superseded measurements of blood flow [SI, appearance time (AT), and mean circulation time (MCT)], arterial pressure, (DP), and UO. When shock was related to drug overdose, parameters reflecting arterial perfusion pressure (SP, MAP) were the most reliable with metabolic deficits indicated by lactate and pH_a, and alterations in heat production and/or loss were reflected in rectal temperature. Among patients with bacterial shock, oxygen consumption emerged as the most reliable single variable for estimating severity and prognosis.

While measurements of arterial pressure are relatively less reliable among patients with myocardial infarction and shock, they have a high level of reliability for estimating severity in patients with drug overdose and those with bacterial shock. However, in patients after shock due to myocardial infarction and in patients with hypovolemic shock, measurements of LAC and SI have a higher reliability than measurements of pressure.

Despite the difference of their relative reliability, some variables had a consistent reliability exceeding 70% for each of the shock groups (myocardial infarction, drug overdose, bacterial infection, and hypovolemia). These included lactate (85%, 76%, 77%, and 84%, respectively), mean arterial pressure (71%, 77%, 89%, and 86%, respectively), and diastolic pressure (71%, 73%, 90%, and 85%, respectively). Consequently, when the cause of shock is not identified, these variables should be regarded as primary references to patient condition.

Recent studies have suggested that measurements of pulmonary artery wedge and left ventricular pressures may provide valuable prognostic information on left-ventricular function, particularly in patients with acute myocardial infarction [4,6,8–10]. Measurements of these variables were available in more recent patients and our observations also point to their potential value for purposes of prognosis. However, the data base was not sufficiently large for purposes of detailed statistical analysis.

Other measurements reflecting cardiac output and pressure, particularly stroke work and to lesser extent, cardiac work, provided a high degree of reliability among patients with myocardial infarction (Table 2). Yet these parameters are derived from more primary measurements of flow and pressure and only provide ease in interpretation of data in the clinical context. The present technique of estimating prognosis takes such relationships between primary variables into account as a matter of course and by more formal statistical procedures. Accordingly, the number and complexity of derived parameters may be curtailed.

Discriminant functions may be readily calculated at the bedside with a conventional and relatively inexpensive calculator. They may therefore be immediately available to facilitate quantitation of responsiveness to treatment when the measurements likely to provide the best discriminant functions are not available. Alternative combinations may be substituted, often with only a relatively small sacrifice in reliability.

Summary

Hemodynamic, respiratory, and metabolic variables, prospectively measured on a repetitive basis in patients in shock due to myocardial infarction, drug overdose, gram-negative bacterial infection, and hypovolemia, are analyzed. The reliabilities of the individual variables for assessing severity for these four groups of patients are computed by the method of multivariate linear discriminant function analysis. Combinations of variables that provide the greatest reliability were identified and they were found to differ among the four groups of patients.

References

1. **Afifi, A. A.**, and **Azen, S. P.** (1972). *Statistical Analysis: A Computer Oriented Approach.* New York: Academic.
2. **Afifi, A. A., Chang, P. C., Liu, V. Y., Luz, P., Weil, M. H.**, and **Shubin, H.** (1974). Prognostic indices in acute myocardial infarction complicated by shock. *Am. J. Cardiol. 33:*826–832.
3. **Afifi, A. A., Sacks, S. T., Liu, V. Y., Weil, M. H.**, and **Shubin, H.** (1971). Accumulative prognostic index for patients with barbiturate, glutethimide and meprobamate intoxication. *New Engl. J. Med. 285:*1497–1502.
4. **Bevegard, S., Blomquist, P.**, and **Hulting, J.** (1972). *Cardiorespiratory Monitoring Indices in Acute Myocardial Infarction.* Stockholm: Karolinska Institute (Rep. Lab. Aviat. Nav. Med.), p. 32.
5. **Chang, P. C., Afifi, A. A., Liu, V. Y., Nishijima, H., Weil, M. H.**, and **Shubin, H.** (1974). Prognostic indices for assessment of patients with gram-negative bacteremia and shock. In: Urbascheck B. (ed.), *Aspects of Biological Reactions to Bacterial Endotoxins,* Vol. 3. Basel: Karger AG.
6. **Cohn, J. N., Khatri, I. M.**, and **Hamosh, P.** (1970). Bedside catheterization of the left ventricle. *Am. J. Cardiol. 25:*66–69.
7. **Dixon, W. J.** (1967). *BMD: Biomedical Computer Programs,* Second edition, Berkeley: University of California Press, p. 214.
8. **Gunnar, R. M.**, and **Loeb, H. S.** (1972). Use of drugs in cardiogenic shock due to acute myocardial infarction. *Circulation 45:*1111–1124.
9. **Parmley, W. W., Diamond, G.**, and **Tomoda, H.** (1972). Clinical evaluation of left ventricular pressure in myocardial infarction. *Circulation 45:* 358–366.
10. **Ratshin, R. A., Rackely, C. E.**, and **Russell, R. O., Jr.** (1972). Hemodynamic evaluation of left ventricular function in shock complicating myocardial infarction. *Circulation 45:*127–139.
11. **Rystrom, L., Weil, M. H.**, and **Shubin, H.** (1971). Technique of measurement of the plasma volume and red cell mass during acute circulatory failure. *Surg. Gynec. Obstet. 133:*621–626.
12. **Shubin, H., Chang, P., Freund, U., Portigal, L., Schriver, J.**, and **Weil,**

M. H. (in preparation). Cumulative prognostic index: Patients with hypovolemic shock.

13. **Shubin, H., Weil, M. H.,** and **Rockwell, M. A., Jr.** (1967). Automated measurement of cardiac output in patients by use of a digital computer. *Med. Biol. Eng. 5:*353–360.
14. **Shubin, H., Weil, M. H.,** and **Rockwell, M. A., Jr.** (1967). Automated measurement of arterial pressure in patients by use of a digital computer. *Med. Biol. Eng. 5:*361–369.
15. **Udhoji, V. N., Weil, M. H.,** and **Sambihi, M. P.** (1963). Hemodynamic studies on clinical shock associated with infection. *Am. J. Med. 34:*461–469.
16. **Weil, M. H.,** and **Afifi, A. A.** (1970). Experimental and clinical studies on lactate and pyruvate as indicators of the severity of acute circulatory failure (shock). *Circulation 41:*989–1001.
17. **Zahn, R. L.,** and **Weil, M. H.** (1966). Central venous blood for monitoring pH and P_{CO_2} in the critically ill patient. *J. Thorac. Cardiovasc. Surg. 52:*105–111.

Disseminated Intravascular Coagulation

ROBERT M. HARDAWAY, III, M.D.
Brigadier General, Medical Corps, U. S. Army,
William Beaumont Army Medical Center, El Paso, Texas

Disseminated intravascular coagulation (DIC) is a new concept in the etiology of disease [3]. It is defined as acute, transient coagulation occurring in the flowing blood throughout the vascular tree which may obstruct the microcirculation. It may or may not result in an accumulation of fibrin but does involve the transformation of fibrinogen into fibrin. It includes the agglutination of platelets and red cells and the sticking of leukocytes.

It has been postulated that coagulation and clot lysis are normally, continuously, and simultaneously going on within the vascular tree. The actual lining of the endothelial layer of the blood vessels may consist of a layer of fibrin, which helps to seal the vessel wall. Electron microscopy has shown fibrin fibrils on the endothelial surface. The implication of this observation is that the blood remains fluid normally in spite of a small but dynamic and continuous clotting of fibrin inside the vascular system. This hypothesis assumes that fibrinogen, which has a half-life under normal conditions of approximately 6 days, disappears from the blood because of its conversion to fibrin by the highly active blood-clotting system. The fibrin then formed is removed by the fibrinolytic enzyme plasmin or fibrinolysin, or by the reticuloendothelial system. The speed of the fibrin accumulation will depend on the concentration of thrombin, and the speed of fibrin dissolution on the concentration of fibrinolysin and the integrity of the reticuloendothelial system. If fibrin is not removed with the same speed as it is formed, an accumulation will occur. It can be seen that changes in this equilibrium may result in the accumulation of fibrin. A great many factors are known to shift this equilibrium toward more intravascular coagulation.

The production of DIC. In significant amounts, this requires two separate factors; neither alone is adequate. These are: (a) stagnant-acid capillary flow and (b) presence of a thrombogenic agent in the blood stream. The stagnant-acid capillary flow may be brought about by nothing more than vasoconstriction produced by factors such as a high catecholamine level, sympathetic stimulation, stress, trauma, and hemorrhage (Fig. 1).

This stagnant flow produces a hypercoagulable blood, which, together with a slow or absent flow, makes it easy for blood to clot [1,2]. However, this alone will not produce DIC. Even severe hemorrhage with shock will not produce DIC alone.

Thromboplastic agents alone cannot produce more than a transient and benign intravascular coagulation. The injection of pure thrombin will produce a transient clotting episode and shock, but unless it is overwhelming and fatal, it does not produce truly disseminated intravascular clotting. Many thrombogenic agents may act in concert with vasoconstriction. These include:

1. Bacterial toxins, both endotoxins and exotoxins.
2. Hemolysis of red cells. This may be due to two separate factors. There is a thromboplastin in red cells first described by Quick in 1954 [4]. Also, the fragments of red cell membranes may act as particulate matter, which is strongly thrombogenic.
3. Tissue juices containing thromboplastin when these are liberated from crushed and injured tissues.
4. Amniotic fluid gaining access to the blood stream. This is strongly thrombogenic due to the cellular debris it contains.
5. Platelet agglutination promotes coagulation. Endotoxin is selectively absorbed by platelets, which causes their clumping and removal from the circulating blood.
6. Malignant tumors as they invade the vascular tree.
7. Ischemic and dead tissue, which may initiate coagulation.
8. Anaphylaxis and antigen–antibody reactions, which initiate coagulation.
9. Trypsin, which has a similar effect as that of thrombin, may be liberated into the blood stream during pancreatitis.
10. Many types of snake venom.
11. Thermal burns.
12. Contact of blood with foreign surfaces during extracorpeal circulation for open-heart surgery and renal dialysis.

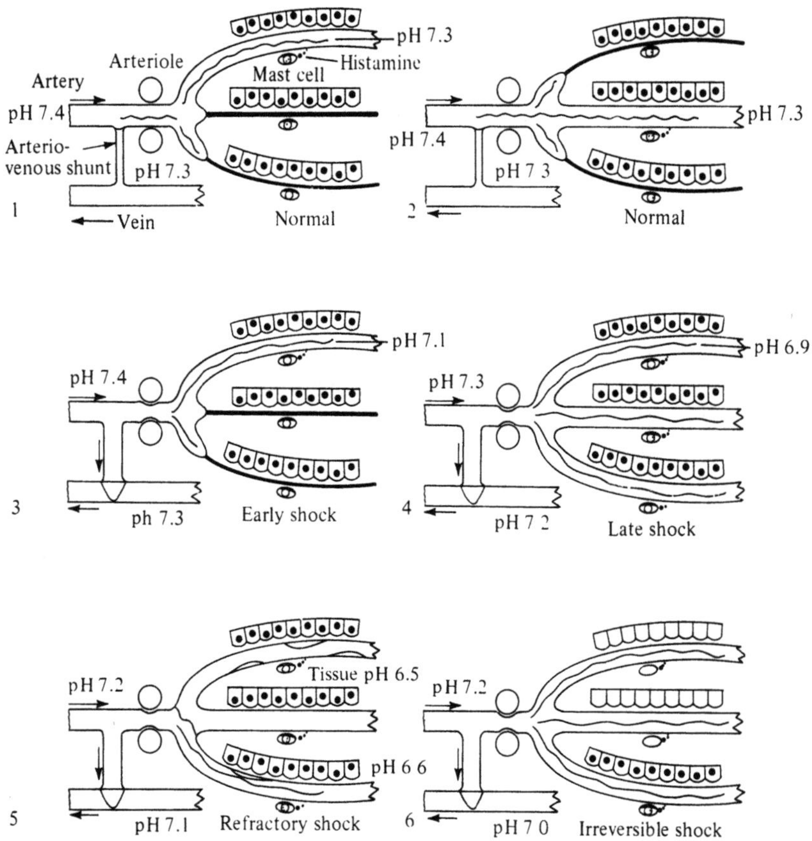

FIGURE 1 Reversible and Irreversible Shock. Shock may also be classified as reversible, refractory, or irreversible depending on its stage of development. The following diagrams illustrate different stages of shock from onset to irreversibility. Each diagram represents a small artery ending in an arteriole with a sphincter-like action. **1.** Normal Condition–Upper Capillary Open. The arteriole is opened quite widely. Only one capillary is being perfused while others rest. Capillaries open in rotation on demand of cells adjacent to them. Histamine secreted by mast cells along the capillaries cause capillary sphincters to open. Constant perfusion is not necessary. Blood flow through the capillaries is rapid; drop in pH along the capillaries is minimal. Cells of middle capillary are becoming slightly anoxic. Arteriovenous shunt is closed. **2.** Normal Condition–Central Capillary Open, Upper Capillary Closed. Center cells have become slightly anoxic and mast cells have secreted histamine, causing central capillary to open. Upper capillary is now closed as mast cells have stopped secreting histamine. Arteriole is still opened quite widely. **3.** Shock, Phase I (Early, Reversible). Elevated catecholamines have caused vasoconstriction. The arteriovenous shunt has opened as a part of the catecholamine action. Poor venous return to the heart may cause a loss of arterial blood pressure. All of these changes cause a slow capillary flow in the upper capillary. **4.** Shock, Phase II (Late, Reversible). Since a long time is required for adequate perfusion of the cells because of the slow capillary flow, all capillaries are now open. Capillary flow is extremely slow and fall in pH along the capillary is marked. This fall in pH is caused by anaerobic metabolism with lactic

The effects of DIC. These may be summarized under three categories: (a) onset of DIC, usually accompanied by a sudden fall in arterial blood pressure and shock, (b) rapid onset of a consumptive coagulopathy (coagulation defect), and (c) focal tissue necrosis and organ failure. DIC and refractory shock usually occur together and are essentially identical (Fig. 1) [1,2]. Refractory shock is defined as shock which does not respond readily to fluid volume administration.

The coagulation defect may appear within a few minutes. It is due primarily to the consumption of all clotting factors leaving the remaining unclotted blood low in clotting factors and incoagulable. It affects all clotting factors and platelets (Table 1). Fibrinogen is usually not affected and generally high except in near-fatal cases and those involving high levels of fibrinolysin. This is due to the rapid replacement rate of fibrinogen. Two other clotting abnormalities are produced secondarily. When fibrinogen is split by thrombin, the resulting split products act as anticoagulants, much like heparin. Also, simultaneous with the body's defense against the clotting process there is the activation of endogenous fibrinolysin. This may be modest or great in amount, with liberation of a large amount of fibrinolysin. This accounts for afibrinogenemia and devastating hemorrhage. The clotting defect may not be clinically detectable except by laboratory testing, or it may be the cause of devastating hemorrhage, particularly in patients who have surgical wounds.

Focal-tissue necrosis is caused by protracted obstruction of capillaries by thrombi. Endogenous fibrinolysin dissolves the thrombi but if fibrinolysis is delayed, necrosis results. This occurs in various vital organs such as the liver, kidney (Fig. 2), lungs (Fig. 3), pancreas, gut, and heart. If pronounced, the necrosis results in organ failure and death.

Diagnosis of DIC. This condition will be missed if it is not looked for. Mild cases produce no clinical symptoms. The sudden onset of a clotting effect in otherwise normally clotting blood is the chief clue. Generalized oozing of blood is a classic sign but it is often absent, especially when there are no surgical wounds. It is necessary to perform laboratory tests. These include platelet count, prothrombin time, partial thromboplastin

---

acid production. **5.** Shock, Phase III (Refractory). This phase is associated with disseminated intravascular coagulation. Stagnant acid blood in the presence of sepsis or tissue injury has begun to coagulate, causing sticking of red cells with occlusion of upper two capillaries. Occlusion stops perfusion in these capillaries completely. Cells nourished by these two capillaries are drying. Blood flow through the lower capillary is sluggish. Circulating blood is incoagulable. Because of the action of endogenous fibrinolysin, clotted blood in upper capillary has started to lyse. **6.** Shock, Phase IV (Irreversible). Cells nourished by the upper and central capillaries have died, producing focal tissue necrosis. Capillary clots have lysed and circulation has been restored. However, large areas of necrosis are producing multiple organ failure with resulting death of the organism.

TABLE 1 Clotting Factor Depletions Noted in 29 Consecutive Cases of Refractory Shock

					CONTROL		FACTOR ASSAYS						
PATIENT	FIBRINOGEN	PLATELETS	PT	PTT	PT	PTT	II	V	VIII	IX	X	XI	XII
1	238 mg%	16,500	19.0	60.4	13.2	38.4							
2	228 mg%	31,000	16.2	72.8	12.5	37.6	46	59	100	57	54		
3	347 mg%	111,000	15.6	49.4	12.5	41.6							
4	359 mg%	102,000	18.0	215.8	13.2	42.5	45	66	48	2	17		95
5	542 mg%	265,000	14.5	120.5	13.0	55.0							
6	318 mg%	24,000	15.8	255.0	12.3	43.0	50	32	10	37			77
7	400 mg%	99,500	15.8	75.0	13.4	47.4	100	86	59	56			48
8	235 mg%	97,500	17.9	71.6	13.9	44.3							
9	280 mg%	16,500	19.3	61.9	14.5	48.2							
10	290 mg%	154,000	120.0	180.0	14.9	42.0							
11	650 mg%	101,500	25.4	93.4	13.5	48.3	100	63	35			26	15
12	320 mg%	8,000	22.0	86.2	12.5	41.0							
13	355 mg%	8,000	19.0	72.6	13.0	44.3	45	35	67			23	90
14	160 mg%	29,000	16.2	132.0	13.6	41.6							
15	165 mg%	3,000	37.0	263.4	13.3	46.2	23	5	3			6	18
16	150 mg%	57,000	17.8	277.0	14.3	55.9							
17	355 mg%	116,000	15.2	49.0	13.7	44.7							
18	184 mg%	13,000	26.4	207.0	13.3	44.9	6	12	54			23	29
19	355 mg%	110,000	15.2	49.0	14.5	44.8							
20	184 mg%	12,500	26.4	207.0	13.5	46.8	6	12	54			23	29
21	50 mg%	18,000	33.0	240.0	14.1	40.5							
22	605 mg%	83,000	14.9	50.5	14.3	46.5							
23	367 mg%	3,500	16.0	116.9	13.1	48.2							
24	240 mg%	15,500	52.5	107.4	12.9	35.7							
25	525 mg%	29,500	16.6	76.6	14.6	48.5							
26	325 mg%	140,000	14.4	44.9	14.2	54.7							
27	465 mg%	3,000	22.2	86.6	12.8	47.1							
28	436 mg%	33,500	17.4	52.0	12.7	47.3							
29	310 mg%	12,000	30.6	94.2	14.5	55.5							
Average	310 mg%	59,000	24.5	119	13.5	43.9	46%	41%	48%	38%	35%	20%	50%

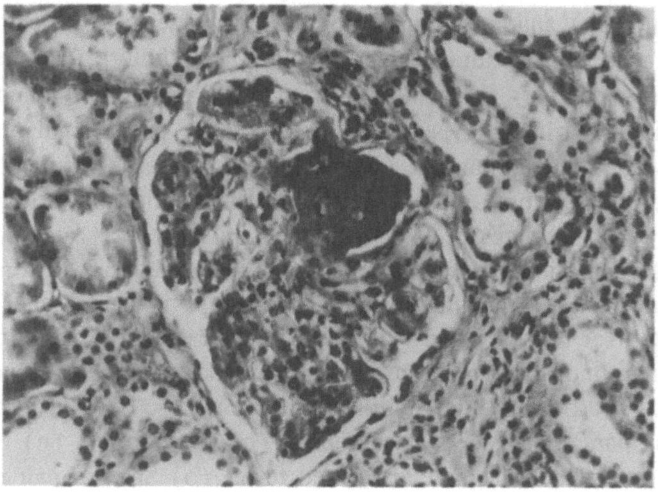

FIGURE 2 Kidney of patient dying from septic shock. Note fibrinthrombus in glomerulus of kidney.

time, and fibrinolytic activity. An increase in fibrin split products is diagnostic.

Occurrence of DIC. This type of coagulopathy occurs with great frequency in a wide variety of medical and surgical conditions. These include: (a)

FIGURE 3 Lung of patient dying of "shock lung" after severe septic shock. Note intravascular thrombi, widened alveolar septa, congestion, edema and proteinacous membrane lining several of the alveoli.

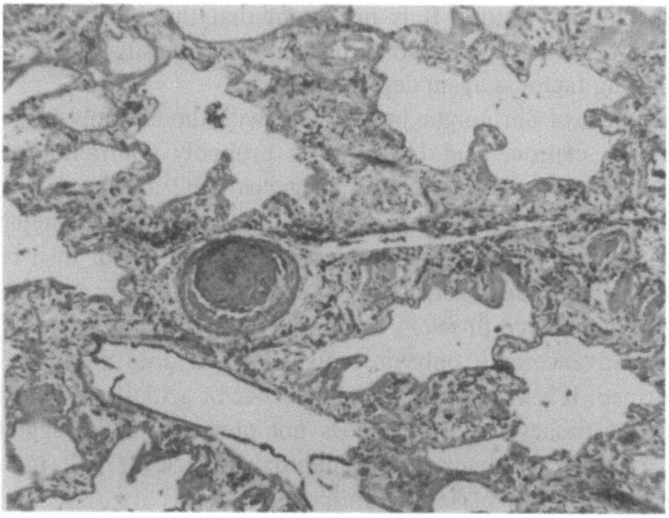

shock (inadequate capillary perfusion): (i) septic, (ii) traumatic (including burns), and (iii) anaphylactic; (b) hemorrhage due to acute clotting defect, (c) acute renal, kidney, lung, liver, or heart failure; (d) hemolytic syndromes; including: (i) hemolytic transfusion reaction or anemic syndrome, (ii) malaria or favism, (iii) trauma, (iv) paroxysmal nocturnal, cold, or March hemoglobinuria, (v) sickle-cell disease, (vi) hemolysis due to hypotonic solution, and (vii) thrombohemolytic thrombocytopenic purpura; (e) syndromes of late pregnancy, including: (i) toxemia, (ii) premature separation of the placenta, (iii) defibrination syndrome, (iv) pituitary necrosis, (v) amniotic fluid embolism, (vi) acute renal failure, (vii) acute liver necrosis, and (viii) sepsis; (f) extracorporeal circulation, (g) clotting abnormalities due to cancer, (h) snake bite, (i) pseudomembranous or necrotizing enterocolitis, (j) hemorrhagic gastritis, (k) acute necrotizing pancreatitis, (l) fat embolism, (m) heat stroke, (n) epidemic hemorrhage or Rocky Mountain spotted fever, (o) Shwartzman reaction, (p) injection of particulate matter, and (q) acute adrenal necrosis (Waterhouse–Friderichsen syndrome).

Treatment of DIC.

1. Promotion of capillary flow by intravenous volume administration to fill the expanded vascular space and promote vasodilation by lowering endogenous catecholamine levels (Fig. 4). Vasodilating agents may be required.
2. Removal of the thrombogenic material by draining abscesses and treating infection with antibiotics.

Treatment of the clotting defect is not usually necessary as it spontaneously resolves with cessation of DIC (Fig. 4). However, if hemorrhage is a problem, the rapid administration of fresh whole blood will replace all clotting factors. It is important that this be given rapidly so that clotting will be accomplished at the hemorrhaging sites before the blood level of clotting factor is again depleted.

The treatment of fibrinolytic hemorrhage with the fibrinolysin antagonist epsilon amino caproic acid (EACA) is probably contraindicated as it interfers with a protective mechanism against DIC and promotes thrombosis and increases DIC. If used, it should be combined with heparin. The use of heparin is a controversial subject. It may be useful in a few cases of continuing DIC. However, it has many disadvantages, as it may complicate the hemorrhage problem and promote further blood loss. It must be given in advance as it only prevents DIC and does not dissolve clots already formed. It is inactivated in the presence of acidosis, which is usually present in the tissues in DIC. It does not prevent platelet agglutination, which is a trigger mechanism for endotoxin shock. It will not prevent coagulation by the coagulase of gram-positive cocci.

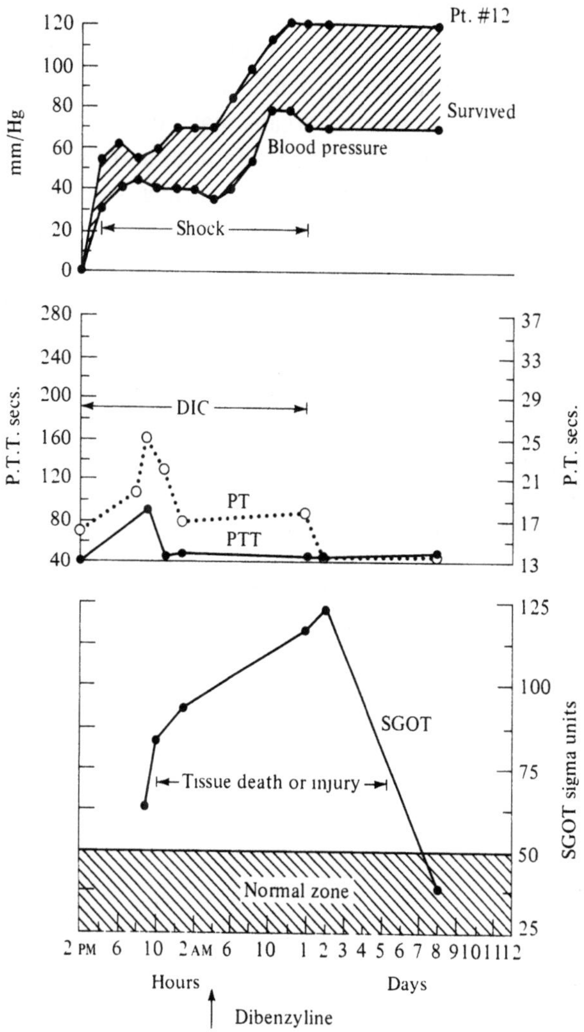

FIGURE 4 This patient was in severe septic shock with unobtainable blood pressure. He rapidly developed a clotting defect. Although volume administration resulted in partial blood pressure return, it was inadequate and vasodilatation was required. This resulted in a return to normal blood pressure and a recovery from shock. Note that an episode of disseminated intravascular coagulation accompanied refractory shock but spontaneously subsided. Note also that while there was considerable tissue death or injury as indicated by the elevated SGOT that this rapidly fell after the shock episode, indicating a good prognosis and relatively mild amount of tissue damage.

Summary

Disseminated intravascular coagulation (DIC) is a common complication in a wide variety of acute medical and surgical conditions. It is caused by a variety of thrombogenic substances (especially bacterial toxins, hemolyzed red cells, and tissue juices) in the blood stream in the presence of a slow capillary blood flow (shock). Diagnosis is by laboratory coagulation studies. A suddenly appearing coagulation deficit with possible hemorrhage and focal tissue necrosis in various vital organs may account for multiple organ failure including renal failure, pulmonary failure, and liver failure, as well as pancreatitis, enteritis, and heart failure. Therapy is centered on promoting capillary flow. Heparin and epsilon amino caproic acid are probably not indicated for routine management.

References

1. **Hardaway, R. M.** (1968). *Clinical Management of Shock.* Springfield, Illinois: Thomas.
2. **Hardaway, R. M.** (1966). *Syndromes of Disseminated Intravascular Coagulation.* Springfield, Illinois: Thomas.
3. **Hardaway, R. M.,** and **McKay, D. G.** (1963). The syndromes of DIC. *Rev. Surg. 20:*297–328.
4. **Qiuck, A. J., Daniels, E. R.,** and **Hussey, C. V.** (1954). Acquired antithromboplastinogenemia. *J. Lab. Clin. Med. 44:*94–103.

Principles of Fluid Challenge for Routine Treatment of Shock

MAX HARRY WEIL, M.D., PH.D.
Shock Research Unit and Center for the Critically Ill, University of Southern California School of Medicine, the Los Angeles County/University of Southern California Medical Center, and the Hollywood Presbyterian Medical Center, Los Angeles, California

A critical reduction of intravascular volume is the most frequent cause of circulatory shock. Clinical and laboratory signs of volume deficit are of limited reliability. Guided by measurements of CVP, pulmonary-artery wedge, or pulmonary diastolic pressures, the major hazard of volume-overload-induced cardiac failure may be avoided.

Bedside cardiac catheterization methods allowing routine monitoring of pressure changes have been simplified. The "fluid challenge" is the evaluation of the effect of infusion of 50–200-ml volumes over 10-min intervals.

Shock-unit studies indicate the need for a systematic approach to the routine management of shock, regardless of cause. Since treatment cannot be delayed and accurate diagnosis is essential, a systematic and diagnostically informative approach is needed during treatment.

Measurement of blood-volume deficits. Volume deficits may be an obvious cause of shock in patients presenting gross evidence of blood loss or dehydration. Less apparent are losses after trauma from a blunt object or with massive infection. An increase of only one inch in the circumference of one thigh may represent extravasation of 50% of the total blood volume. After blood loss the laboratory measurement of hemoglobin and hematocrit values is sometimes misleading, particularly when there has not been enough time for transcapillary refill and, consequently, compensation by hemodilution. Measurements of blood volume by radioisotopic or dye-dilution methods may be helpful under these circumstances if rigorous techniques are used, including multiple sampling over a period of ≧35 min to assure complete mixing of the indicator. However, this technique is time-consuming and requires specialized technical staff [4].

Measurement of central venous and pulmonary-artery wedge or diastolic pressure. The measurement of CVP and, more recently, of pulmonary artery and pulmonary-artery wedge pressures (PAWP), which permits the clinician to detect limitations in cardiac competence, provides a practical guide for fluid repletion (Fig. 1). Since congestive heart failure is the only immediate hazard of fluid challenge, the PAWP and CVP provide a reliable indication of the capability of the heart to accept the additional volume load.

The technique of central venous and pulmonary-artery catheterization by way of the arm vein or by direct subclavian or internal jugular puncture is easily mastered. The importance of its routine use to guide management of shock is established [1–3,5,7,9,10].

Measurements of PAWP provide a more precise indication of left-

FIGURE 1 Simultaneous measurement of arterial, arterial venous (right atrial), and pulmonary-artery pressure. Following inflation of the balloon, the catheter advances into wedge position with typical decline in pressure and pulse contour. After deflation of the balloon, pulmonary-artery pressure is once again recorded.

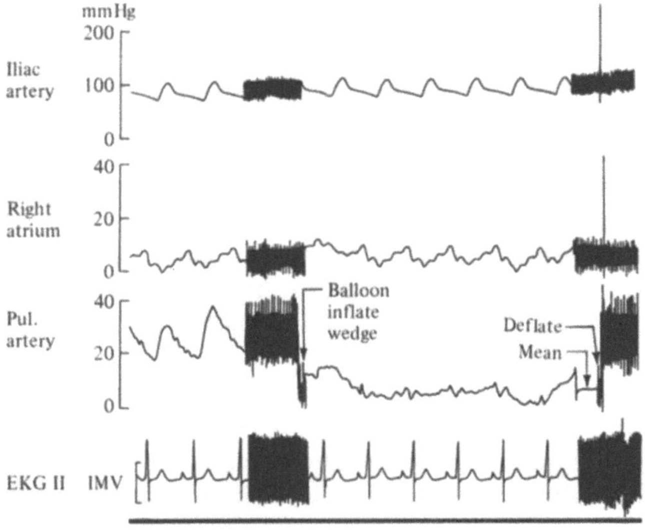

ventricular function than do CVP measurements [5]. The development of a flow-directed, balloon-tipped catheter [7] has greatly facilitated the introduction of the catheter into the pulmonary artery. The catheter is inserted percutaneously or by surgical cut down into a peripheral vein and advanced into the proximal superior or inferior vena cava. In our own Center for the Critically Ill, the flow-directed catheter is now routinely inserted by percutaneous puncture of the vein with the aid of a catheter introducer (Figs. 2 and 3). Antecubital, internal jugular, femoral, and supraclavicular subclavian routes are preferred because of the risk of pneumothorax with the intraclavicular subclavian approach. After the catheter has been advanced into the vena cava, the balloon at the tip is inflated with carbon dioxide or air and the catheter is advanced through the right atrium and ventricle into the pulmonary artery. Arrhythmias are surprisingly infrequent and most often limited to the brief interval when the catheter is advancing through the right ventricle. In approximately 70% of patients the catheter tip can be floated into a peripheral pulmonary vessel and pulmonary capillary pressure obtained. Since this measurement closely approximates the

FIGURE 2 Methods of inserting central venous and pulmonary-artery catheters are illustrated. In each instance, percutaneous guide-wide techniques may be utilized after the vein has been punctured with a suitable needle. A percutaneous catheter introducer includes a spring guide, a thin-walled sheath, and an optimally tapered perforating catheter. After the catheter introducer is in place, the spring guide and the perforating catheter are withdrawn, leaving the sheath in place. The central venous or pulmonary-artery catheter is then advanced through the sheath, after which the sheath is withdrawn over the catheter. The same technique may be used for placement of a temporary transvenous pacemaker. Published by permission of the American Medical Association, from Weil and Shubin, *JAMA 207*:338, 1969.

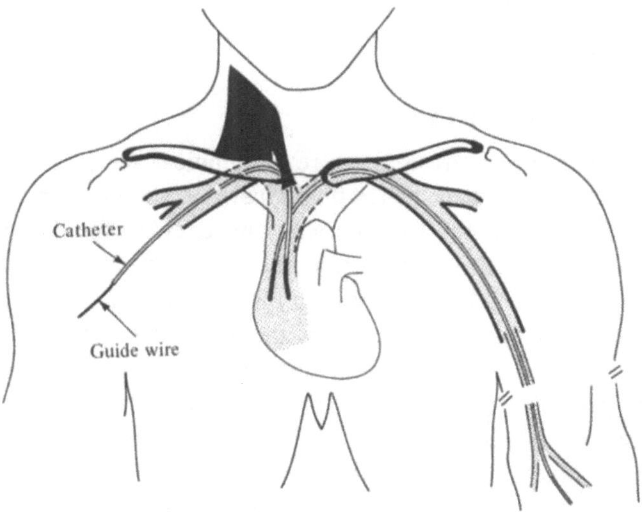

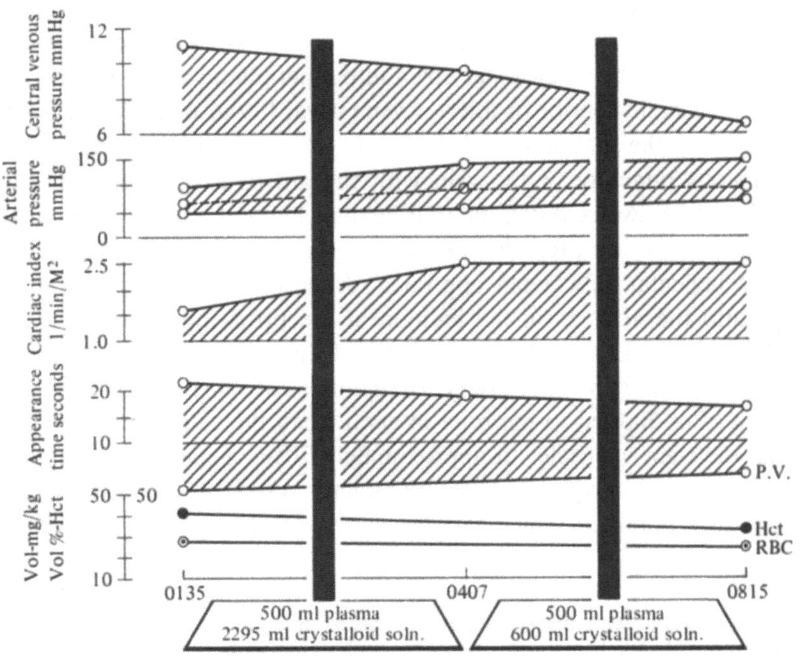

FIGURE 3 Decline in CVP during infusion of almost 4 l of fluid over an 8-hr period was part of a favorable clinical and hemodynamic response to treatment of an 81-year-old patient in shock after perforation of peptic ulcer. *Legend:* PV = plasma volume, RBC = red blood cell mass; Hct = arterial hematocrit; and appearance time = interval (circulation time) between injection of indocyanine green dye into right atrium and its arrival in brachial artery. Published by permission of the American Medical Association, from Weil and Shubin, *JAMA 207*:339, 1969.

left-ventricular end-diastolic pressures, it serves as a measure of left-ventricular function.

Rationale of Volume Repletion

If there is evidence of perfusion failure and clinical signs of shock, hypovolemia should be assumed; hence fluid challenge should be performed on a routine basis. This should be done with awareness of the colloid osmotic pressure (COP) [6,8]. It has been recently demonstrated by our group that in some patients the PAWP is normal in the presence of clinical and radiographic signs of pulmonary edema. In these patients the COP had been reduced from a normal value of 26 torr to <17 torr. Consequently, the hydrostatic pressure in the pulmonary capillaries, although in a normal range, may have exceeded the colloid osmotic (oncotic) pressure with consequent extravasation of fluid into the pulmonary interstitium or alveoli. In the clinical assessment of such patients, a reduction in the partial pressure of oxygen in arterial blood and signs of pulmonary congestion provide evidence that pulmonary edema is due to causes other than left ventricular failure. The routine measurement of COP is now feasible and greatly facilitates diagnosis of oncotic defects.

In the assessment and management of the patient with suspected hypovolemia, PAWP monitoring usually provides a reliable indicator of the safety of fluid repletion. Serial CVP measurements provide comparable information but are less sensitive when left-ventricular function is selectively impaired, as in acute myocardial infarction. Insertion of a pulmonary-artery catheter would therefore appear to be preferable, provided it can be accomplished expeditiously and without undue complications by a trained operator. Some additional dexterity and experience are required to properly position the pulmonary-artery catheter. Its routine use is warranted in those patients in whom left ventricular competence is most likely to be an issue, particularly in patients with known heart disease.

Neither CVP nor PAWP alone can indicate hypovolemia. In fact, these pressures may be increased after massive blood or fluid loss, particularly in elderly patients having limited cardiac reserve. Reductions in blood volume account for a decline in venous return to the heart; this accounts for a fall in cardiac output and arterial blood pressure and a critical reduction in the blood supply to the coronary arteries. If deprived of coronary blood flow, the contractile power of heart muscle is likely to be reduced, and ventricular end-diastolic volume, PAWP, and CVP are consequently increased. When cardiac output, arterial pressure, and coronary blood flow are restored to more normal values, the CVP, and less often the PAWP, may decline. In other words, the PAWP and CVP do not reflect the vascular volume alone but indicate the relationship between the volume that enters the heart and the effectiveness with which the heart pumps it out [3].

The Standard Fluid Challenge

For assessment of both volume deficits and pump failure, aliquots of 50–200 ml of crystalloid fluid (isotonic saline or dextrose solution) or colloid (5% albumin solution) are administered in a systematic manner. Measurements of either pulmonary artery wedge (PAWP) or pulmonary-artery diastolic pressure (PADP) are obtained during a 10-min observation period. Fluid is then administered through an intravenous route other than that used for pulmonary artery or central venous monitoring. If the PAWP or PADP is <11 torr, the fluid is infused at a rate of 20 ml/min for a 10-min period. If the PAWP or PADP range is 11–18 torr, 10 ml/min are administered; if >18 torr, we employ fluid challenges of 5 ml/min. If, during infusion, the PAWP or PADP increases at any time by >7 torr above the initial pressure and remains at this level for more than 1 min, the infusion is discontinued. When the pressure increases by >3 torr but <7 torr, infusion is discontinued after 10 min. In most cases, the PAWP or

PADP will decline to ±3 torr of the starting pressure. If this occurs, an additional aliquot of 200, 100, or 50 ml of fluid is administered over the next 10 min. The process is repeated until the pressure values during any given 10-min period increase to >7 torr or by >3 torr without decline during the 10-min waiting period. Often several liters of fluid may be required to restore effective circulation. Consequently, the full attention of a well-trained physician or nurse clinician may be required for up to 8 hr.

If the PAWP and PADP are both unavailable, the CVP may be used instead as a guide. Baseline measurements of CVP are obtained over a 10-min period. Fluid is then administered by a route other than that used for monitoring. If the CVP is <12 cm H_2O (9 torr), the fluid is infused at a rate of 20 ml/min for a 10-min period. If the CVP increases by >5 cm H_2O (4 torr) above the initial pressure during the 10-min infusion, fluid challenge is discontinued. If the CVP increases by more than 2 but no more than 5 cm H_2O (2–4 torr), the infusion is discontinued for 10-min. Fluid challenge is resumed after the 10-min delay if CVP declines to within 2 cm of the initial measurement during that interval. The procedure is then repeated in the manner illustrated in Fig. 4. In each instance the pressure

FIGURE 4 Technique of fluid challenge. Upper panel shows response of patient with primary fluid deficit. Decline in PAWP during fluid administration indicates improvement in cardiac competence. Lower panel shows limitation in cardiac competence with progressive rise in PAWP or PADP during infusion. Cardiac competence is restored after treatment with digitalis or phlebotomy.

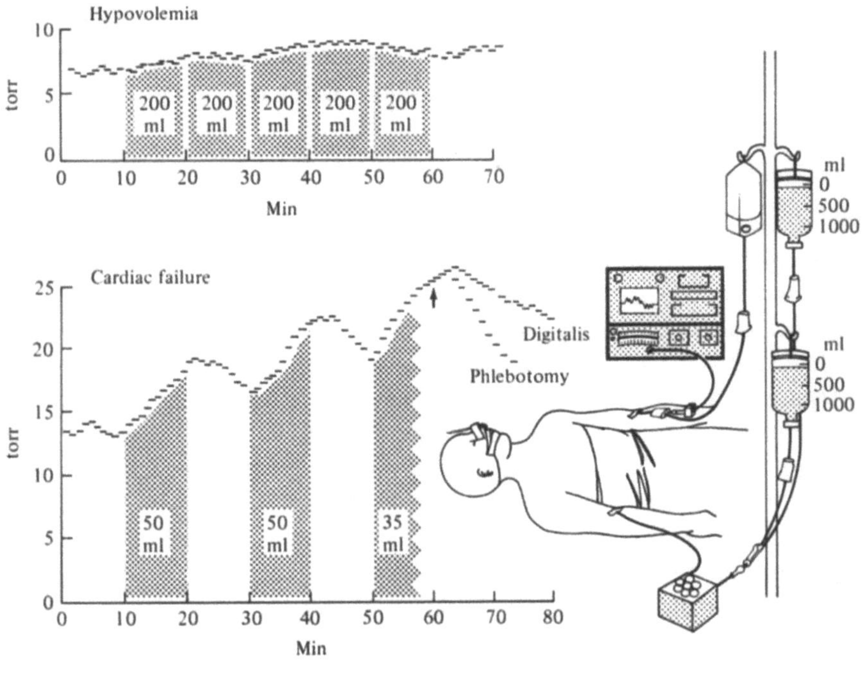

value immediately preceding the 200-, 100-, or 50-ml infusion serves as the reference measurement. Fluid challenge is discontinued as soon as hemodynamic signs of shock are reversed. Central venous and pulmonary-pressure measurements are indices not of shock reversal but only of limitation in cardiac competence in instances where fluid repletion must be curtailed prior to optimal reversal of the shock rate due to threat of acute heart failure.

The volume of fluid contained in the venous circuit may be increased as much as threefold with relatively little pressure change. Veins are highly distensible vessels, acting as reservoirs, and the venous system functions as a capacitance bed. Its behavior is different from that of the arterial system, which acts as a resistance bed in which pressure increases in direct relationship to the volume ejected into it.

A progressive increase in PAWP or CVP, especially following fluid challenge, may terminate in acute life-threatening pulmonary edema. However, withdrawal of fluid is likely to be curative. An immediate phlebotomy may be performed in such instances; this is done with disarming ease by simply attaching the central venous catheter to a standard evacuated blood-collection bottle. We advise that such a unit be routinely kept at the bedside for this purpose.

We emphasize the importance of routine volume repletion, which has so greatly improved management of shock states in the past 15 years. Even when the initial PAWP or CVP is increased, fluid challenge should be undertaken if the patient is in shock. Care must be taken to confirm the patency and proper location of the catheter tip, since this is such a critical issue in the use of these pressure measurements to guide volume repletion.

A corollary measurement to the adequacy of volume repletion is the response of the CVP to abdominal pressure (hepatojugular reflux). A sustained increase in CVP exceeding 8 cm H_2O (5 torr) while pressure is applied over the right upper quadrant suggests that further augmentation of venous return may not significantly increase cardiac output. When the pressure of the examiner's hand on the abdomen triggers a Valsalva response, a transient increase in both CVP and arterial pressure represents a misleading response. Consequently the measurement should be made during quiet inspiration and expiration.

Summary

A standardized technique for administration of fluid for resuscitation of patients with volume deficits is described. During infusion of specific aliquots of fluid, quantitative changes in central venous pulmonary artery wedge, and/or pulmonary diastolic pressure are monitored. Specific rules (algorithms) are provided by which the capability of the heart to accept the fluid load is assessed. This technique makes it possible to administer fluids, even in large amounts, and yet greatly minimizes the risk of inducing cardiac failure.

References

1. **Cohn, J. N.** (1967). Central venous pressure as a guide to volume expansion. *Ann. Intern. Med. 66:*1283–1287.
2. **Crexells, C., Chatterjee, K., Forrester, J., Dikshit, K.,** and **Swan, H. J. C.** (1973). Optimal level of filling pressure in the left side of the heart in acute myocardial infarction. *New Engl. J. Med. 289:*1263–1266.
3. **MacLean, L. D.** (1964). Blood volume versus central venous pressure in shock. *Surg. Gynec. Obstet. 118:*594–595.
4. **Rystrom, L., Weil, M. H., Shubin, H.,** and **Palley, N.** (1971). Technique of measurement of the plasma volume and red cell mass during acute circulatory failure. *Surg. Gynec. Obstet. 133:*621–626.
5. **Shubin, H.,** and **Weil, M. H.** (1974). Routine central venous catheterization for management of critically ill patients. In: Ingelfinger, F. J., Ebert, R. V., Finland, M., and Rolman, A. S. (eds.), *Controveries in Internal Medicine.* Philadelphia: Saunders, pp. 177–184.
6. **Stein, L., Beraud, J. J., Cavanilles, J. M., da Luz, P., Weil, M. H.,** and **Shubin, H.** (1974). Pulmonary edema during fluid infusion in the absence of heart failure. *J. Am. Med. Assoc. 109:*61–64.
7. **Swan, H. J. C., Ganz, W., Forrester, J., Marcus H., Diamond, G.,** and **Chonette, D.** (1970). Catheterization of the heart in man with the use of a flow, directed, balloon-tipped catheter. *New Engl. J. Med. 283:*447–451.
8. **Weil, M. H., Morissette, M., Michaels, S., Bisera, J., Boycks, E., Shubin, H.,** and **Jacobson, E.** (1974). Routine plasma colloid osmotic pressure measurements. *Crit. Care Med. 3:*229–234.
9. **Weil, M. H., Shubin, H.,** and **Rosoff, L.** (1965). Fluid repletion in circulatory shock. Central venous pressure and other practical guides. *J. Am. Med. Assoc. 192:*668–674.
10. **Wilson, J. N., et al.** (1962). Central venous pressure in optimal blood volume maintenance. *Arch. Surg. 85:*563–578.

The Diagnosis and Treatment of Anaphylactic Shock

JOHN DE ANGELIS, M.D.
Department of Anesthesiology
University of California at Los Angeles
Cedars-Sinai Medical Center
Los Angeles, California

The dynamic effects of anaphylactic shock can be categorized into two phases. Phase I begins with a person's exposure to a foreign substance, the antigen. A variety of substances such as proteins, polysaccharides, and simple organic chemicals can act in the capacity of an antigen [15]. This exposure to the antigen initiates the production of immunoglobulin antibodies. These newly formed antibodies are specific for the antigen and fix themselves to the surface of mast cells and basophils [10]. Those organ systems which harbor the greatest number of antibodies become the primary target sites during Phase II. Phase II begins as the antigen reappears and immediately has a shattering interaction with the antibodies. This interaction triggers the release of at least three mediators: (a) histamine, (b) bradykinin, and (c) slow-reacting substance. The mediators have a profound systemic effect.

Histamine, the most prominent of the mediators, constricts the bronchioles (Fig. 1). As a consequence of this intense bronchospasm, ventilation–perfusion inequalities ensue and severe hypoxemia and hypercarbia may appear. At the same time, another target site, the small veins, is affected. Dilation of the venules results, thus expanding the vascular space and creating a relative hypovolemia. The venous return to the heart is reduced

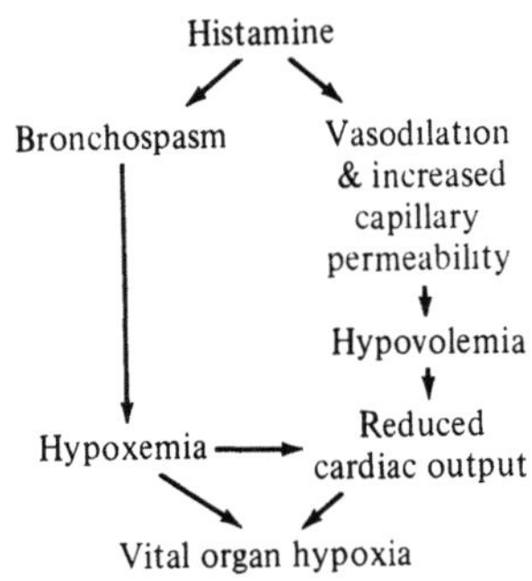

FIGURE 1 Mechanism by which histamine release during anaphylaxis propagates cardiorespiratory failure with vital organ hypoxia.

with a consequent reduction in cardiac output. Histamine elicits an increase in capillary permeability, leading to a loss of intravascular fluid, further compounding the hypovolemia and reduction in cardiac output. As a consequence of a low cardiac output and hypoperfusion, there is hypoxia of vital organs.

Bradykinin also attacks the capillaries, thereby increasing permeability and loss of plasma volume (Fig. 2). There is an abrupt increase in hemoglobin and the hematocrit as well. The loss of plasma volume results in hypovolemia, and the repercussion of this is a further step down in cardiac output. There is vital-organ hypoxia as a result of perfusion failure. Bradykinin may act directly on the myocardium, severely impairing its functional capability. One of the most threatening of the bradykinin actions is its effect on the upper airway. Angioedema, a consequence of increased capillary permeability, leads to airway obstruction and eventual hypoxemia. The slow-reacting substance also affects the lung, further eliciting bronchospasm and leading to what is by this time a common pathway to hypoxemia (Fig. 3) [12].

FIGURE 2 Mechanism by which bradykinin release during anaphylaxis propagates cardiorespiratory failure with vital organ hypoxia.

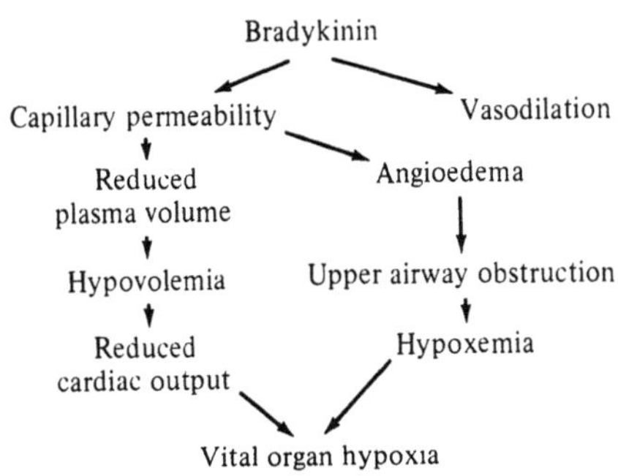

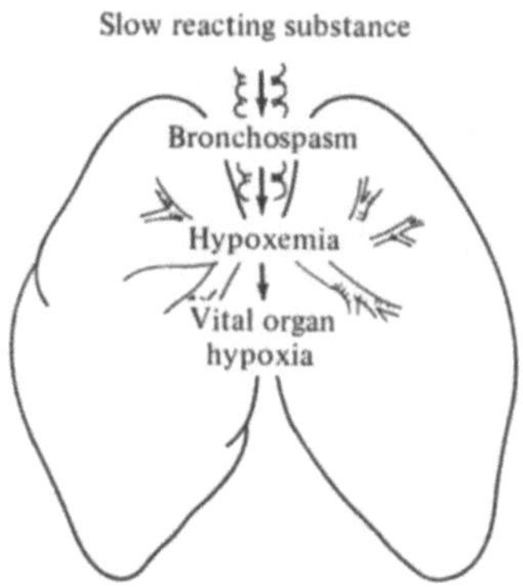

FIGURE 3 Mechanism by which release of slow reacting substance propagates respiratory failure and vital organ hypoxia.

The effects of the histamine, bradykinin, and slow-reacting substance potentiate each other, thereby provoking the extreme circulatory and respiratory defects that characterize anaphylactic shock.

CLINICAL PRESENTATION

Patients may be alert or may have mental obtundation. Those patients who are alert at the onset of anaphylaxis are apprehensive, perspire profusely, have extreme itching, exhibit both erythema and urticaria, and may complain of marked weakness. There is often a striking air hunger. Fecal and urinary incontinence may occur. Unless treatment is rapidly initiated, syncope and coma ensue [13].

When the patient becomes comatose, other features provide a clue as to what is happening. A survey of the literature reveals 11 reported cases of thiopental (pentothal) anaphylaxis. We added one additional case from the U.S.C. Center for the Critically Ill. In this group of patients, the sensorium was obtunded at the time of insult. The abnormal findings are listed in order of decreasing frequency. Hypotension was the most common finding, followed by an absent pulse and erythema. Cyanosis, urticaria, and bronchospasm were important findings and were followed in frequency by laryngospasm and cough [1–9,11,14].

Differential diagnosis of anaphylaxis is usually not difficult because of the rapid onset of signs and symptoms immediately following exposure to the antigen. However, when confronted with a hypotensive patient admitted through the emergency room, anaphylaxis is merely one of several possibilities. A history of a recent insect sting, the administration of a drug, or the recent ingestion of food would suggest a systemic allergic reaction. Accompanying signs of facial edema, urticaria, rash, and bronchospasm would further suggest anaphylaxis. Anaphylaxis should be suspected in a

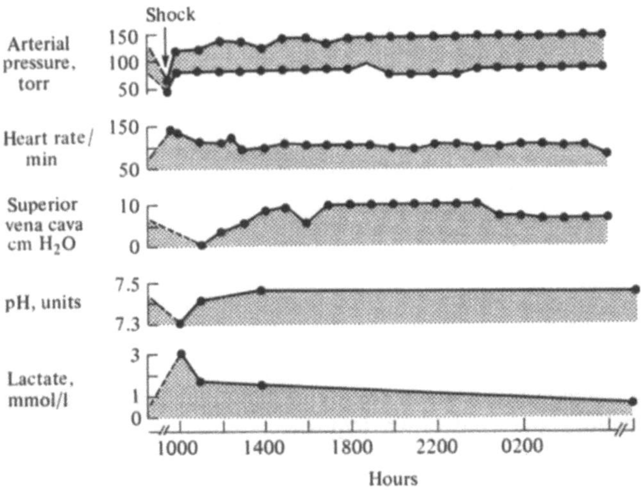

FIGURE 4 Hemodynamic and metabolic observations in a 29-year-old woman who had an immediate reaction with clinical signs of anaphylaxis following thiopental.

child or young adult presenting with sudden hypotension with peripheral vasoconstriction, whereas the same set of circumstances occurring in an older patient would imply other causes [15].

Figure 4 summarizes the case of a 29-year-old woman who experienced an anaphylactic reaction from thiopental (pentothal). Five minutes after receiving 300 mg of thiopental intravenously she was found to be pulseless. External cardiac massage, epinephrine, sodium bicarbonate, and fluid challenge were used to successfully resuscitate her. Severe hypotension with disappearance of the pulse were noted at 1000 hrs. A marked acceleration in the heart rate took place following epinephrine. Central venous pressure within the superior vena cava decreased to zero. The patient became acidemic, attributable to a high lactate reflecting anaerobic metabolism. Coincident with the initial severe decrease in blood pressure there was an abrupt increase in the hemoglobin and hematocrit (Fig. 5). Increases in hemoglobin and hematocrit reflect the loss of plasma due to increased capillary permeability mediated by histamine and bradykinin. The elevated hematocrit occurred despite the administration of large volumes of crystalloids and albumin, as shown in the lower part of the graph.

PRINCIPLES OF TREATMENT

When anaphylactic shock is suspected, there must be immediate therapeutic intervention. The patient may either be salvaged by an immediate and effective counterattack or may die within 30 min or less. The patient

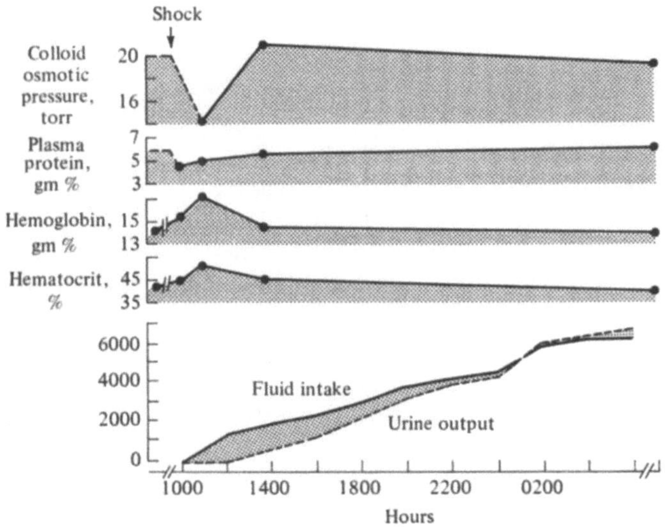

FIGURE 5 Reduction of colloid osmotic pressure and plasma protein with concurrent increase in hemoglobin and hematocrit following anaphylaxis caused by thiopental in the same patient presented in Figure 4. The difference between fluid intake and urine output provides an estimate of temporary loss of plasma water due to increases in capillary permeability.

is placed in a supine position and his neck is extended, thus facilitating ventilatory exchange and chest accessiblity in the event that cardiopulmonary resuscitation is necessary. Epinephrine is given intravenously as an aqueous 1:1000 solution in a 0.5-cc bolus. If it is not possible to readily administer the epinephrine intravenously, the cricothyroid membrane may be entered with a needle attached to a syringe containing the epinephrine. The epinephrine is injected rapidly and the needle promptly removed. Another site for injection of epinephrine is under the tongue. This area has a rich vascular supply and quickly delivers the drug into the systemic circulation. Under circumstances of circulatory failure (shock), absorption from an intramuscular site may be slow and totally ineffective in reversing the rapidly progressive circulatory and respiratory failure.

If the anaphylaxis stems from an intramuscular drug injection or insect sting of an extremity, a tourniquet is applied proximal to the site, and 0.5 cc of 1:1000 acqueous epinephrine is injected into the involved area. This maneuver delays further absorption of the antigen [13].

Subsequent therapy is selected as specific needs arise and is guided by continuous monitoring of the patient's sensorium, his facility for breathing, and his hemodynamic status. Progressive laryngeal edema, manifested by stridor and retraction of the anterior chest, supraclavicular, and subcostal

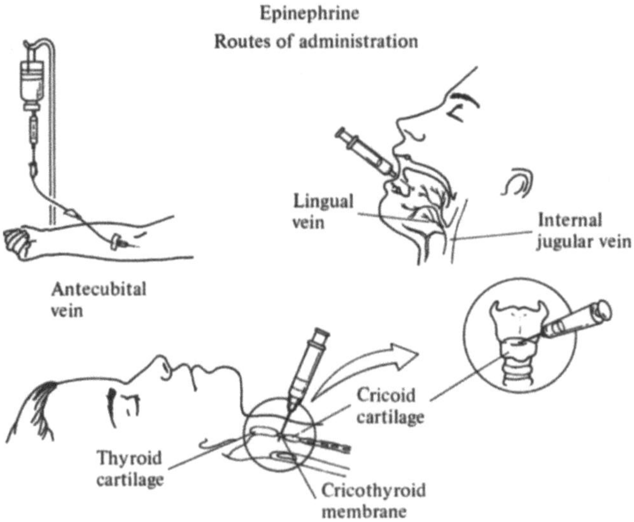

FIGURE 6 Options for emergency administration of epinephrine during anaphylactic shock.

areas, requires an atraumatic endotracheal intubation. However, this is not always possible. When the degree of upper airway obstruction precludes tracheal intubation from the oral or nasal route, tracheostomy becomes mandatory. A skilled surgeon has little difficulty in performing the classic tracheostomy as an emergency measure. Others may elect to use an easier, but more temporary cricothyrotomy as a stopgap procedure.

One or more angiocatheters of 12-gauge size or of similar large bore may be inserted over a guide needle through the cricothyroid membrane (Fig. 6). The needle is then removed leaving the catheter within the tracheal lumen. A tracheostomy oxygen mask is then applied to deliver oxygen to the catheter. This relatively easy procedure will provide an additional 10–20 min of safety until the surgeon arrives. When endotracheal intubation is carried out, a low-pressure cuffed tube is used to safeguard the airway from aspiration of gastric contents. This is particularly necessary in patients with tracheal reflex obtundation, in coma, or in those in whom external cardiac massage is employed. The pressure of external cardiac massage frequently regurgitates the gastric contents into the esophagus.

Since there is marked loss of fluid from the intravascular into the extravascular space, a fluid challenge is also started immediately, utilizing crystalloid solutions supplemented by colloids if necessary. Large volumes of fluid may be required, and this poses the threat of overloading the patient. Placement of a central venous line and a pulmonary-artery catheter with measurement of PAWP and CVP provides an objective basis for assessing the capacity of the heart to accept these large fluid loads. After resolving these rather urgent problems, diaphenhydramine (Benadryl) may be administered intravenously in a dose of 50–75 mg over a 3-min interval.

Aminophylline may be necessary for the control of persistent bronchospasm. A dose of 250–500 mg diluted in 500 ml of crystalloid solution may be delivered by intravenous infusion over 20–30 min.

Although usually given to a patient with anaphylactic shock, steroids do not seem to play a significant role during the acute phase of anaphylaxis [13]. Dexamethasone, 25 mg, or methylprednisolone, 125 mg injected intravenously as a bolus, may be advantageous for subsequent therapy.

Summary

Anaphylactic shock is a biophysical encounter of antibody with antigen. This cellular level reaction provokes an explosion in miniature unleashing chemical mediators capable of multisystem insult. Prompt recognition with immediate countermeasures are necessary to sustain life. Epinephrine is the first line of defense and can be administered by intravenous, transtracheal or sublingual route. Subsequent therapy is selected as specific needs arise and is guided by continuous monitoring of the patient's sensorium, the ease with which he is able to breathe, and his hemodynamic status.

References

1. **Anderton, J. M.,** and **Hopton, D. S.** (1968). Thiopentone anaphylaxis. *Anaesth. 23:*90–93.
2. **Barjenburch, K. P.,** and **Jones, J.** (1972). Thiopental anaphylaxis. A Case Report. *Anesth. Analg. 51:*113–116.
3. **Carrie, L. E. S.,** and **Buchanan, R. L.** (1967). Thiopentone anaphylaxis. *Anaesth. 22:*290–295.
4. **Clark, M. M.,** and **Cockburn, A.** (1971). Anaphylactoid response to thiopentone. Case Report. *Brit. J. Anaesth. 43:*185–189.
5. **Cole, F.** (1968). Sensitivity to thiopental. *Nebr. Med. J. 53:*478.
6. **Currie, T. T., Whittingham,** and **S. Erbringer, A.** (1966). Severe anaphylactic reaction to thiopentone. Case Report. *Brit. Med. J. 1:*1462–1463.
7. **Davis, J.** (1971). Thiopentone anaphylaxis. Case Report. *Brit. J. Anaesth. 43:*1191–1193.
8. **Fox, G. S., Wilkinson, R. D.,** and **Rabow, F.** (1971). Thiopental anaphylaxis. A case and a method for diagnosis. *Anesthesiol. 35:*655–657.
9. **Hayward, J. R.,** and **Keister, G. L.** (1957). Severe allergic reaction during thiopental sodium anesthesia. Report of a Case. *J. Oral Surg. 15:*61–63.
10. **Kelly, J. F.** (1973). The treatment of anaphylaxis. *Ration. Drug Ther. 7:*1–5.
11. **Kivalo, I., West, A.,** and **Mustakallio, M.** (1960). Anaphylactic shock in thiopental anesthesia. *Duodecim 76:*509–512.
12. **Pruzansky, J.** (1972). Immunologic and cellular aspects of immediate

hypersensitivity. In: Patterson, R. (ed.), *Allergic Diseases*. Philadelphia: Lippincott, pp. 31–61.
13. **Queng, J. T.,** and **McGovern, J. P.** (1974). When every second counts. In Cohen, I. J. (ed.), *Touching All Basics*. New York, EM Books, pp. 3–6.
14. **Strunk, H. A.** (1962). Reaction to thiopental. *Anesthesiol.* 23:271.
15. **Weiszer, I.** (1972). Allergic emergencies. In: Patterson, R. (ed.), *Allergic Diseases*. Philadelphia: Lippincott, pp. 327–340.

Indications for Use of Corticosteroid Agents in Treatment of Shock

WILLIAM SCHUMER, M.D.
Professor and Chairman, Department of Surgery,
University of Health Sciences, The Chicago Medical School,
Chicago, Illinois

The use of steroids in the treatment of shock is indicated in early septic shock, in late refractory hypovolemic shock, and in post-traumatic pulmonary insufficiency.

SEPTIC SHOCK

Glucocorticoids have been shown to protect several species–including rat, dog, and monkey–against endotoxic or bacterial shock. These agents are capable of reversing the microcirculatory perfusion changes in these types of shock. They increase both cardiac output and microcirculatory perfusion. Furthermore, they can reverse the metabolic changes in the septic shocked animal and obviate the gluconeogenic block. Experimental evidence has also supported an immunologic effect of glucocorticoids: they have been shown to interfere with the endotoxin–antibody–complement reaction during septic shock [5]. Finally, our retrospective and prospective studies of human septic shock [6], as well as those of Lillehei and associates [3] and Weil and Shubin [7], have indicated that steroids exert a significant, protective effect.

REFRACTORY HYPOVOLEMIC SHOCK

The use of corticosteroids in this type of shock is more difficult to support, since controlled studies are almost impossible in such critically ill patients. However, in the rat, dog, and monkey, studies of profound hypovolemic shock have indicated protection and an improved survival rate with the use of these agents. Whether this protective effect is partially due to either a decrease of the myocardial depressant factor described by Lefer [2] in all types of shock or to the toxic phase of late hypovolemic shock as described by Fine is not altogether certain. The later toxic phase is postulated to be due to the anoxic changes in the mucosal-cell membrane barrier, allowing either bacteria, its endotoxin, or its exotoxin to enter the blood. Steroids are postulated to decrease the myocardial depressant factor and to protect the mucosal cell membrane by decreasing permeability.

POST-TRAUMATIC PULMONARY INSUFFICIENCY

The use of steroids in post-traumatic pulmonary insufficiency is also controversial. Motsay and Lillehei previously reported that corticosteroids protect pulmonary capillary membranes during endotoxic shock [4]. They further found that steroids minimized the elevation of precapillary and postcapillary resistances in dogs during endotoxic shock. Corticosteroids have been shown to decrease the level of pulmonary extravascular lung water in hemorrhagic shock. These studies supported the use of steroids in post-traumatic pulmonary insufficiency; however, the derivation of clinical support is difficult; thus the use of steroids in this syndrome is still questionable. James [1] and Wilson [8] have separately reported a marked decrease in the incidence of human pulmonary insufficiency after steroid administration. Additional studies in this area are needed to prove statistical significance.

THERAPEUTIC REGIME

Steroids should be administered as follows. A single bolus of either 3 mg/kg of dexamethasone or 30 mg/kg of methylprednisolone is given as soon as a diagnosis of either septic shock, refractory hypovolemic shock, or post-traumatic pulmonary insufficiency is made. This dose may be repeated after 4 hr if no beneficial clinical response is apparent. No additional steroids are infused unless there is another discrete episode of septic shock or pulmonary insufficiency.

Summary

Corticosteroid agents protect against the lethal effects of bacterial endotoxin, increase cardiac output and microcirculatory perfusion, and interfere with the endotoxin–antibody–complement reaction during septic shock. Indications for the use of corticosteroids for the treatment of hypovolemic shock and post-traumatic pulmonary insufficiency following hemorrhage is less secure. Present practice testifies to the use of a single bolus of dexamethasone or methlyprednisolone for the immediate treatment of septic shock, refractory hypovolemic shock, or post-traumatic pulmonary insufficiency.

References

1. **James, P. M.** (1974). Response of patients in shock to treatment with corticosteroid. In: Glenn, T. M. (ed.), *Steroids and Shock*, Baltimore: University Park Press, p. 420.
2. **Lefer, A. M.** (1970). Role of a myocardial depressant factor in the pathogenesis of circulatory shock. *Fed. Proc. 29:*1836.
3. **Lillehei, R. C., Longerbeam, J. K., Block, J. H.,** and **Manax, W. G.** (1964). The nature of irreversible shock; experimental and clinical observations. *Ann. Surg. 160*:682.
4. **Motsay, G. J., Alho, A., Jaeger, T., Dietzman, R. H.,** and **Lillehei, R. C.** (1970). Effects of corticosteroids on the circulation in shock: experimental and clinical results. *Fed. Proc. 29:*1861.
5. **Schumer, W., Erve, P. R., Earnest, W., Miller, B.,** and **Nichols, R. L.** (1974). Glucocorticoid effect on complement fixation. *J. Surg. Res. 16:*13.
6. **Schumer, W.,** and **Nyhus, L. M.** (1969). The role of corticoids in the management of shock. *Surg. Clin. N. Amer. 49:*147.
7. **Weil, M. H., Shubin, H.,** and **Nishijima, H.** (1974). Corticosteroid therapy in circulatory shock. In: Glenn, T. M. (ed.), *Steroids and Shock*, Baltimore: University Park Press, p. 351.
8. **Wilson, R. F.,** and **Fisher, R. R.** (1968). The hemodynamic effects of massive steroids in clinical shock. *Surg. Gynec. Obstet. 127:*769.

Hemodynamic Defects Underlying Shock with Indications for Treatment: An Appraisal of Vasopressors and Vasodilators

MAX HARRY WEIL, M.D., PH.D.
Center for the Critically Ill and the Shock Research Unit, University of Southern California School of Medicine, the Los Angeles County/University of Southern California Medical Center, and the Hollywood Presbyterian Medical Center, Los Angeles, California

Until the sphygmomanometer came into wide use after 1910, the character and rate of the pulse served as the primary objective measure of severity of circulatory failure. Subsequently, blood pressure became an index for both the diagnosis and estimation of severity of the shock state. In the search for therapy by which hypotension could be reversed, the clinician was attracted to drugs restoring blood pressure to more normal levels. This led to the early use of epinephrine and the subsequent use of its adrenergic analogs. Beginning in the 1940s synthetic adrenergic drugs came into wide use for treatment of shock states. Unlike epinephrine, phenylephrine and methaxamine increased blood pressure but more often decreased the heart rate. Except for the relatively conservative use of fluids, blood, blood components, and blood substitutes, vasopressor drugs were until recently the mainstay of therapy for shock, regardless of cause.

During World War II hemodynamic studies of hemorrhagic shock in patients prompted applications of cardiac catheterization and measurements of cardiac output and intravascular pressures by Andre Cournand and his famed group [4]. In the early 1960s shock-research units were evolved and in-depth studies were initiated on patients in shock due to diverse causes. It soon became apparent that the heart rate, blood pressure, and even the cardiac output constituted secondary indicators of the underlying circulatory defect. The primary disturbance was perfusion failure rather than blood-pressure inadequacy.

On the basis of clinical and physiologic studies, an etiologic classification of shock states was adapted by our group. When it was first organized in 1960, seven categories of shock were defined: (a) hypovolemic, (b) cardiogenic, (c) bacterial (spetic), (d) hypersensitivity (anaphylactic), (e) neurogenic, (f) obstructive, and (g) endocrinologic [17]. Although now obsolete, this classification helped to establish the usefulness of objective criteria for the diagnosis of mechanisms as a basis for planning treatment.

HEMODYNAMIC MECHANISMS

For purposes of defining primary hemodynamic mechanisms of circulatory shock and implications for treatment, conceptualization of a simple working model of the circulatory system is probably helpful. Five primary components may be identified (Fig. 1). The first component, a resistance circuit that includes the arteries and arterioles, is the mainstream by which blood is carried to the capillary exchange beds. The second component is the capillary bed, which constitutes a passive circuit. Blood flow through the capillary bed and fluid filtration between the intravascular and interstitial fluid compartments are regulated by humoral, neurogenic, and hydrostatic controls on: (a) precapillary arterioles and postcapillary venules, (b) the colloid osmotic pressure gradient, and (c) the characteristics of the

FIGURE 1 Primary components of the circulation including the resistance circuit, the capillary exchange vessels, the venous capacitance vessels, and the heart. Not shown is the fifth component, which is the volume contained within the intravascular compartment. From Weil and Shubin, DIAGNOSIS AND TREATMENT OF SHOCK, Williams and Wilkins, 1967, p. 312.

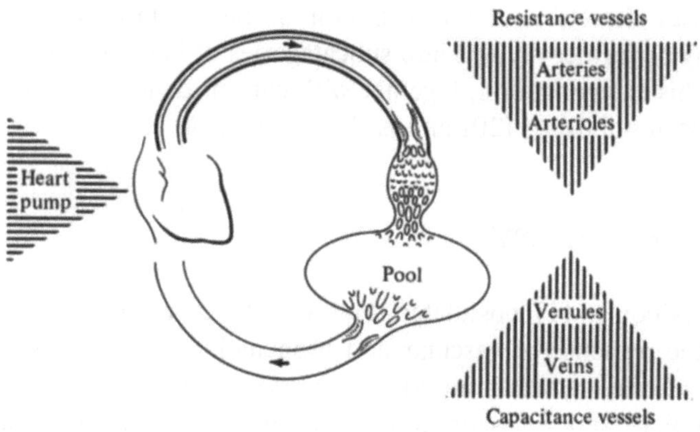

vascular endothelium. The third component is the venous capacitance bed. Some metarterioles bridge the arterial resistance and postcapillary venous vessels, and blood may be shunted from the resistance to the capacitance circuits, thereby allowing bypass of capillary-exchange vessels. In some instances, metabolic or membrane defects impair capillary exchange of oxygen and other substrates that represent the physiological equivalent of arteriovenous shunting. The capacitance bed acts as the major reservoir for blood. Approximately 80% of the total blood volume is contained within this portion of the circuit. Changes in capacitance regulate "circulating volume" and hence the volume of blood returned to the heart. The fourth component is the heart. It is the pump that provides the hydraulic power for circulation.

Excessive resistance in the arterial circuit, shunting of blood through arteriovenous communications, excessive resistance in the postcapillary venous bed, pooling of blood in a dilated venous capacitance bed, a reduction in blood volume, failure of the heart to serve as an effective pump, or on obstruction to the mainstream of flow through the system constitute seven major defects that account for acute perfusion failure and the clinical signs of shock.

The cardiac output represents the net effect of arterial resistance, venous capacitance, and blood volume and the competence of the heart to expel that volume. Arterial pressure is best viewed as the product of the cardiac output and arterial resistance. Although it serves as an index of hemodynamic status, it should be considered a secondary rather than primary hemodynamic variable. The potential value of vasoactive drugs for treatment may then be evaluated on the basis of their actions on the five primary components of the circulatory system and in relationship to the seven major defects identified in terms of these components.

These are the considerations that prompted a revision of the earlier classification of shock states [18]. Hypovolemia, cardiac failure, and vascular obstruction identify three of the seven major defects. For purposes of simplification, alterations in arterial resistance, shunting, postcapillary resistance, and venous pooling are combined into a single category that encompasses defects in the distribution of blood flow. The distributive defect may be further divided into subcategories of high- and low-resistance defects. This categorization, together with current concepts of therapy, has recently been published [20] and is shown in Table 1.

PHARMACOTHERAPY

In 1948 Ahlquist [1] postulated that two types of adrenergic receptor regulate the response of vascular and bronchiolar smooth muscle and the response of the myocardium to epinephrine and its analogs. These he termed alpha- and beta-adrenergic receptors. Consequently, adrenergic drugs were categorized as alpha-adrenergic receptor agonists and beta-adrenergic receptor agonists. With the synthesis of alpha- and beta-adrenergic receptor blocking agents, impressive evidence was at hand supporting this hypothesis of receptor sites even though they had not been automatically identified.

Alpha-adrenergic receptor agonists. Phenylephrine hydrochloride (Neo-synephrine) and methoxamine hydrochloride (Vasoxyl) are vasopressor agents that have primarily alpha-adrenergic receptor activity. They increase arterial pressure by increasing arterial vasoconstrictor action and this increases the arterial resistance and the workload of the heart. At the same time, they increase resistance in the postcapillary-capacitance bed, which accounts for a net increase in capillary hydrostatic pressure and a net loss of fluid into the interstitial space [5]. This loss of intravascular volume may in itself propagate the shock state. As arterial pressure is increased, carotid and aortic baroreceptors are stimulated and vagal bradycardia ensues. No indications for the use of these drugs for treatment of shock are presently recognized, except during a selective type of cardiogenic shock in which they may be employed to induce hypertension and reflex vagotonus for reversal of the low-output syndromes that are due to supraventricular tachycardias.

Beta-adrenergic receptor agonists. Isoproterenol (Isuprel) hydrochloride is regarded as a selective beta-adrenergic receptor agonist. Mephentermine (Wyamine), isoxsuprine (Vasodilan) hydrochloride, and nylidrin hydrochloride (Arlidin) also have primary beta-adrenergic actions. This group of drugs has inotropic and chronotropic actions by which strength of myocardial contraction and heart rate are increased. Spontaneous ventricular-rhythmicity is augmented. Ectopic ventricular beats appear because isoproterenol accelerates spontaneous depolarization of pacemaker cells. Arterial vasodilatory actions are particularly prominent in the skeletal muscle and in the mesenteric vascular beds and therefore account for a decline in peripheral resistance. The size of the capacitance bed is reduced with a consequent increase in the return of venous blood to the heart. This increase in preload, the inotropic and chronotropic actions on the heart, and the decrease in afterload all serve to increase cardiac output without increase in left ventricular end-diastolic pressure. Effects on arterial pressure are variable. Contingent on cardiac output, the reduction in resistance may be without decline in arterial pressure because of a substantial increase in cardiac output (see Fig. 2).

Beta-adrenergic receptor agonists are employed for treatment of shock states. Cardiac and peripheral actions of these agents provoke increases in metabolic rate and a disproportionately high requirement for oxygen. Hence, blood flow is augmented but at the price of substantially increased

TABLE 1 Classification of Shock States and Related Concepts of Management

TYPE OF SHOCK	PRIMARY MECHANISM	CLINICAL CAUSES	PRIMARY THERAPY	SECONDARY THERAPY
Hypovolemic	Volume loss	Exogenous Blood loss due to hemorrhage Plasma loss due to burn, inflammation Fluid and electrolyte loss due to vomiting, diarrhea, dehydration, osmolal diuresis (diabetes) Endogenous Extravasation due to inflammation, trauma, tourniquet, anaphylaxis, snake venom, and adrenergic stimulation (pheochromocytoma)	Fluid repletion: crystalloid, electrolyte, colloid, blood infusion	Dexamethasone sodium phosphate,* methylprednisolone sodium succinate* α-adrenergic blockade* β-adrenergic agonist*
Cardiogenic	Pump failure	Myocardial infarction	Maintain diastolic coronary perfusion pressure, fluid challenge, reduce afterload	
		Heart failure	Inotropic agent (digitalis), diuretic	α-β-adrenergic agonist Counterpulsation Coronary revascularization
		Dysrhythmia	Antiarrhythmia pharmacotherapy, cardioversion, pacemaking	

Distributive (vasomotor dysfunction)				
(1) High or normal resistance	Expanded venous capacitance (pooling)	Bacterial shock due to Gram-negative enteric bacillemia	Control infection: antibiotic, surgical drainage or excision Fluid challenge Glucocorticoid analog	β-adrenergic agonist* α-adrenergic blockade
		Ganglionic blockade, spinal shock, and autonomic blockade	Body supine, elevate lower extremities, fluid challenge	α-β-adrenergic agonist
		Sedative overdose	Fluid challenge	Diuresis, alkalinization, hemodialysis
(2) Low resistance	Arteriovenous shunting	Pneumonia, peritonitis, abscess, reactive hyperemia, hepatorenal syndrome	Control infection Fluid challenge	α-β-adrenergic agonist*
Obstructive	Obstruction to main channel of blood flow	Vena cava obstruction (supine hypotensive syndrome)	Mechanical relief (body position)	
		Pericarditis (tamponade)	Aspiration, surgical drainage	α-β-adrenergic agonist Cardiopulmonary bypass Thrombolysis Surgical bypass
		Intracardiac ball valve thrombus	Open heart surgery	
		Pulmonary embolism	Anticoagulation	
		Dissecting aneurysm of aorta (exclusive of coronary obstruction)	Induced hypotension Surgical repair	

*Potentially beneficial.

Published by permission of the American Medical Association, from Weil *et al.*, *JAMA 231*:1281, 1975.

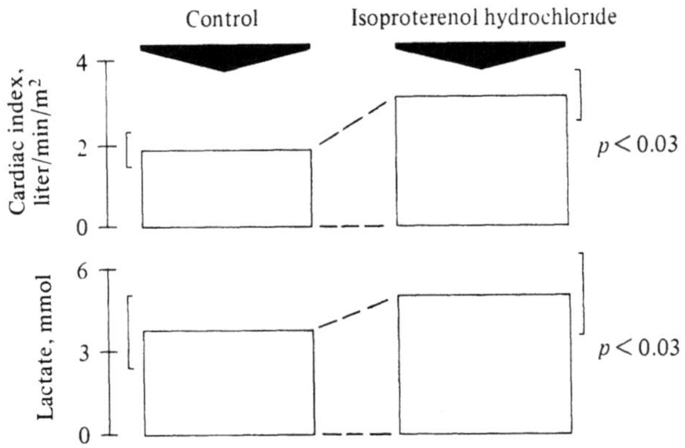

FIGURE 2 Increases in cardiac index after treatment with isoproterenol hydrochloride over an average of 220 min are associated with significant increases in blood lactic acid, indicating persistence of anoxic metabolism. Published by permission of the American Medical Association, from Weil *et al.*, *JAMA 231*:1283, 1975.

oxygen need. Heart rate, ventricular ejection velocity, cardiac pressure, and diastolic volume are increased and ventricular filling pressure is decreased. These are presumably beneficial hemodynamic actions in patients with reduced venous return or impaired myocardial contractility. However, a progressive and statistically significant increase of lactic-acid content in coronary venous and arterial blood indicates that the increase in oxygen requirement is even greater than the increase in blood flow available to meet this need. Consequently, anaerobic metabolism signals a continuing and often augmented deficit in oxygen availability, particularly in the coronary circuit. There is also evidence of increased arteriovenous shunting after treatment with isoproterenol so that increases in total blood flow do not predictably accrue to the benefit of improved capillary perfusion, thereby further accentuating the deficit in oxygen delivery.

Alpha–beta-adrenergic agonists. The sympathomimetic drugs most widely used for treatment of shock, namely epinephrine, norepinephrine, and metaraminol, have both alpha- and beta-adrenergic receptor actions. Epinephrine has a prominent beta-adrenergic action. In small doses, a biphasic effect is observed with initial arterial vasoconstriction and subsequent vasodilation. Inotropic and chronotropic effects predominate with prominent increases in systolic pressure and heart rate. Epinephrine is specificially indicated for treatment of anaphylactic shock. Both epinephrine and isoproterenol may be used as inotropic drugs for treatment of low output states due to heart failure in the absence of ischemic heart disease, especially after cardiac surgery.

The prototype of vasopressor agents is norepinephrine [i.e., levarterenol (Levophed) bitartrate]. It is identical to the endogenous ardenal medullary hormone and also to the neurotransmitter substance released at post-ganglionic sympathetic nerve endings. In small doses, norepinephrine has primarily beta-adrenergic inotropic actions and in larger amounts, alpha-adrenergic arterial and venous constrictor activity; the balance of alpha and beta adrenergic actions accounts for minimal effects on heart rate. Intense localized vasoconstriction provoked by this drug can result in tissue necrosis and sloughing with ischemic necrosis in skin and viscera. These effects are obviated by concurrent administration of small doses of an alpha-adrenergic receptor antagonist such as phentolamine. Metaraminol bitartrate, which acts, in part, by releasing norepinephrine, is less potent but has a more persistent action [16]. These drugs augment cardiac output but tend to reduce renal cortical blood flow [2]. As they increase arterial resistance and the workload on the heart, simultaneous increases on coronary blood flow and inotropic actions on the myocardium may favor increased perfusion of myocardium after myocardial infarction [6,10].

Norepinephrine and metaraminol have substantial venoconstrictor actions with increases in capillary hydrostatic pressure, which account for decreases in intravascular volume. This, in part, accounts for refractoriness and difficulty in "weaning." These effects were confirmed by sequential measurements of plasma volume in the studies performed by our group (see Fig. 3).

Dopamine hydrochloride (Intropin), a naturally occurring precursor of norepinephrine, is now available for clinical use. Its relative alpha- and beta-adrenergic actions, like those of norepinephrine, are dose related. In addition to its adrenergic effects, it has a direct vasodilator action on resistance

FIGURE 3 Reduction in measured plasma volume in six patients during treatment of shock with metaraminol bitartrate and levarterenol bitartrate, in comparison to a control group observed during the same interval. Increases in plasma volume with subsequent fluid repletion are also shown. Published with permission of the American Medical Association, from Weil *et al., JAMA 231:*1284, 1975.

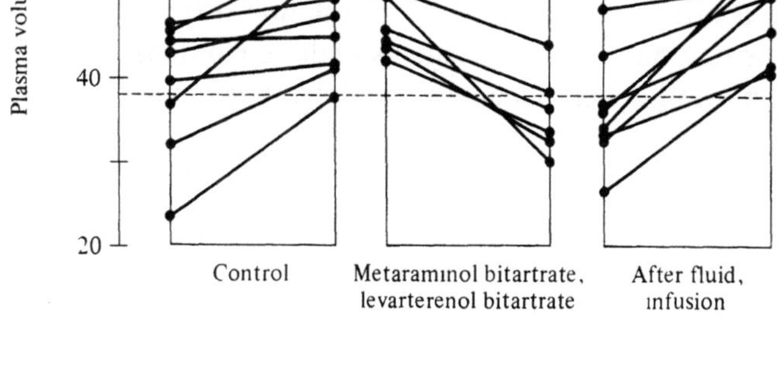

vessels by which visceral blood flow and particularly renal and mesenteric blood flow are increased. In contrast to isoproterenol, however, blood flow to the skeletal muscles is reduced by its alpha-adrenergic actions, thereby favoring preferential perfusion of viscera. Clinical reports currently favor the use of dopamine in place of isoproterenol because of lesser effects on myocardial oxygen consumption, peripheral resistance, and heart rate [9,14].

Nonadrenergic vasopressor agents. Angiotensin amide (Hypertensin) increases arterial resistance and hence the workload of the heart, decreases visceral blood flow, but increases skin and muscle blood flow. Although this polypeptide is a potent pressor agent, no evidence of improvement in perfusion may be anticipated from its clinical use [3].

Lypressin is a synthetic analog of the neurohypophyseal octapeptide. Experimentally, its actions favor normalization of arteriolar and especially venular tone [7], but data are presently inadequate for assessment of its clinical value.

Alpha- and beta-adrenergic receptor blocking agents and ganglionic blockade. Nickerson [11] was among the first to recognize the detriments to nutrient flow that stem from endogenous or exogenous alpha-adrenergic constrictor actions on the arterial resistance and postcapillary venous vessels. Adrenergic receptor blockade with haloalkyamines and especially phenoxybenzamine hydrochloride (Dibenzyline) or the imidazoline, phentolamine (Regitine) hydrochloride, reduce arterial and venular resistance and thereby increase flow through capillary-exchange channels. Since volume pooled in venous capacitance vessels is mobilized, venous return may be augmented provided that the blood volume is sufficiently large to adequately fill the capacitance bed [5]. This increase in preload and the decrease in arterial resistance account for increases in cardiac output. Arterial-perfusion pressure is usually reduced, although this effect is minimized by augmentation of intravascular volume. Visceral blood flow is increased.

These drugs, like beta-adrenergic isoproterenol, dilate arterial resistance vessels in skeletal muscle, increase heart rate, and augment peripheral blood flow. However, in contrast to the effects of isoproterenol, oxygen consumption is not disproportionately increased [15], nor is there evidence of increased arteriovenous shunting. Substantial experimental and clinical evidence favors the use of these agents under conditions when considerable increases in arterial resistance and consequent reduction in perfusion constitute the critical issue of survival. Lillehei, Motsay, and their colleagues [8] view a similar role for high-dosage glucocorticoid therapy.

Ganglionic blocking agents, such as hemamethonium chloride, and autonomic blockade following spinal anesthesia or spinal injury create a more general form of autonomic blockade. Arterial resistance is reduced and venous capacitance is increased. Venous return to the heart, cardiac output, and arterial pressure all decline. Phenothiazines, such as chloropromazine, have effects that simulate ganglionic blockade. In contrast to more selective receptor blockade, however, the end-organ response to epinephrine is usually increased.

Beta-adrenergic receptor blocking agents such as propranolol hydrochloride (Inderal) may be indicated for the conservative treatment of dissecting aortic aneurysm, and for otherwise uncontrollable and life-threatening ectopic ventricular rhythms. However, there is no rationale for use of these agents for treatment of acute perfusion failure.

CLINICAL THERAPY

Hypovolemic shock. The primary treatment for hypovolemia, which accounts for more than 75% of all shock cases encountered in general hospitals, is a fluid challenge guided by quantitative measurement of central venous, or preferably, PAWP (see the chapter by Weil entitled "Principles of Fluid Challenge for Routine Treatment of Shock"). When safe limits of fluid challenge are exceeded and perfusion failure persists, a trial of therapy with isoproterenol or phentolamine is warranted in the absence of ischemic heart disease. Isoproterenol hydrochloride may be infused in amounts of 0.05–0.2 μg/kg/min diluted in 5% dextrose in water injection. Its use would be best avoided in patients with obstructive coronary or peripheral arterial disease.

Phentolamine is likely to be effective for the treatment of patients with severe arterial vasoconstriction characterized by great increases in peripheral arterial resistance and clinically identifiable by considerable mottling and cyanosis of toes, nose, or fingertips. Amounts of 10–20 μg/kg/min of phentolamine hydrochloride diluted in 5% dextrose in water injection are infused, preferably by infusion pump. When a decline in CVP and PAWP values is observed, fluid challenge is resumed. Substantial volumes of fluid may then be infused as the capacitance is expanded. Vasoactive drugs with alpha-adrenergic action are contraindicated as they are likely to increase ischemic injury to viscera.

When a profound decline in arterial blood pressure and major disturbances in cardiac rhythm threaten immediate survival, the administration of norepinephrine, 0.03–0.15 μg/kg/min; bitartrate metaraminol, 1.5–10 μg/kg/min; or dopamine hydrochloride, 2–30 μg/kg/min is justified. Dopamine is currently viewed as the agent of choice. The infusion is adjusted to increase systolic arterial pressure to a level of approximately 90 mm Hg or 30 mm less than the estimated "normal" value for the individual patient. This should be regarded as a temporary maneuver pending fluid challenge. If perfusion failure is not reversed, drugs that reduce arterial resistance, such as sodium nitroprusside or phentolamine mesylate, are administered for purposes of reducing the workload on the heart. Isoproterenol is contraindicated because it is likely to increase oxygen demands and therefore ischemic injury of the myocardium. Methoxamine hydrochloride, phenylephrine hydrochloride, and angiontension amide are also contraindicated, for these drugs severely increase arterial resistance and therefore the workload on the heart.

Distributive Defects

For treatment of the shock state that follows bacteremia due to gram-negative enteric bacteria, practices comparable to those presented for treatment of hypovolemic shock are advised. Isoproterenol is potentially useful but the increases in metabolic rate and oxygen requirements that follow treatment with adrenergic agonists may intensify rather than reverse the perfusion deficit. Moreover, the striking increases in cardiac output and the lowering of peripheral resistance do not necessarily imply improved tissue perfusion, since arteriovenous shunting is increased. Although we discourage its routine use, there is experimental laboratory evidence that isoproterenol may increase survival and clinical observations, suggesting occasional reversal of the shock state. Ischemic heart disease constitutes a major contraindication to its employment. If this agent is administered, we further advise that moderate doses be used for a brief period, usually not exceeding 1 hour.

Both norepinephrine and metaraminol have been widely used for treatment of bacterial shock states. Arteriolar and venoconstrictor actions associated with their pressor actions may reduce effective tissue perfusion. In instances in which the pressor effect is sought to reverse critical reductions in coronary or renal arterial-perfusion pressures, employment of these agents for brief periods may be justified. We do not favor their routine use since our own experience suggests that these agents may decrease rather than increase survival [19].

For treatment of circulatory failure due to ganglionic blockade, spinal injury, or spinal (caudal or epidural) anesthesia, placing the patient in supine position with lower extremities elevated is likely to reverse perfusion failure. Systemic fluid challenge has also proven effective in patients with such capacitance defects.

Alpha-adrenergic or beta-adrenergic agonists, including methoxamine, phenylephrine, metaraminol, and ephedrine, are frequently used as vasopressor agents during anesthesia [12]. Arterial resistance is increased and thereby the arterial perfusion pressure is elevated. This is only rarely justified to sustain perfusion of the fetus during labor or delivery, or perfusion of the coronary circulation in patients with ischemic heart disease or cerebrovascular insufficiency. Ephedrine in bolus injections, 10–50 mg, is the preferred drug for maintaining uterine blood flow during delivery.

There is no evidence that adrenergic vasopressor agents increase survival when employed for treatment of shock after sedative overdose. On the contrary, current data indicate that they increase mortality [13].

Arteriovenous shunting with considerable increases in cardiac output is characteristically observed in patients with liver or kidney failure. Metaraminol reportedly reduces cardiac output and increases renal blood flow. However, there is presently inadequate evidence favoring the clinical use of adrenergic agents for treatment of the low-resistance type of distributive shock.

Obstructive shock. Due to their inotropic effects, epinephrine, norepinephrine, or metaraminol increase ventricular emptying. In addition, these agents temporarily increase cardiac filling pressure and thus increase cardiac output during pericardial tamponade. Volume expansion with augmentation of cardiac filling alone constitutes an important option for temporary support and complements the use of the adrenergic amines. This may be lifesaving. With this exception, there is presently no indication for the employment of vasopressor or adrenergic blocking agents for treatment of shock when a central blood pathway is obstructed.

Summary

Epinephrine is specifically indicated for the treatment of anaphylactic shock, but there is no indication for the routine use of alpha- or beta-adrenergic agonists such as levarterenol, meteraminol, or dopamine for the treatment of shock. Vasopressor agents may increase blood pressure and even cardiac output, but nutritive flow is not necessarily improved. The place of alpha-adrenergic receptor blocking agents is under active study. However, selective effects on the heart and on the resistance, exchange, and capacitance vessels may be advantageous when these agents are used as an interim and complementary measure for the treatment of shock states. Dopamine has emerged as the alpha–beta-adrenergic agonist of choice in view of complimentary nonadrenergic actions by which perfusion of striated muscle is decreased in favor of augmented visceral (including renal) blood flow. Since vasoactive drugs frequently intensify the fundamental defect accounting for perfusion failure, their selective rather than routine employment is mandatory.

References

1. **Ahlquist, R. P.** (1948). A study of adrenotropic receptors. *Am. J. Physiol. 153:*586–600.
2. **Carriere, S.** (1969). Effect of norepinephrine, isoproterenol and adrenergic blockers upon the intrarenal distribution of blood flow. *Can. J. Physiol. Pharmacol. 47:*199–208.
3. **Cohn, J. N.,** and **Luria, M. H.** (1965). Studies in clinical shock and hypo-

tension: II. Hemodynamic effects of norepinephrine and angiotension. *J. Clin. Invest. 44:*1494–1504.
4. **Cournand, A., et al.** (1943). Studies of the circulation in clinical shock. *Surg. 13:*964–995.
5. **da Luz, P. L., et al.** (1974). Plasma volume prior to and following volume loading during shock complicating acute myocardial infarction. *Circulation 49:*98–105.
6. **Gunnar, R. M., et al.** (1967). Ineffectiveness of isoproterenol in shock due to acute myocardial infarction. *J. Am. Med. Assoc. 202:*1124–1128.
7. **Hershey, S. G., et al.** (1964). Influence of a synthetic analogue of vasopressin on survival after hemorrhagic shock in rats. *Proc. Soc. Exp. Biol. Med. 115:*325–328.
8. **Lillehei, R. C., Longerbeam, J. K.,** and **Bloch, J. H.** (1964). The nature of experimental irreversible shock with its clinical implications. In: Hershey, S. G. (ed.), *Shock.* Boston: Little, Brown, pp. 139–205.
9. **Loeb, H. S., Winslow, E. B. J.,** and **Rahimtoola, S. H.** (1971). Acute hemodynamic effects of dopamine in patients with shock. *Circulation 44:* 163–173.
10. **Mueller, H. S., et al.** (1970). Hemodynamics, coronary blood flow and myocardial metabolism in coronary shock. *J. Clin. Invest. 49:*1885–1902.
11. **Nickerson, M.** (1955). Factors of vasoconstriction and vasodilation in shock. *J. Mich. Med. Soc. 54:*45–49.
12. **Shnider, S. M., Lorimier, A. A.,** and **Hefferson, J. L.** (1970). Vasopressors in obstetrics: III. Fetal effects of metaraminol infusion during obstetrical spinal hypotension. *Am. J. Obstet. Gynec. 108:*1017–1022.
13. **Shubin, H.,** and **Weil, M. H.** (1971). Shock associated with barbiturate intoxication. *J. Am. Med. Assoc. 215:*263–268.
14. **Talley, R. C., et al.** (1969). A hemodynamic comparison of dopamine and isoproterenol in patients in shock. *Circulation 39:*361–378.
15. **Taylor, S. H., et al.** (1965). The circulatory effects of intravenous phentolamine in man. *Circulation 31:*741–754.
16. **Weil, M. H.** (1955). Clinical studies on a vasopressor agent: Metaraminol (Aramine). II. Observations on its use in the management of shock. *Am. J. Med. Sci. 230:*357–369.
17. **Weil, M. H.,** and **Shubin, H.** (1967). *Diagnosis and Treatment of Shock.* Baltimore: Williams and Wilkins, p. 10.
18. **Weil, M. H.,** and **Shubin, H.** (1972). Proposed reclassification of shock with special reference to distributive defects. In: Hinshaw, L. B., and Cox, B. G. (eds.), *The Fundamental Mechanisms of Shock.* New York/London: Plenum, pp. 13–23.
19. **Weil, M. H., Shubin, H.,** and **Biddle, M.** (1964). Shock caused by gram-negative microorganisms: Analysis of 169 cases. *Ann. Intern. Med. 60:* 384–400.
20. **Weil, M. H., Shubin, H.,** and **Carlson, R.** (1975). Treatment of circulatory shock: Use of sympathomimetic and related vasoactive agents. *J. Am. Med. Assoc. 231:*1280–1286.

III

NEUROLOGIC CRISES AND OPPORTUNISTIC INFECTIONS

Brain Monitoring and Homeostasis in Comatose, Critically Ill Patients[1]

PETER SAFAR, M.D.
Professor and Chairman, Department of Anesthesiology/Critical Care Medicine, University Health Center of Pittsburgh, Pittsburgh, Pennsylvania

Preservation of brain function should be the pivotal concern in the management of critically ill or injured patients, for the status of the brain will determine the quality of life subsequent to recovery. Acute focal or total cerebral anoxic–ischemic, traumatic, inflammatory, metabolic, hemorrhagic, or neoplastic insults may result in coma, cerebral edema, total or regional cerebral blood flow (CBF) disturbances, and permanent cerebral metabolic derangements. Various insults to other organ systems may also ultimately jeopardize cerebral functioning. The initial insult is often followed by secondary (postresuscitative) cerebral changes that can be either ameliorated or prevented. With the use of titrated therapy aimed at restoring cerebral homeostasis, the chance for neuronal recovery may be enhanced [65]. The present chapter summarizes information on cerebral pathophysiology and some current therapeutic recommendations.

[1] Adapted from Safar, P.: (a) (1970–1975) Brain homeostasis in critical care. Lecture synopses, CCM Symposia, University of Pittsburgh; (b) American Society of Anesthesiologists Refresher Course Synopsis, 1973; and (c) Chapter 5, in: Schwartz, G. (ed.), *Principles and Practice of Emergency Medicine*, Saunders, Philadelphia: in press, 1978.

Acknowledgment: Dr. Nancy Caroline helped with editing this manuscript.

PATHOPHYSIOLOGY AND MONITORING

The human brain, with its 10 billion neurons, 100 billion glial cells, and 500 trillion synapses, makes up only about 2% of the body weight but accounts for about 20% of the total oxygen consumption and requires 15% of the cardiac output. The brain is the most vulnerable organ for several reasons, such as its: (a) high energy and blood-flow requirements, (b) dependency on aerobic glucose metabolism, (c) probable need for protein synthesis during learning and memory function, and (d) anatomic limitation imposed by a rigid cranium, especially during swelling due to injury.

Sudden total cessation of cerebral circulation results in unconsciousness within 10 sec (after which brain oxygen stores are depleted); a flat electroencephalogram within about 20–30 sec; dilated, fixed pupils within about 60 sec; and irreversible neuronal damage within about 5 min (using conventionally applied therapeutic measures after the resumption of perfusion). Anaerobic glucose metabolism, which produces only 2 mole of ATP per mole of glucose, in contrast to aerobic metabolism, producing 38 moles of ATP per mole of glucose, is inadequate to sustain consciousness and, for more than a few minutes, the integrity of neuronal cells [50]. When brain ATP is decreased to $\leqslant$20% of nórmal levels, within about five minutes of circulatory arrest [42], glucose stores are depleted and lactic-acid production and accumulation cease. This coincides with the duration of circulatory arrest required to produce irreversible neuronal damage [9].

The cranium is a closed box (Munro-Kellie doctrine), the total volume of which is almost constant. Its contents are essentially noncompressible and consist of brain fluid (65%), solids (25%), cerebrospinal fluid, (7%), and capillary blood (3%) [61,62]. This excludes large-vessel volume. Total intracranial blood volume, i.e., blood in capillaries, arteries, and veins constitute about 10% of total intracranial volume. Small volume changes result in large intracranial pressure (ICP) changes.

Cerebral neurons are "sheltered" by: (a) glial cells, (b) the blood–brain barrier (BBB), (c) the choroid plexus, and (d) extracellular fluid (ECF), which comprises about 10–20% of brain volume. The ECF bathes brain cells and is contiguous with cerebrospinal fluid (CSF).

Hypercarbia and hypoxemia, which increase CBF, as well as increased venous and arterial pressure, all increase intracranial blood volume and hence ICP. Some of these alterations may also result in cerebral edema, particularly if they are prolonged and the integrity of the BBB is disturbed.

Cerebrospinal Fluid

This is formed at a rate of about 0.5 ml/min, about 70% by the choroid plexus and 30% via brain ECF, and is absorbed mainly through the arachnoid villi (Table 1). Normal CSF is low in protein and has electrolyte concentrations similar to those in plasma. However, plasma electrolyte

TABLE 1 Composition of CSF in Man

Normal Values

VARIABLE	PLASMA (OR ARTERIAL BLOOD)		CSF
pH	7.4		7.3
Pa_{CO_2}, torr	35 – 45		>45
Pa_{O_2}, torr	75 – 100		<75
Bicarbonate, meq/l	23 – 26 (art.)		22 – 25
Lactate, μmole/ml	0.5– 1.0 (art.)	cf.[a] 9.0	1.5 – 2.0
mg/100 ml	4.5– 9.0 (art.)		14 – 18
Cell count			0.5/mm^3
Total osmolality, meq/l	280 – 295		280 –295
Sodium, meq/l	135 – 145		142 –147
Potassium, meq/l	3.5– 5.0		2.8 – 3.1
Magnesium, meq/l	1.5– 2.5		2.23
Calcium, meq/l	2.1– 2.6		2.28
Chloride, meq/l	100 – 106		120 –130
Bromide, meq/l	0		0.9
Inorganic phosphate, meq/l	1.0– 1.5		1.0
Protein, mg/100 ml	6000 –8000		15 – 45
Albumin, mg/100 ml	4000 –5000		12 – 36
Globulins, mg/100 ml	2000 –3000		3 – 9
Glucose, μmole/ml	3.9– 5.6	cf. 0.05551	2.8 – 4.2
mg/100 ml	70 – 100		50 – 75
Amino nitrogen, μmole/ml	2.1– 3.9		0.8
Bilirubin, total μmole/l	<12.0	cf. 17.1	0
mg/100 ml	<0.7		0
Phospholipids, μmole/ml	2.9– 5.2	cf. 0.3229	0.11
mg/100 ml	9.4– 16.8		0.35
Glutamic oxalacetic transaminase, (GOT), μMO/hr/ml	1.0		0.66
Lactic dehydrogenase (LDH), mU/ml	60 – 120		60 –120

[a] cf = correction factor.

changes are reflected only slowly in the CSF. And, while CSF in the cerebral ventricles and supracorticaltentorial spaces equilibrates with cisternal CSF within minutes, equilibration with lumbar CSF occurs only after 1–2 hr of a change in composition.

The cerebrospinal fluid plays both mechanical and chemical roles. It protects the brain and spinal cord within a rigid enclosure and adapts its volume, within limits, to changes of intracranial blood volume and brain volume. The chemical function of the CSF is mediated principally through changes in acid–base balance; CSF pH is normally 7.3 at a $Pa_{CO_2} = 40$ torr and is more finely regulated than blood pH. This is due to a system of balances among blood and CSF CO_2, brain CO_2 production, CSF bicarbonate concentration, and CSF lactate, the latter being normally slightly higher than arterial lactate. Rate of arterial pH change reflected in the CSF varies with the respiratory or metabolic nature of this change. Carbon dioxide readily crosses the BBB, but charged ions such as hydrogen or bicarbonate cross more slowly. Therefore, hypocarbia rapidly increases and hypercarbia rapidly decreases brain and CSF pH, while in metabolic alkalemia or acidemia, CSF pH is maintained near normal over a wide range of blood-pH values for some time.

In acute systemic acid–base disturbances, brain pH and not arterial pH determines the level of consciousness [56]. Sampling of CSF provides a valuable means of assessing cerebral pH balance which, for the reasons mentioned above, is not always accurately reflected in arterial samples. Samples for pH and P_{CO_2} must be entirely bubble-free and cleared of deadspace, since even a small loss of CO_2 into a bubble or by diffusion through plastic catheters can cause a measured P_{CO_2} lower and pH higher than actual values. Use of a low-deadspace connecting catheter with mobile stopcock and glass syringe facilitates accurate CSF sampling. For calculation of CSF bicarbonate from pH and P_{CO_2}, the Severinghaus sliderule is recommended [70]. CSF P_{O_2} values, unless extremely low, are of little value in guiding therapy.

The pH level in CSF significantly influences both respiration and cerebral blood flow. In its respiratory actions, low CSF pH stimulates the medullary surface chemoreceptors and thereby increases respiratory efforts. A decrease in CSF pH may thus be the principal cause of hyperventilation in patients with head trauma. The effects of CSF pH on cerebral blood flow are believed to occur through relaxation of cerebral arterioles when the smooth muscle of the arteriolar walls is bathed in an ECF of high hydrogen-ion concentration [13]. In addition, CSF P_{O_2} and P_{CO_2} values, normally ranging between those of arterial and cerebral venous pressure, tend to decrease and increase, respectively, in areas surrounding ischemic lesions [19,20]. Thus, local hypoxia and hypercarbia further lower the pH in ischemic areas, contributing to arteriolar dilatation and CBF augmentation.

Cerebrospinal lactate, the product of anaerobic metabolism, is increased following brain hypoxia, ischemia, or trauma. The presence of blood in the subarachnoid space also results in vasospasm and CSF lactacidosis. In patients with head injury, there appears to be a correlation between CSF lactate concentration and prognosis—with lactate values of >15 μmole/ml (>10 times normal) and rarely associated with recovery of consciousness. However, the diagnostic and prognostic values of CSF enzyme elevations and cytologic examinations for sloughed cells have not yet been established.

Cerebral Edema and Intracranial Pressure

Data on brain edema, primarily from studies of histologic changes, brain impedance, and wet:dry-weight ratios, are confusing, as the results vary with different experimental techniques. Abnormal H_2O imbibition by the brain may increase intracellular or extracellular fluid, or both. Cerebral edema following head trauma, for example, seems to be both intra- and extracellular, as there is injury to the BBB. However, following ischemia or anoxia (e.g., cardiac arrest), accumulation of excess fluid in the brain seems to be primarily intracellular. Cessation of brain perfusion appears to result immediately in a shift of sodium and water from the extracellular into the intracellular space because of failure of the cell membrane sodium pump, increase in brain tissue osmolality, and other factors [59,74]. Also, swelling of glial, neuronal, and endothelial cells may pinch capillaries and impair perfusion. Even focal ischemic or other types of brain lesion are surrounded by a "trouble zone" of edema.

Cerebral edema may at first increase the pressure within brain tissue without increasing ICP, as the swelling brain first displaces CSF and blood. As intracranial compliance decreases, however, even slight arterial or venous hypertension (e.g., coughing, straining, hypercarbia, and hypoxemia) or further increase in edema can increase ICP greatly. *Intracranial pressure* is controlled by many factors: (a) distensibility, volume, and pressures of arteries and veins; (b) venous outflow rate; (c) rate of formation and absorption of CSF; (d) osmotic gradients between CSF, brain, and plasma; and (e) intracranial bleeding.

Cerebral electric impedance to a weak, high-frequency test current is a promising but still experimental, relatively noninvasive method for monitoring shifts of extracellular fluid into the intracellular space. There are unidentified errors from current spread outside the brain and from brain or blood displacing CSF. Techniques, apparatus, and interpretations have yet to be worked out. In general, intracellular edema increases brain impedance.

With the patient in horizontal position, normal ICP and lumbar CSF pressure are 0–15 cm H_2O ($\leqslant$11 torr); a pressure of $>$20 cm H_2O lumbar CSF in this position is abnormal. In the sitting position, ICP is negative and lumbar CSF pressure is about 50 cm H_2O. Pressure should be measured before fluid displacement with either a water manometer or strain gauge. Lumbar subarachnoid puncture or catheterization is hazardous in patients with signs of a tentorial pressure cone as it may provoke brain herniation; however, it is not absolutely contraindicated in the presence of papilledema, provided a thin needle is used and rapid CSF drainage is avoided [3]. Lumbar puncture or catheterization is probably safe in patients with diffuse brain pathology without suspected ICP rise.

Increased ICP damages the brain primarily but not exclusively by decreasing cerebral perfusion pressure (CPP); CPP is calculated as mean (systemic) arterial pressure (MAP) minus mean ICP or jugular-vein pressure, whichever is higher. Therefore MAP and CPP should be monitored together with ICP; both arterial pressure and ICP strain gauges must be set at zero at midcranium and all pressures recorded in torr units. Increased ICP in the "healthy" brain elicits compensatory vasodilation; however, when CPP is reduced from a normal value of about 80 torr to about $\leqslant$50 torr,

CBF declines. Although occasionally patients remain conscious or semiconscious until CPP decreases to <10–20 torr, an ICP rise of >20 torr and a CPP decrease of <50 torr in the "injured" brain should be reversed if possible. Direct pressure on the brain, as from retractors in neurosurgery, of >20 torr produces hemorrhagic cerebral necrosis, particularly in the presence of arterial hypotension (Albin, personal communication). When ICP equals $\overline{\text{MAP}}$, CBF is zero (brain death).

A sustained increase in ICP to values of >50 torr is sometimes associated with decreased consciousness, even without CPP decrease. This is more likely in the presence of focal lesions that cause brain distortions than with diffuse, evenly distributed ICP rise [31]. A key factor in the vicious cycle of ICP rise seems to be compression of the small veins of the arachnoid villi draining into the sinuses. When baseline ICP is elevated to >20 torr, ICP waves, probably caused by cerebral blood-volume variations, are seen unexpectedly [34,35]. These plateau waves of 50–100 torr may last 5–20 min and occasionally hours and are terminated either spontaneously or by therapy. There seems to be some correlation between duration and degree of ICP rise and outcome in terms of mortality and morbidity in patients suffering from head injury.

An increase in ICP does not invariably cause systemic arterial hypertension and bradycardia (the Cushing reflex) [55]. For example, supratentorial mass lesions that expand produce sequential changes in breathing, circulation, and eye signs as the diencephalon, midbrain, pons, and finally the medulla progressively fail. The Cushing reflex is more common with posterior fossa lesions or rapidly expanding supratentorial lesions (e.g., epidural hemorrhage). Cerebral ischemic anoxia may produce arterial hypertension, even when ICP is normal [48].

In supratentorial space-occuping lesions, the clinician must try to recognize and reverse an ICP rise before the diencephalic changes (Cheyne–Stokes breathing, drowsiness, localizing signs such as contralateral hemiplegia and homolateral stiffening, and pupil constriction) lead to compression and displacement of the midbrain [55]. The latter is suspected when there are hyperventilation, dilated, fixed pupils of medium size, and disappearing ciliospinal reflex, oculovestibular reflex (caloric test), and oculocephalic reflex ("doll's eye" phenomenon). Accompanying motor derangements may be reflected in decorticate rigidity. This includes: (a) flexion of arms, wrists, and fingers; (b) extension, internal rotation, and plantar flexion of the lower extremity due to interruption of the corticospinal pathways (provoked by vigorous external stimuli); and (c) progression to decerebrate rigidity from midbrain transsection [with (i) opisthotonous and arms extended, adducted, and pronated, (ii) legs extended with plantar flexion, and (iii) shivering and increased respiratory rate]. Finally, tentorial herniation due to supratentorial ICP rise causes axial displacement, either symmetrically or by herniation of the brain across the falx and one side of the tentorium with unilateral lesions. This axial displacement results in the pontine and medullary changes of hypoventilation (sighs or gasps), tachycardia, progressive arterial hypotension, maximally dilated pupils, and finally, apnea. A unilaterally dilating pupil is the principal early sign of herniation of the uncus over the edge of the tentorium, compressing the third nerve. This can result in immediate midbrain transsection because of direct compression. All of this is accompanied by a progressive decrease in consciousness from drowsiness to stupor to coma.

Subtentorial lesions can also increase ICP and cause herniation, both downward through the foramen occipitale magnum and upward through the tentorium. Such lesions, when they involve the reticular formation, cause coma. Those not involving the reticular formation may produce the peculiar clinical picture of an awake patient who is tetraplegic, apneic, and aphasic.

Usually, ventricular and cisternal ICP and lumbar CSF pressures change in the same direction and to the same degree. However, localized brain lesions may cause ICP pressure gradients between these compartments. Tissue pressure (e.g., pressure in the cortex underlying a subdural hematoma) may be higher than mean supratentorial ICP. Cranial extradural pressure may exceed ICP, for instance, in extradural hematoma, because of the dura's elasticity. Localized or diffuse brain injury, with or without hemorrhage, may result in a vicious cycle of edema–hypoperfusion–impaired venous drainage–edema, which after displacement of CSF increases ICP. A mass lesion (but not intracranial fluid injection) may cause tentorial brain herniation with compression of the brain stem and finally medullary herniation, both resulting in ICP differences between supratentorial, infratentorial, and lumbar CSF spaces.

Any space-occupying intracranial lesion decreases CSF volume and thereby decreases the margin for blood or brain-volume expansion without an associated rise in ICP. Normally, intraventricular or supracortical injection of 0.5–1.0 ml of isotonic saline will not result in a sustained rise of monitored ICP, while in the presence of edema or a space-occupying lesion, this "intracranial compliance test" will cause a sustained ICP rise.

It should be noted that not all intracranial pathology is associated with elevated ICP. Arterial hypotension, ischemia (e.g., cardiac arrest), hypoxemia, or hypoglycemia sufficiently long and severe to produce neurohistologically detectable neuronal cell damage may, for example, result in scattered focal areas of cerebral edema, hypoperfusion, and locally increased tissue pressure, without an overall rise in ICP [34,74].

Nonetheless, ICP rise is common, and ICP monitoring is indicated in head injury [31,35,72] and in certain types of metabolic brain failure, for instance, Reye's syndrome [12,37]. Monitoring of ICP is also indicated in selected patients with coma of unknown etiology, since intracranial hypertension cannot be recognized reliably without direct measurement of ICP. Even serious increases in ICP may escape clinical detection [31,35,44,72].

Monitoring of ICP is probably not needed following transient ischemic-anoxic insults [74], since ICP usually increases only after very severe insults, when brain death develops [48]. After cardiac arrest, postresuscitative measures aimed at blood-flow promotion [67] and metabolic depression [8] seem more promising than those aimed at ICP reduction (e.g., osmotherapy).

We recommend wide use of ICP monitoring for clinical studies in comatose patients who may have increasing ICP, as a guide to both titrate measures for ICP reduction (CSF drainage, hyperventilation, osmotherapy, barbiturate loading, and hypothermia) and possible termination of measures that may increase ICP (e.g., therapeutic increase in arterial pressure, tracheal suctioning, and continuous positive pressure ventilation).

Direct continuous ICP monitoring has become feasible and safe [31,79]. Much experience has been gained with the insertion of an intraventricular catheter through a drill hole in the skull into the anterior horn of the lateral ventricle of the nondominant hemisphere [31,35]. Such a catheter permits ICP monitoring, chemical analysis of the CSF, and therapeutic CSF removal for decreasing ICP, either by intermittent withdrawal or by continuous drainage.

In the supracortical subarachnoid space or the cranial epidural space, fluid-filled soft catheters, micro strain gauges, and hollow skull screws are used for ICP monitoring. The hollow fluid-filled screw [79] is inserted first through a drill hole in the skull and then through a small opening in the dura into the supracortical subarachnoid space. The hollow screw is a popular means of monitoring ICP but does not permit CSF drainage and sampling.

Cerebral Blood Flow and Metabolism

Cerebral blood flow (CBF) (Table 2) is normally about 50 ml/100 g brain weight per minute. It decreases when cerebrovascular resistance increases. Cerebrovascular resistance (CVR) is CPP divided by CBF. Flattening of the EEG seems to occur in brain regions where CBF is reduced to $\leqslant$20 ml/100 g. Cerebrospinal fluid decreases during hypocarbia (levels off at about 50% of normal with a Pa_{CO_2} of 15–20 torr) and increases during hypercarbia (normally levels off at about 200% of normal at a Pa_{CO_2} of 80–100 torr). Due to autoregulation CBF normally remains unchanged when CPP ranges between 50–150 torr; but it decreases with decrease in CPP to about $\leqslant$50 torr and increases with a rise in CPP to $\geqslant$150 torr. However, hypoxemia, ischemia, and trauma [33] diminish or abolish this CBF autoregulation and, to a lesser extent, the changes in CBF due to changes in Pa_{CO_2} as well. Thus, the already impaired CBF in the postanoxic brain may be drastically reduced with even moderate arterial hypotension [32,33,47].

Recent research data suggest it is multiple, spotty focal microcirculatory changes rather than the overall degree of CBF reduction that largely determines the amount of damage to neurons in critically ill or injured patients. After an ischemic–anoxic insult, for instance, reperfusion of brain

TABLE 2 Cerebral Variables

VARIABLES	ABBREVIATION	APPROXIMATE NORMAL VALUES (a) RECOMMENDED UNITS	(b) TRADITIONAL UNITS	CONVERSION FACTOR (a) TO (b)
Cerebral blood flow	CBF	0.50 ml/g brain per min	50 ml/100g per min	× 100
Cerebrovascular resistance CPP/CBF	CVR	200 torr/ml per g per min	2.0 torr/ml per 100 g per min	÷ 100
Cerebral arteriovenous O_2 content difference	cer(a-v)O_2	3.0 μmole/ml blood	6–7 ml/100 ml = vol. %	× 2.24
Cerebral arteriovenous glucose difference	cer(a-v)G	0.5 μmole/ml blood	9.0 mg/100 ml = mg %	× 18.0 (MW gluc. 180)
Cerebral arteriovenous lactate difference	cer(a-v)L	−0.05 μmole/ml blood	−0.45 mg/100 ml = mg %	× 9.0 (MW lact. 90)
Cerebral metabolic, rate for oxygen (O_2 consumption): CBF × cer(a-v)O_2	$CMRO_2$	1.50 μmole/g per min	3.36 ml/100 g per min	× 2.24
Cerebral metabolic rate for glucose (gluc. consumption): CBF × cer(a-v)G	CMRG	0.25 μmole/g per min	4.5 mg/100 g per min	× 18.0
Cerebral metabolic rate for lactate (− production + consumption). CBF × cer(a-v)L	CMRL	−0.023 μmole/g per min	−0.21 mg/100 g per min	× 9.0
Mixed cerebral venous P_{O_2}	cvP_{O_2}	35–45 torr		
Intracranial pressure	ICP	<20 torr	<26 cm H_2O	× 1.3
Cerebral perfusion pressure[a]	CPP	>80 torr		

[a] Systemic arterial pressure minus jugular vein pressure or ICP, whichever is higher.

capillaries is impaired at first because of local capillary pinching from tissue-cell edema and plugging from blood-cell aggregates [4,17,18] and later perhaps because of other factors such as vasospasm. Notably, total brain ischemia from normovolemic arrest (e.g., ventricular fibrillation and asphyxial asystole) seems to result in vascular changes and greater neurologic deficit than the same period of total brain ischemia with brain vessels empty (e.g., exsanguination cardiac arrest or intracranial hypertension). This observation could be explained by greater impairment of reflow after blood has been stagnant in capillaries, which seems to occur in all organs after cardiac arrest and also during the resuscitative phase from shock states without cardiac arrest [30,78].

Monitoring of CBF is still predominantly a research technique, utilizing brain saturation or desaturation curves of an inert gas [29]. Cerebral bloodflow can be measured by experts at the bedside with the use of expensive equipment, including a portable gamma camera, computer, and surface probes (single probe for hemispheric CBF; multiple probes for regional CBF) [33,76] and techniques such as intracarotid, venous, or inhaled administration of radioactive xenon [51].

Cerebral angiography or brain scanning does not give information on CBF except in brain death from intracranial hypertension when nonfilling of intracranial arteries indicates zero CBF.

Monitoring of CBF gives more relevant information if combined with the use of a superior jugular bulb catheter to obtain arterial and mixed cerebral venous contents of oxygen, glucose, and lactate. When arterial blood hemoglobin is fully saturated with oxygen and cerebral oxygen consumption is constant, a decrease in CBF results in a decrease in mixed cerebral venous P_{O_2}, i.e., $\overline{cv}\ P_{O_2}$, and mixed cerebral venous oxygen content ($\overline{cv}\ C_{O_2}$); i.e., an increase in cerebral arteriovenous oxygen-content difference. Conversely, an increase in CBF causes an increase in $\overline{cv}\ P_{O_2}$. These estimates of changes in CBF from changes in cerebral venous oxygen content or tension or from arteriovenous oxygen content difference are the "CBF equivalent." They reflect overall CBF changes only when cerebral oxygen consumption does not change. Localized CBF reduction, as in stroke, may not decrease $\overline{cv}\ P_{O_2}$, cerebral venous oxygen content difference, or total CBF values.

The above limitations complicate clinical CBF measurements in the intensive care unit. Moreover, the usefulness of the information gained from total CBF monitoring in guiding therapeutic intervention is limited at present. Hemispheric or regional CBF values may not change when there are multiple areas of focal hypoperfusion, as is common after ischemic–anoxic, metabolic, or infectious brain insults, unless these areas are extensive. Also, CBF determinations are discontinuous, and ICP waves, often occurring suddenly and unexpectedly, may be missed.

The cerebral metabolic rates for oxygen ($CMRO_2$, cerebral oxygen consumption), glucose (CMRG, glucose uptake), and lactate (CMRL, lactate production) are calculated from CBF times cerebral arteriovenous gradients of oxygen, glucose, and lactate, respectively (Table 2). During consciousness $CMRO_2$ is remarkably constant (~3–5 ml/100 g^{-1} min; $CMRO_2$) but $CMRO_2$ increases during convulsions, in hyperthermia, or with epinephrine, and decreases during anesthesia, coma, severe hypercarbia, or hypothermia. Changes in $CMRO_2$, particularly persistently low levels (decreases to <2 ml/100 g min^{-1}) may have prognostic value in determining the irreversibility of coma in the absence of depressant drugs or hypothermia [7].

Superior jugular bulb catheterization, performed percutaneously via a catheter inserted into the internal jugular vein in the neck, or with fluoroscopic guidance, from an arm vein, permits monitoring of mixed cerebrovenous blood oxygen, glucose and lactate, and jugular vein pressure. A decrease of $\overline{cv}\,P_{O_2}$ from the normal value of 30–40 torr to about 10–27 torr gives evidence of anaerobic metabolism in the brain and indicates need to increase CBF. A normal $\overline{cv}\,P_{O_2}$, however, does not rule out focal areas of hypoperfusion. Cerebral arteriovenous oxygen, glucose, and lactate gradients theoretically permit estimation of the degree of brain anaerobiosis without the need for CBF measurement, by determining in molar values oxygen–glucose index (OGI) and the lactate–glucose index (LGI):

$$OGI = \frac{\text{a-vO}_2}{6 \times \text{a-vG}} \times 100 \qquad LGI = \frac{\text{a-vL}}{2 \times \text{a-vG}} \times 100$$

Normally, the brain burns only about 5% of glucose to lactate (LGI) and 95% to oxygen (OGI). These indexes should total 100%. The accuracy, and thus clinical value of OGI/LGI determinations, however, are limited by difficult analytical methods and small concentration gradients [11].

Cerebral Electrical Activity

In general, high CO_2 (low pH) and severe hypoxemia exert a depressant effect, while mild hypoxemia exerts a stimulating effect, on the electrical activity of cerebral cortical neurons. Clinically, cerebral electrical activity monitored from surface electrodes reflects primarily the electrocorticogram. In the assessment of critically ill patients, the EEG is widely used to detect brain death and convulsions in curarized patients. Less well developed is EEG monitoring in critically ill or injured patients without electrocortical silence. Multiple EEG tracings can be analyzed by computer for average voltage and frequency, enabling assessment of the depth of CNS depression, perhaps more reliably than is possible from clinical signs [7,57].

Monitoring of average cortically evoked EEG potentials, recorded via scalp electrodes and elicited by somatosensory, auditory, and/or visual stimuli, can enable early detection of deterioration and thus early surgical or pharmacologic intervention. Equipment for this is expensive and includes an averaging computer with memory. Unilateral lesions cause a decrease in the amplitude of evoked potentials on the affected side, while the latency remains unchanged. Demyelinization or compression of pathways increases the latency and renders the normally polyphasic evoked wave form monophasic. Unconsciousness is associated with decreased amplitude, even in the absence of mass lesions. Recovery is associated with improved amplitude of evoked potentials.

PATIENT MANAGEMENT

Clinical Observations

Clinical monitoring of patients with brain failure [55] should focus on the state of consciousness, respiratory patterns, cranial-nerve function, and, when they can be assessed, sensory- and motor-function integrity. Furthermore, periodic examination of the eye grounds is indicated to assess hemorrhage, edema, and perfusion defects. Papilledema usually develops slowly, after about 2 days of increased ICP, and persists after normalization of ICP. Cerebral edema is suspected when there is a decrease in consciousness, pupillary dilatation, convulsions, or papilledema. Cerebral edema cannot be proven clinically. The charges accompanying rostrocaudal compression, axial displacement, or unilateral herniation of the temporal lobe include unconsciousness, unilateral or bilateral pupillary dilatation, hyperventilation–hypoventilation, hypertension–hypotension, and bradycardia–tachycardia. Such changes must be detected immediately, since prompt surgical intervention may be required.

General Measures

In comatose patients, extracranial changes and general life-supporting measures can greatly influence intracranial dynamics [65,81]. General monitoring requires at a minimum arterial and central venous catheters, as well as a bladder catheter. Variables to be monitored and optimized include: (a) arterial and central venous pressures; (b) ECG findings; (c) urine volume; (d) Pa_{O_2}, Pa_{CO_2}, pH, and base excess; (e) blood glucose and hematocrit, and (f) serum electrolytes, albumin, oncotic pressure, and osmolality. General therapeutic measures (given below) should begin as soon as possible after the emergency is recognized.

Airway control. Personnel involved in the care of critically ill patients must be experienced and skillful with rapid intubation at risk of aspiration ("crash intubation") [75]. Such intubation must be accomplished with sufficient rapidity so as to avoid even brief periods of hypoxemia or hypercarbia. Furthermore, coughing and straining (bucking) should be minimized, as these struggles increase CVP, ICP, and arterial pressure, produce hypoxemia, and promote intracranial bleeding. The need for pulmonary clearing and the jeopardy to the airway from aspiration must, in each instance, be weighed against these hazards.

Control of arterial P_{O_2}, P_{CO_2}, pH, and base deficit. Adequate cerebral oxygenation is critical to maintenance of neurologic integrity, and thus even brief episodes of hypoxemia must not occur. Arterial P_{O2} should be maintained above 100 torr to allow a margin of safety and thereby protect against hypoxemic episodes during convulsions, hypoventilation, or apnea. An adequate Pa_{O_2} is best achieved by administration for several hours of 80–100% oxygen, decreasing if possible to $\leqslant$60% after no longer than 12–24 hr, to prevent pulmonary oxygen toxicity. If Pa_{O_2} cannot be maintained above 100 torr with 60% oxygen, some form of continuous positive-pressure breathing is indicated. However, this should be adjusted to enable optimal oxygenation without undue CVP increase. The use of hyperbaric oxygenation in various acute cerebral states needs reevaluation [27].

Control of neurogenic pulmonary edema. This type of edema may interfere with maintenance of high arterial P_{O_2} and its mechanisms are not fully understood. In the experimental setting, acute, isolated cerebral hypoxia results in pulmonary edema in normal innervated but not denervated lung, [45,46]. Pulmonary venospasm has been postulated as a mechanism in this disorder, but definitive proof is lacking. Acute pulmonary edema in coma is sometimes preceded or accompanied by a severe increase in systemic peripheral vascular resistance, which may or may not be triggered by ICP rise; in these situations, control of arterial hypertension may reverse the pulmonary edema. In any event, adequate Pa_{O_2} control and early detection of pulmonary edema require periodic 100% oxygen tests, which demonstrate pulmonary shunting earlier than do clinical signs and roentgenograms.

Control of hypercarbia. In addition to hypoxemia, hypercarbia also threatens cerebral homeostasis. At the slightest suspicion of hypoventilation (Pa_{CO_2} >35 torr), artificial ventilation with IPPV should be started. Most patients with acute brain failure hyperventilate spontaneously, mainly because of moderately increased ICP or CSF lactacidosis. Moderate prolonged controlled hyperventilation (aiming at a Pa_{CO_2} of 25–35 torr) seems indicated when the patient does not hyperventilate alone or becomes exhausted from doing so. Intermittent mandatory ventilation may well be the most easily controllable ventilatory pattern, combining the benefits of spontaneous and controlled ventilation.

Control of intracranial hypertension. When, in the presence of monitored ICP, intracranial hypertension does not yield to CSF drainage, hyperventilation to values of <25 torr can often transiently reduce ICP. However, Pa_{CO_2} values of about <20 torr are not recommended on a long-term basis, as extreme degrees of hypocarbia may produce severe spasm in reactive circulatory channels. Arterial pH values over 7.6 should be avoided if possible. Ideally, ventilation volumes should be adjusted to normalize CSF pH. Additional steps for ICP normalization are osmotherapy [31,44] barbiturate [8,37,64,72], and hypothermia [61].

Pa_{CO_2} normalization in emphysema. Controlled ventilation to normal Pa_{CO_2} (40 torr) in stuporous or comatose patients with decompensated chronic obstructive lung disease, where the levels of bicarbonate and Pa_{CO_2} are high, can result in alkalotic brain failure with reduced CBF [63]. In these patients, oxygenation should be prompt, but Pa_{CO_2} normalization gradual. Should coma or convulsions occur in the presence of a high arterial or CSF pH, acetazolamide (Diamox), 0.5 g IV, is indicated as this carbonic anhydrase inhibitor can acidify the brain rapidly [66].

Control of circulation. Mean systemic arterial pressure should be maintained within about 80–120 torr in a previously normotensive patient (higher in a hypertensive person), higher than normal following brain ischemia, and slightly lower than normal following head injury or in suspected intracranial hemorrhage. Arterial pressure can be raised by volume expansion and short-term infusion of a vasopressor and lowered by a vasodilator, such as nitroprusside or trimethaphan (Arfonad). Increasing $\overline{MAP}$ moderately (120–140 torr) with plasma expansion and vasopressors may improve the cerebral microcirculation and ameliorate brain damage following cardiac arrest [67]. However, when the ICP is found to be elevated, measures to lower ICP should have priority over those aimed at increasing $\overline{MAP}$, since the elevated $\overline{MAP}$ may itself increase ICP further and since, as well, ICP rise over about 40–50 torr, even with maintained CPP, can depress consciousness. Raising $\overline{MAP}$ is contraindicated in brain lesions with vascular damage (from head injury) as it may increase bleeding, edema, and ICP. In focal ischemia (stroke), therapeutic hypertension treatment is controversial. In comatose patients both arterial hypotension and severe hypertension should be avoided.

Control of total cardiac output and blood volume. This is of less importance to the brain than to extracranial organs that participate in compensatory vasoconstriction in shock (splanchnic and renal vessels), but these variables should nonetheless also be maintained at optimal levels. Cardiac arrhythmias, which may disturb cerebral circulation, should be monitored, recognized, and controlled.

Control of posture. Attention to the patient's position is a matter of some importance. The Trendelenburg position should be avoided, as it increases arterial, venous, and intracranial pressures. The supine position is preferred over the sitting position, as the latter may produce postural hypotension and cerebral hypoperfusion. Flexion or torsion of the neck should be avoided, as it may cause neck-vein compression.

Control of blood variables. Hematocrit level should be 30–40% and lower when deliberate hemodilution is sought. In experimental animals, normovolemic hemodilution during or immediately following reperfusion after an ischemic–anoxic insult, in addition to other measures, reverses or prevents brain damage, particularly if $\overline{MAP}$ is maintained normal or high [18,47,67]. However, this approach has not yet been tested in clinical trials. Likewise, heparinization, which may promote reperfusion after an ischemic–anoxic insult [67], needs further investigation and is contraindicated following trauma or other insults associated with BBB damage.

Control of serum variables. Serum-electrolyte concentration should be normalized. Oncotic pressure should be maintained near normal and albumin levels at about ⩾2.5 g%. Changes in serum and CSF osmolality may also exert profound effects on cerebral homeostasis and thus warrant monitoring in comatose patients [39]. In acute hyperosmolar states, coma may develop when serum osmolality increases acutely from a normal value of 290 to about ⩾340 mosmole/l. In some hyperosmolar states, such as infant hypernatremia and hyperosmolality from concentrated feeding formulas, brain petechial and subarachnoid hemorrhages have been observed [36]. In acute hypo-osmolar states, with serum osmolality reduced acutely to about ⩽250 mosmole/l, cerebral edema, convulsions, and coma may occur. Treatment of coma due to such extreme fluctuations in serum osmolality includes pharmacologic control of convulsions, general life-supporting measures, correction of the cause, and corrective fluid therapy (0.45% sodium chloride IV in hyperosmolality, 3% sodium chloride, sodium bicarbonate, potassium, glucose, and a diuretic in water intoxication).

Fluid balance and alimentation. Dehydration should be avoided, as well as administration of salt-free dextrose 5% in water. Since glucose transport across the BBB may be impaired, dextrose administration is essential. Therefore, continuous infusion of 10% dextrose in 0.25–0.5% sodium chloride (30–50 ml/kg/24 hr in adults and children and 100 ml/kg/24 hr in infants), with potassium added as needed, should be started as soon as possible. Additional fluid may be necessary to correct for increased diuresis. Except in the case of brain death, patients with head injury usually have high caloric requirements (3000–5000 cal/24 hr/70 kg) and considerable catabolism [10,22]. This calls for early institution of parenteral alimentation and a switch to gastric feeding as soon as the bowel is active. Monitoring should include daily measurements of body weight.

Control of body temperature. Hyperthermia, common in patients with hypothalamic lesions, calls for rapid normalization of body temperature, since permanent neurologic damage is added to the existing injury by body (brain) temperatures of about ⩾41°C (105°F). Hypothermia is better tolerated and, under some circumstances, may be desirable in moderate degree as a means of decreasing cerebral metabolic rate.

Control of convulsions. Prompt control of seizures is essential to minimize cerebral oxygen and metabolic demands. Seizure control is accomplished initially by the use of a muscle relaxant. This facilitates ventilation and oxygenation but may be discontinued intermittently to permit periodic neurologic assessment. Cerebral electric hyperactivity, however, should also be suppressed, using diazepam (Valium) or thiopental for short-term management and, for long-term, diphenylhydantoin (Dilantin), phenobarbital, or pentobarbitol.

Anesthesia. In acutely brain-damaged, comatose patients, anesthetic management must include the above principles of general life support. With coma, general anesthetics are rarely needed, or only in very low concentrations. Immobilization with a muscle relaxant and controlled ventilation with oxygen are favored. Many anesthesiologists prefer nitrous oxide/oxygen, 50/50%, barbiturates, narcotics, and relaxants over the use of other inhalation anesthetics (e.g., halothane) and ketamine, since the latter agents impair autoregulation of CBF and may increase ICP.

Special Brain-oriented Therapy

Monitoring of ICP, CPP, CSF chemistry, and EEG is indicated in most patients with potentially reversible coma from causes that may increase ICP (see above). Monitoring of cerebrovenous blood oxygen, CBF, CMR, and cerebral electric impedance is still considered semiexperimental.

Steroids. The use of steroid therapy for treatment of suspected cerebral edema is popular, but its value has not yet been proven [5,6,53,58,59]. Therapeutic doses of steroids activate the sodium/potassium pump, enabling a reduction in intracellular sodium concentration (and water volume) and an increase in intracellular potassium. These changes result in membrane hyperpolarization and an increase in the electric-shock seizure threshold. In addition, steroids may stabilize mitochondria and also lysosomal membranes, preventing release of lytic enzymes. Since steroid medication has not been implicated as the sole cause in the only life-threatening complication associated with its short-term use, namely, stress ulceration of the gastrointestinal tract, a reasonable compromise in patients with suspected cerebral edema is the administration of pharmacologic doses of dexamethasone (0.2 mg/kg) or methylprednisolone (1 mg/kg) every 6 hours until there is an improvement in the state of consciousness, but not longer than 3–4 days.

Osmotherapy. This is the most popular treatment for suspected cerebral edema. It reduces brain size during craniotomies and usually can ameliorate or entirely reverse elevated intracranial pressure in various types of brain failure. Osmotherapy may increase CBF even when overall ICP is not increased [31], perhaps by decongesting the swollen cells that pinch the capillaries. For reversal of acute increases of ICP, osmotherapy should be used in combination with CSF drainage and hyperventilation. Osmotherapeutic solutions raise serum osmolality and thereby draw water from the intracellular and interstitial compartments into the vascular compartment. However, this mechanism provides only a symptomatic reduction of edema, as osmotherapeutics remove water from brain cells temporarily and do not restore membrane integrity. The reduction in cerebral edema and intracranial pressure is followed by rebound brain swelling when the osmotic agent equilibrates back into cells. This rebound is most marked with urea, less following mannitol, and least following glycerol [15,40,49,77]. The latter does not pass the BBB and is almost entirely metabolized. A mild osmotherapeutic effect is produced also by hypertonic glucose, dextrans, and albumin. The efficacy of rapidly acting intravenous diuretics for reducing cerebral edema is under investigation. Commonly used intravenous osmotherapeutic techniques include: (a) mannitol 0.5–1.0 g/kg body weight in one dose, followed by 0.3 g/kg/hr for continuous intravenous infusion and (b) glycerol in isotonic saline solution, in the form of 0.5–1.0 g/kg bolus over 30 min. The glycerol may be given about every 6 hours or in the form of a continuous infusion, preferably titrated according to monitored ICP values in doses ranging from about 1 g/kg/24 hr to 1 g/kg every 2 hr. Ideally, osmotherapy should be titrated by adjusting infusion rates intermittently according to monitored ICP. If osmotherapy is considered essential, glycerol may be safer than other agents [44]. However, all osmotherapeutic agents complicate fluid balance and can produce excessive degrees of hyperosmolality. Glycerol, furthermore, may produce hemolysis. Thus, "blind" administration of osmotherapeutic agents is discouraged. Serum osmolality should be monitored during osmotherapy; for while osmolality usually increases only 3–5%, at times it may rise to dangerous levels (350 mosmole/l), unless care is taken to assess osmolar changes.

Hypothermia. Hypothermia decreases cerebral oxygen consumption (to about 50% at 28°C central body temperature), CBF, cardiac output, and heart rate. Furthermore, hypothermia decreases the brain's inflammatory response to injury, diminishes edema formation, and may also protect enzyme activity. Experimentally, hypothermia results in smaller focal ischemia or focal traumatic brain lesions, more so when cooling is induced prior to than following insult [61–62]. Prolonged controlled hypothermia following total brain ischemia–anoxia has not yet been satisfactorily evaluated in terms of neurologic outcome and histopathologic changes. Therapeutic hypothermia is a hazardous and complex technique requiring an experienced intensive-care team, including an anesthesiologist. Uncontrolled hypothermia with unchecked shivering and vasoconstriction increases ICP and oxygen consumption and is arrhythmogenic, particularly in aged patients and in those with cardiac disease. At about 25–28°C cardiac (esophageal) temperature, asystole or ventricular fibrillation usually develops. Hypothermia also increases blood viscosity and decreases defense mechanisms against infection. Hypothermia is usually produced by surface cooling; poikilothermia (vasodilation and hypothalamic depression) and inhibition of shivering are produced by drugs. In the young and previously healthy patient with acute traumatic, inflammatory, or ischemic–anoxic brain damage, and perhaps even with metabolic brain damage and deep, persistent coma, induction of hypothermia (the earlier the better) may be justified, particularly in cases of intractable ICP rise. The ICP-reducing effect of hypothermia is augmented by barbiturate [72].

Some of the other therapeutic approaches described here may reverse the neurologic deficit due to *spinal-cord injury* if applied immediately but *local* hypothermia, involving surgical exposure of the injured spinal cord, appears especially promising [2,52,82]. All patients with spinal-cord injury should be taken immediately to the nearest spinal-cord injury center. Hypothermia in experimental stroke may worsen the outcome [43].

Barbiturate loading. Short-acting barbiturates decrease cerebral oxygen consumption, CBF, and ICP and, when given before or during the insult, reduce postanoxic brain damage. In experimental animals with focal brain ischemia, large doses of thiopental or pentobarbital have reduced infarct size when given before the insult and also when given after the insult [25,73]. In patients with head injury, thiopental or pentobarbital, particularly when combined with hypothermia, have been effective in rapidly controlling intractable intracranial hypertension [1,72]. In our laboratory, large doses of thiopental given to monkeys *immediately after* total brain ischemia of 16 min and reperfusion dramatically prevented or reduced postischemia brain damage [8]. Optimal doses and duration of administration have not been determined. The mechanism of this protective action of barbiturate has not yet been clarified. One may speculate that the barbiturate has a beneficial effect on intracranial blood-flow distribution, that it reduces ICP and neuronal metabolism, and that it mops up free radicals which damage membranes postischemia [8,68,72,80]. Barbiturate loading, now undergoing clinical trials, appears promising immediately after cardiac arrest of over 5 min [64,68] and in end-stage metabolic-infectious coma [37], i.e., Reye's Syndrome [12,60].

Cranial decompression. Wide surgical decompression has been effective in a few cases for diffuse cerebral edema with severely elevated ICP following traumatic, metabolic, or other types of brain injury, when the patient approaches brain death [28]. Salvage has been reported when surgical intervention was carried out within about 30 min after the onset of apnea and dilating pupils.

Brain-death Certification [21,23,24]

Clinical death is the period of apnea and cessation of circulation with brain function suspended, but with complete neurologic recovery still possible if

TABLE 3 Guidelines for Diagnosis of Brain Death [21]

Presbyterian-University Hospital, Pittsburgh, Pa. 15213; 1971, revised 1977.

Two clinical examinations must be performed; the second no sooner than 2 hours after the first.	Date of examination: ______ ______ Time of examination: ______ ______		
		(yes, no)	(yes, no)
A. Absence of induced hypothermia and absence of central nervous system depressant drugs.		______	______
Body temperature should be recorded.		______	______
B. Generalized flaccidity, no spontaneous movements, and no evidence of postural activity or shivering (all in the absence of muscle relaxants)		______	______
C. Cranial-nerve reflexes and responses			
1. Pupils dilated and light-fixed		______	______
2. Absent corneal reflexes		______	______
3. Unresponsiveness to intensely painful stimuli (e.g., supraorbital pressure)		______	______
4. Absent response to upper and lower airway stimulation (e.g., pharyngeal and endotracheal suctioning)		______	______
5. Absent ocular response to head turning (no ocular movement)		______	______
6. Absent ocular response to irrigation of the ears with 10-20 ml ice water (no ocular movement)		______	______
D. Isoelectric EEG, recorded in part at full gain.		______	______
Date and time of tracings must be recorded.		______	______
E. Absence of spontaneous breathing movements for 3 min (in absence of hypocarbia and muscle relaxants). $PaCO_2$:			
F. Comments:			

Certification

Having considered the above findings, we hereby certify the death of:

____

Pittsburgh. Date: ______________ Time: ______________

Physician's Signature: ______________ ______________

Names Printed: ______________ M.D. ______________ M.D.

This document should be signed by two licensed physicians, who must not be the physicians of a proposed organ recipient.

spontaneous circulation and oxygen transport are restored. If reoxygenation is delayed, the outcome may be permanent neurologic deficit with or without coma ("coma prolongé") or persistent apnea and coma with cerebral cortical silence, namely, brain death ("coma depassé").

Brain-death determination and certification must be carried out according to strict rules. Clinical criteria (including apnea, dilated fixed pupils, absence of spontaneous movements, and deteriorating circulation) are as important as an isoelectric EEG. Opinion regarding the minimal time of EEG silence required for brain-death certification varies and is not based on scientific data. A recent multi-institutional study revealed that the usual brain-death certification criteria, including EEG silence for 2 hours or more, were never associated with recovery of consciousness. The author's institution uses 2 hours of EEG silence, in addition to the clinical criteria (Table 3).

Summary

Physicians and others involved in the care of acutely ill patients in critical care units should familiarize themselves with the pathophysiology of acute brain failure and newer therapeutic approaches to restoration of intracranial homeostasis. The breakthroughs in respiratory resuscitation in the 1950s and cardiovascular resuscitation in the 1960s are now being followed by breakthroughs in the resuscitation of the arrested brain, with control and reversal of rising ICP by CSF drainage, hyperventilation, osmotherapy, barbiturates, and hypothermia. The previously sacrosanct 4–6-min limit of clinical death is being challenged by experimental studies in which dramatic amelioration or prevention of postischemic brain damage has been achieved after 12–16 min of cessation of circulation [8,67]. Studies have shown chemical and electrical recovery of some neurons in cats after 60 min of circulatory arrest [26]. This gives hope for cardiopulmonary-cerebral resuscitation.

References and Selected Readings

1. **Albin, M.** (1977). Anesthetic management of the patient with head injury. *International Anaesthesiology Clinics*. Boston: Little, Brown and Company, *15/3:*297–307.
2. **Albin, M. S., White, R. J.,** and **Locke, G. E.** (1965). Treatment of spinal cord trauma by selective hypothermic perfusion. *Surg. Forum 16:*423–424.
3. **Alexander, E.** (1971). Medical management of closed head injuries. *Clin. Neurosurg. 19:*240.
4. **Ames, A., Wright, R., Kowada, M., Thurston, J.,** and **Majno, G.** (1968). Cerebral ischemia. II. The no-reflow phenomenon. *Am. J. Pathol. 52:*437.
5. **Bartko, D., Reulen, H. J., Koch, H.,** and **Schurmann, K.** (1972). Effect of dexamethasone on the early edema following occlusion of the middle cerebral artery in cats. In: *Steroids and Brain Edema*. New York: Springer-Verlag.
6. **Bauer, R. B.,** and **Tellez, H.** (1973). Dexamethasone as treatment in cere-

brovascular disease. 2. A controlled study in acute cerebral infarction. *Stroke 4:*547.
7. **Bergamasco, B., Bergamini, L., Doriguzzi, T.,** and **Fabiani, D.** (1968). EEG sleep patterns as a prognostic criterion in post-traumatic coma. *Electroenceph. Clin. Neurophysiol. 24:*374.
8. **Bleyaert, A. L., Nemoto, E. M., Safar, P., Stezoski, S. W., Moossy, J., Rao, G. R.,** and **Mickell J.:** Thiopental amelioration of postischemic encephalopathy in monkeys. (a) *The Physiologist 18:*145, 1975 (abstract); (b) *Acta Neurol. Scand. 56,* suppl. *64:*144, 1977 (synopsis); (c) *Anesthesiology,* 1978, accepted for publication.
9. **Brierley, J. B., Meldrum, B. S.,** and **Brown, A. W.** (1973). The threshold and neuropathology of cerebral "anoxic–ischemic" cell change. *Arch. Neurol. 29:*367.
10. **Bryan-Brown, C. W., Savitz, M. H., Elwyn, D. H.,** and **Shoemaker, W. C.** (1973). Cerebral edema unresponsive to conventional therapy in neurosurgical patients with unsuspected nutritional failure. *Crit. Care Med. 1:* 125–129.
11. **Cohen, P.** (1972). The metabolic function of oxygen and biochemical lesion of hypoxia. *Anesthesiol 37:*148.
12. **Cook, D. R., Mickell, J. J., Painter, M. J., Reigel, D. H.,** and **Safar, P.** (in press). Resuscitation of the brain in metabolic failure. Experience with Reye's syndrome. Proceedings of the International Symposium on Intensive Therapy, Rome, 1975. *Excerpta Medica.*
13. **Cotev, S.,** and **Severinghaus, J. W.** (1969). Role of cerebrospinal fluid in management of respiratory problems. *Anesth. Analg. 48:*42.
14. **DeLong, G. R., et al.** (1974). Citrulline for Reye's syndrome. *New Engl. J. Med. 290:*1488.
15. **DeSouza, S. W., Dobbing, J.,** and **Adlard, B. P. F.** (1973). Glycerol in treatment of cerebral œdema. *Lancet 1:*835.
16. **Dohrmann, G. J.** (1972). Experimental spinal cord trauma. *Arch. Neurol. 27:*468.
17. **Fischer, E. G.** (1973). Impaired perfusion following cerebrovascular stasis. *Arch. Neurol. 29:*361.
18. **Fischer, E. G.,** and **Adelbert, A., III.** (1972). Studies on mechanisms of impairment of cerebral circulation following ischemia: Effect of hemodilution and perfusion pressure. *Stroke 3:*538.
19. **Gordon, E.** (1971). Controlled respiration in the management of patients with traumatic brain injuries. *Acta Anaesth. Scand. 15:*193.
20. **Gordon, E.** (1971). The acid–base balance and oxygen tension of the cerebrospinal fluid and their implications for the treatment of patients with brain lesions. *Acta Anaesth. Scand. Suppl. 39:*7.
21. **Grenvik, A.** (1978). Discontinuance of life support in brain death and vegetative state. *Crit. Care Med.* in press.
22. **Haider, W., Lackner, F., Schlick, W., Benzer, H., Gerstenbrand, F., Irsigler, K., Korn, A., Krystof, G.,** and **Mayrhofer, O.** (1975). Metabolic changes in the course of severe acute brain damage. *Europ. J. Int. Care Med. 1:*19.
23. **Harp, J. R.** (1974). Criteria for the determination of death. *Anesthesiol. 40:*391.

24. Harvard Medical School Ad Hoc Committee to Examine the Definition of Brain Death (1968): A definition of irreversible coma. *J.A.M.A. 205:* 337.
25. **Hoff, J. T., Smith, A. L., Hankinson, H. L.,** and **Nielsen, S. L.** (1975). Barbiturate protection from cerebral infarction in primates. *Stroke 6:*28.
26. **Hossmann, K. A.,** and **Kleihues, P.** (1973). Reversibility of ischemic brain damage. *Arch. Neurol. 29:*375.
27. **Ingvar, D. H.,** and **Lassen, M. A.** (1964). Focal cerebral ischemia treated with hyperbaric oxygen. *Nord. Med. 72:*1352.
28. **Kerr, F. W. L.** (1968). Radical decompression and dural grafting in severe cerebral edema. *Mayo Clin. Proc. 43:*852.
29. **Kety, S. S.** (1950). Circulation and metabolism of the human brain in health and disease. *Am. J. Med. 8:*205.
30. **Kovach, A. G. B.,** and **Sandor, P.** (1976). Cerebral blood flow and brain function during hypotension and shock. *Ann. Rev. Physiol. 38:*571.
31. **Langfitt, T. W.** (1973). Increased intracranial pressure. In: Youmans, J. R. (ed.), *Neurologic Surgery,* Vol. I, Chapter 18. Philadelphia: W. B. Saunders.
32. **Lassen, N. A.,** and **Ingvar, H. D.** (eds.) (1977). Cerebral Function, Metabolism and Circulation. *Acta Neurol. Scand.* 64, 56.
33. **Lassen, N. A.** (1959). Cerebral blood flow and oxygen consumption in man. *Physiol. Rev. 39:*183.
34. **Lind, B., Snyder, J.,** and **Safar, P.** (1975). Total brain ischemia in dogs. Cerebral, physiologic, and metabolic changes after 15 minutes of circulatory arrest. *Resuscitation 4:*97.
35. **Lundberg, N.** (1960). Continuous recording and control of ventricular fluid pressure in neurosurgical practice. *Acta Psychiat. Neurol. Scand. 36:* Suppl. 149.
36. **Luttrell, C. N., Finberg, L.,** and **Drawdy, L. P.** (1959). Hemorrhagic encephalopathy induced by hypernatremia. II. Experimental observations on hyperosmolarity in cats. *Am. Med. Assoc. Arch. Neurol. 1:*153.
37. **Marshall, L. F., Shapiro, H. M., Rausch, A., and Kaufman, N. M.** (1978). Pentobarbital therapy for intracranial pressure in metabolic coma (Reye's syndrome). *Crit. Care Med. 6:*1.
38. **Martin, S. H.,** and **Bloedel, J. R.** (1973). Evaluation of experimental spinal cord injury using cortical evoked potentials. *J. Neurosurg. 39:*75.
39. **Mattar, J. A., Weil, M. H.,** and **Shubin, H.** (1973). A study of the hyperosmolal state in critically ill patients. *Crit. Care Med. 1:*293.
40. **Meyer, J. S., Charney, J. Z., Rivera, V. M.,** and **Mathew, N. T.** (1971). Treatment with glycerol of cerebral edema due to acute cerebral infarction. *Lancet 2* (part 2):993.
41. **Michenfelder, J. D., Milde, H. J.,** and **Sundt, T. M.** (1976). Cerebral protection by barbiturate anesthesia. Use after middle cerebral artery occlusion in Java monkeys. *Arch. Neurol. 33:*345.
42. **Michenfelder, J. D.,** and **Theye, R. A.** (1970). The effects of anesthesia and hypothermia on canine cerebral ATP and lactate during anoxia produced by decapitation. *Anesthesiol. 33:*430.
43. **Michenfelder, J. D.** (1977). Failure of prolonged hypocapnia, hypother-

mia, or hypertension to favorably alter acute stroke in primates. *Stroke 8:*87.

44. **Mickell, J. J., Reigel, D. H., Cook, D. R., Binda, R. E., and Safar, P.** (1977). Intracranial pressure: monitoring and normalization therapy in children. *Pediatrics 59:*606.
45. **Moss, G., Staunton, C.,** and **Stein, A. A.** (1973). The centrineurogenic etiology of the acute respiratory distress syndromes: Universal, species independent phenomenon. *Am. J. Surg. 126:*137.
46. **Moss, G.,** and **Stein, A. A.** (1975). Cerebral etiology of the acute respiratory distress syndrome: Diphenylhydantoin prophylaxis. *J. Trauma 15:*39.
47. **Nemoto, E. M., Synder, J. V., Carroll, R. G.,** and **Morita, H.** (1974). Global ischemia in dogs. Cerebral vascular CO_2 reactivity and autoregulation. *Stroke 6:*425.
48. **Nemoto, E. M., et al.** (1975; 1977; 1977]. Global brain ischemia. A reproducible monkey model. (a) *Fed. Proc. 34:*384; (b) *Stroke 8:*558; (c) *Acta Neurol. Scand. 56:*142.
49. **Newkirk, T. A., Tourtellotte, W. W.,** and **Reinglass, J. L.** (1972). Prolonged control of increased intracranial pressure with glycerin. *Arch. Neurol. 27:*95.
50. **Nilsson, B., Norberg, K.,** and **Siesjö, B. K.** (1975). Biochemical events in cerebral ischemia. *Brit. J. Anaesth. 47:*751.
51. **Obrist, W. D., Thompson, K. H., King, C. H.,** and **Wang, H. S.** (1967). Determination of regional cerebral blood flow by inhalation of ^{133}Xenon. *Circ. Res. 20:*124.
52. **Osterholm, J. L.** (1974). Special review. The pathophysiological response to spinal cord injury. *J. Neurosurg. 40:*5.
53. **Pappius, H. M.,** and **McCann, W. P.** (1969). Effects of steroids on cerebral edema in cats. *Arch. Neurol. 20:*207.
54. **Plum, F.** (ed.) (1973). Symposium on the threshold and mechanisms of anoxic–ischemic brain injury. *Arch. Neurol. 29:*359.
55. **Plum, F.,** and **Posner, J. B.** (1972). *The Diagnosis of Stupor and Coma.* Second Edition, Philadelphia: F. A. Davis.
56. **Posner, J. B., Swanson, A. G.,** and **Plum, F.** (1965). Acid–base balance in cerebrospinal fluid. *Arch. Neurol. 12:*479.
57. **Prior, P. F., Maynard, D. E., Scheaff, P. C., Simpson, B. R., Strunin, L., Weaver, E. J. M.,** and **Scott, D. F.** (1971). Monitoring cerebral function: clinical experience with new device for continuous recording of electrical activity of brain. *Brit. Med. J. 2:*736.
58. **Ransohoff, J.** (1972). The effects of steroids on brain edema in man. In: Reulen, H. J. (ed.), *Steroids and Brain Edema.* New York: Springer-Verlag.
59. **Reulen, H. J.** (ed.) (1972). *Steroids and Brain Edema.* New York: Springer-Verlag.
60. **Reye, R. D. K., Morgan, G.,** and **Baral, J.** (1963). Encephalopathy and fatty degeneration of the viscera: A disease entity in childhood. *Lancet 2:*749.
61. **Rosomoff, H. L., Shulman, K., Raynor, R.,** and **Grainger, W.** (1960). Experimental brain injury and delayed hypothermia. *Surg. Gynec. Obstet. 110:*27.

62. **Rosomoff, H. L.**, and **Zubide, F. P.** (1963). Distribution of intracranial contents in experimental edema. *Arch. Neurol. 9:*26.
63. **Rotheram, E. B., Safar, P., and Robin, E. D.** (1964). CNS disorder during mechanical ventilation in chronic pulmonary disease. *J.A.M.A. 189:* 993.
64. **Safar, P.** (ed.) (1977). Advances in Cardiopulmonary Resuscitation (the Wolf Creek Conference). New York: Springer-Verlag. Chapters 27 (Safar, P. et al); 28 (Nemoto, E. et al); and 29 (Safar, P.).
65. **Safar, P.** Maintenance of brain homeostasis in critical care: (a) Proceedings of Annual Symposia on Critical Care Medicine, University of Pittsburgh, May, 1970–1975; (b) Am. Soc. Anesthesiol. meeting, October 1973, refresher course synopsis.
66. **Safar, P., Nemoto, E. M.**, and **Severinghaus, J. W.** (1973). Pathogenesis of central nervous system disorder during artificial hyperventilation in compensated hypercarbia in dogs. *Crit. Care Med. 1:*5.
67. **Safar, P., Stezoski, W.**, and **Nemoto, E. M.** (1975). Amelioration of brain damage following 12 minutes of cardiac arrest in dogs. *Fed. Proc. 34:*384 (Abstract #932); *Arch. Neurol.* (in press, 1975).
68. **Safar, P.** (ed.), **Nemoto, E., Langfitt, T., Hoff, J., Breivik, H., Grenvik, A., Albin, M., Brennan, R. et al.** (1978). Symposium on brain resuscitation. *Crit. Care Med.* (Symposium Issue), in press.
69. **Secher, O.**, and **Wilhjelm, B.** (1968). The protective action of anesthetics against hypoxia. *Canad. Anaesth. Soc. J. 15:*423–440.
70. **Severinghaus, J. W.** (1966). Blood gas calculator. *J. Appl. Physiol. 21:* 1108.
71. **Shalit, M. N., Doller, A. J., Feinsod, M., Drapkin, A. J.**, and **Cotev, S.** (1970). The blood flow and oxygen consumption of the dying brain. *Neurology 20:*740.
72. **Shapiro, H. M.** (1975). Intracranial hypertension: Therapeutic and anesthetic considerations. *Anesthesiology 43:*443.
73. **Smith, A. L., Hoff, J. T., Nielsen, S. L.**, and **Larson, C. P.** (1974). Barbiturate protection in acute focal cerebral ischemia. *Stroke 5:*1.
74. **Snyder, J. V., Nemoto, E. M., Carroll, R. G.**, and **Safar, P.** (1975). Global ischemia in dogs: Intracranial pressures, brain blood flow and metabolism. *Stroke 6:*21.
75. **Stept, W.**, and **Safar, P.** (1970). Rapid induction–intubation for prevention of gastric content aspiration. *Anesth. Analg. 49:*633–636.
76. **Sveinsdottir, E.**, and **Lassen, N. A.** (1975). A 254-detector system for measuring regional cerebral blood flow. In: Langfitt, T. W., McHenry, Reivich & Wollman (eds.), *Cerebral Circulation & Metabolism.* New York: Springer-Verlag.
77. **Tourtellotte, W. W., Reinglass, J. L.**, and **Newkirk, T. A.** (1972). Cerebral dehydration action of glycerol. I. Historical aspects with emphasis on the toxicity and intravenous administration. *Clin. Pharm. Ther. 13:*159.
78. **Vranova, Z., Keszler, H.**, and **Vrana, M.** (1968). Oxygen tension in the cerebral cortex of dogs in haemorrhagic shock and its changes after oxygen therapy. *Acta Anaesth. Scand. 12:*171.
79. **Vries, J. K., Becker, D. P.**, and **Young, H. F.** (1973). A subarachnoid screw for monitoring intracranial pressure. *J. Neurosurg. 39:*416.

80. **Wechsler, R. L., Dripps, R. D.,** and **Kety, S. S.** (1953). Blood flow and oxygen consumption of the human brain during anesthesia produced by thiopental. *Anesthesiology 12:*308–320.

81. **Weiss, M. H.** (1974). Head trauma and spinal cord injuries: Diagnostic and therapeutic criteria. *Crit. Care Med. 2:*311.

82. **White, J.,** and **Albin, M. S.** (1970). Spine and spinal cord injury. In: Gurdjian, Lange, Patrick, and Thomas (eds.), *Impact Injury and Crash Protection.* Springfield, Illinois: C. C. Thomas.

83. **Yatsu, F. M., Diamond, I., Graziano, C.,** and **Lindquist, P.** (1972). Experimental brain ischemia: Protection from irreversible damage with a rapid-acting barbiturate (Methohexital). *Stroke 3:*726.

Neurologic Monitoring

JOHN MCRAE, M.D.
Assistant Clinical Professor of Surgery (Neurological),
University of Southern California School of Medicine,
Los Angeles, California

Monitoring of the critically ill patient suffering a neurological event can be equated to the support of a patient in coma. The available monitors comprise a formidable display of available techniques to assure optimum physiology of the cardio-pulmonary, renal, and metabolic processes. Additional techniques to specifically monitor the response of the central nervous system to disorder are the subject of this chapter.

In a specialized intensive care unit for neurologic disorders, protocols can be established for the routine monitoring of patients with subarachnoid hemorrhage, stroke syndrome, head or spinal trauma, or following cranial surgery. It is probable that in the general intensive care unit, the frequency of encountering specific neurological disorders is such that a protocol approach is impractical, being either too general for excellent care of the neurologic patient or too specific and infrequently used to be practical from a human engineering viewpoint. In practice, monitoring of the neurologic patient in the general intensive care unit means a specialized, or custom protocol, individualized for each patient.

Neurological monitoring begins with the clinical examination, which remains the sine qua non of the monitoring system. In clinical neurology, history taking provides the nature of the pathology; the neurological examination provides information as to the site and severity of central nervous system involvement. Laboratory testing is specifically ordered to confirm clinical diagnosis, to evaluate secondary diagnostic possibilities, as well as to establish baseline values as the starting point for monitoring trends.

The timing of the initial neurological examination is determined by the neuroclinician following telephone contact with the physicians and nurses who receive the patient in the intensive care unit. If the neuroclinician were a computer, the software programing for the initial neurological examination might problem solve the following queries: (a) what has happened [pathology: (i) inflammatory (infectious vs. autoimmune), (ii) toxic (exogenous vs. endogenous), (iii) traumatic (blunt vs. penetrating), (iv) neoplastic (primary vs. metastasic), and (v) infarction (hypoxic, ischemic, hypoglycemic)]; (b) which organ has failed (primary vs. secondary CNS); (c) should this be treated (severity and prognosis); and (d) what will go wrong next (trends to be monitored)? Without such a beginning, monitoring of a critically ill patient is like planning a journey without knowing the location of the departure point, the destination, or the time of travel. The reader not convinced that all this can be accomplished at bedside by examination is referred to the classic monograph of Plum and Posner [8].

Once clinical orientation to the patient's pathology is achieved, specific monitors can be designed to measure trends of the patient's response to disease and to measure the effect of treatment. The first monitor is direct measurement of the intracranial pressure. The second parameter, that of cerebral metabolism, can be measured only indirectly.

MONITORING INTRACRANIAL PRESSURE

The Munro-Kellie doctrine [3] states that the neurocranium is a closed box containing noncompressible liquids and gels consisting of brain tissue, blood and blood vessels, and spinal fluid. The capacity of the closed box is finite, and the volume of its contents exerts a pressure. As brain bulk increases in volume, as in brain swelling, intracranial pressure rises, and a compensatory reduction in spinal fluid volume occurs. When brain volume is increased by a mass lesion such as a hematoma or tumor, the focal increase of brain bulk causes internal herniations within the cranial cavity, the cerebral hemisphere herniating beneath the falx cerebri, and then through the tentorial notch. Ultimately the brain stem and cerebellar tonsils become impacted in the foramen magnum. When these herniations of brain are severe, the circulation of spinal fluid from the infratentorial to the supratentorial compartments is blocked so that pressure compensation by further absorbtion of spinal fluid can no longer occur. In this situation, there is a pressure differential between supratentorial and infratentorial compartments, and the lumbar pressure does not reflect intracranial pressure. Ultimately intracranial pressure will rise to the level of blood pressure, and arrest of cerebral blood flow ensues.

Intracranial pressure is measured by inserting a catheter into the lateral ventricle of the brain, or inserting a cannula in continuity with the subarachnoid space, using a device such as the Richmond cranial screw [4]. The device must be aseptically and atraumatically inserted, and a watertight seal must be achieved to ensure valid recording. Infection remains a hazard, and the risk of establishing such an intracranial-pressure monitor must be balanced against the importance of the information derived. The catheter or cannula is connected to a pressure transducer to enable the direct reading of intracranial pressure in millimeters of mercury (torr). With simultaneous recording of the mean systemic arterial pressure, the difference between these two measurements represents the cerebral-perfusion pressure. Generally, it is desired to maintain a cerebral-perfusion pressure of 60 torr, with clinical problems being evident when the cerebral perfusion pressure falls below 40 torr, and ischemic brain damage almost assured when the pressure is below 20 torr.

Return to the Munro-Kellie doctrine and consider the linear relationship between volume and pressure. Since intracranial contents are noncompressible, there are limits of compensation for increase in any one component. A volume–pressure curve can be derived displaying the volume zone in which compensation occurs, and the critical volume zone which exceeds pressure-compensating mechanisms. The patient with an intracranial pressure of 20–40 torr can be periodically challenged by introducing 1 cc of saline via the intraventricular catheter, and the pressure change to this increased volume determined 1 sec later. When the pressure change is <3 torr, it is known that the patient is still within the compensatory zone of the volume–pressure curve. If, however, the pressure response to a 1-cc saline challenge is greater than 3 torr, this patient is in danger of decompensating from increased intracranial pressure, and treatment should be undertaken to reduce intracranial volume into the safe range [6].

Patients with intracranial pressure above 20 torr who fall into the decompensated zone frequently will spontaneously show transient increases in intracranial pressure to >50 torr lasting for 5–30 min. These so called Lundberg "plateau" waves appear to be consequent to increased blood volume within the brain and represent a poorly understood partial failure of cerebral blood flow autoregulation. The clinical significance of the plateau wave is that the patient has used up his compensatory reserve for tolerating an increase in intracranial volume. Often, symptoms of clinical decompensation such as increased headache, altered consciousness, or decerebration accompany plateau waves [3,5].

Clinical determination of decompensation of intracranial pressure mechanisms is made by detecting the various syndromes of internal herniation of the brain. With herniation of a cerebral hemisphere under the falx cerebri, increasing headache, increasing hemiparesis, and frequently conjugate tonic deviation of the eyes toward the swollen hemisphere are seen. With tentorial-notch herniation there are alterations of consciousness in the form of either confused, combative, and irritable behavior, or decreasing alertness and responsiveness, accompanied by sighing, yawning, and eventually Cheyne–Stokes periodicity of respiration. When herniation through the tentorial notch occurs eccentrically, either to the right or to the left, an ipsilateral third-nerve palsy is recognized by dilitation of the pupil, altered light responsivity, and finally failure of inturning of the involved eye together with ptosis. The contralateral cerebral peduncle and posterior cerebral artery can be compromised against the rigid tentorium producing a hemiparesis, and homonymous visual-field defect ipsilateral to the swollen hemisphere. With herniation of the brain stem and cerebellar tonsils through the foramen magnum, deep coma is produced, accompanied by ataxic respirations and finally respiratory arrest, cardiac arrhythmias, and ultimate loss of blood pressure with death. The nursing staff of the intensive care unit should be familiar with these syndromes and recognize the significance of the neurological change observed.

When decompensating from increased intracranial pressure, treatment can either be definitive or temporizing. Definitive treatment is dependent upon recognizing the pathophysiology of the process. All information derived from monitoring systems is assessed:

1. Is venous drainage from the head impaired? Elevate the head of the bed, straighten the patient's neck, clear the airway, and determine CVP.
2. Is ventilation adequate? Check the integrity of the ventilator, endotracheal tube, and ventilatory effort of each hemithorax. Obtain the arterial blood gasses, since hypercapnia of >45 torr or hypoxia <50 torr greatly increases intracranial pressure via cerebral vasodilation.
3. Is cardiac output adequate? The classic Cushing response to increasing intracranial pressure is a rising blood pressure and slowing pulse rate. Cardiac output can fail because of reduced blood volume, arrhythmias consequent to altered sympathetic or parasympathetic cardiotonia, or pump failure. Since severe brain damage can produce pulmonary edema, the CVP is not an adequate index of left-heart function, and PAWP may be required.
4. Is serum hypotonicity present? Check serum osmolality and electrolyte content. Severe hypotonicity, or low colloid pressure, can produce cerebral edema. A serum osmolality of >280 mosmole, a serum sodium of >130 meq, and a serum albumin of >3 g is desired.
5. Is spinal-fluid circulation obstructed, producing acute hydrocephalus? Immediate treatment is spinal-fluid drainage via the ventricular catheter until the need for spinal-fluid shunting can be determined.
6. Is there a mass lesion requiring immediate neurosurgical decompres-

sion or malignant cerebral edema requiring cranial decompression? With the full spectrum of cardiopulmonary monitoring available, modern neuroanesthesia has vastly decreased the risk of even major neurosurgical procedures in the most critically ill patient.

The temporizing measures for lowering increased intracranial pressure provide time for the diagnostic procedures necessary to allow for definitive treatment. The use of high doses of dexamethasone can dramatically decrease cerebral edema, particularly the focal variety of cerebral edema surrounding neoplasms, through a mechanism of stabilizing cell membranes and mitochrondrial physiology. Steroids can act within 24–72 hours, and even though intracranial pressure may not be lowered, the challenge technique will often show that steroids have moved the volume-pressure response into the safe zone [1,6].

Hyperosmotic agents such as mannitol or urea will dramatically lower intracranial pressure within 1 hr by means of extracting water from edematous brain tissue. The beneficial effect will last for 6–8 hr, and repetition produces a lesser response. Immediate lowering of intracranial pressure can be achieved by ventricular fluid drainage. However, as soon as the ventricle is drained, in malignant situations, the intracranial pressure will rise within minutes. Hyperventilation producing hypocapnia to 25 torr will reduce cerebral blood flow and decrease intracranial pressure, the response being immediate.

MONITORING CEREBRAL METABOLISM

The indirect monitoring of cerebral metabolism at present is most unsatisfactory in caring for the critically ill comatose patient. Repeated accurate clinical neurologic examination in demonstrating the intactness of the induced and spontaneous reflexes associated with the central nervous system remains the most useful and practical monitor of cerebral metabolism.

The EEG trace is quite sensitive to alterations in the metabolism of the cerebral cortex, and to a lesser extent of the reticular activating system of the brain stem. With a depressed cerebral cortex the resting alpha rhythm of 9–14 Hz gives way to focal or generalized slowing, first in the theta range (5–7 Hz), and then in the delta range (1–3 Hz), and ultimately to the isoelectric trace of brain death (0 Hz). Continuous EEG monitoring has long been employed as an adjunct to neuroanesthesia and has proven monitoring sensitivity [9]. More recently, the signal-averaging ability of the digital computer has been coupled with the EEG to provide an automatic printout of dominant rhythm [2]. These devices have been slow to gain clinical acceptance, because of expense, the complexity of the technology required, and the tribulations of maintaining scalp electrode integrity in the frequently moved and often sweating patient. Although the information derived from such continuous EEG monitoring is quite sensitive and lends itself to the feedback logic of a completely automated monitoring system, at present the information derived from such techniques is more readily obtained with lesser expense by the careful clinical observation of the patient. A derivitive of the signal-averaging ability of the digital computer is the special technique of extracting an evoked response from the background EEG trace. Although still experimental because of cost and complexity, such evoked responses hold great promise for the future in that the clinician would be able to circuit trace within the CNS, accurately identifying intact and deficit circuits, in a manner not now possible by clinical examinaton.

The measurement of cerebral blood flow also remains largely an experimental technique. At present, this is accomplished by arranging an array of gamma detectors next to the head and introducing a radioactive inert gas, xenon-133, via direct carotid injection, intravenous bolus, or inhalation. Washout curves are constructed and it is possible through computer analysis to differentiate blood flow in the scalp from that within the gray matter, and, within the white matter from that core of brain within the focus of each gamma detector [7]. Since measurement of cerebral blood flow does consume minutes of time, and since cerebral blood flow can vary from moment to moment, many extrapolations are inherent in the technique. A cerebral blood flow of 50 ml/min/100 g brain weight is considered normal, and when the cerebral blood flow falls below 20 ml/min/100 g, ischemic damage to nervous tissue results [9]. The principal value of cerebral blood-flow monitoring is that it has contributed greatly to the understanding of cerebral blood-flow autoregulation in various pathologic states. By autoregulation is meant the peculiar ability of the brain to demand a constant blood flow through a relatively wide range of cardiac outputs, blood pressures, and pulse rates. Cerebral vascular resistance reflexly lessens to increase blood flow when the brain suffers from hypoxia, hypercapnia, or ischemia. Cerebral vascular resistance increases to protect the brain against overload from hypertension, hyperoxia, or hypocapnia. The most important stimulous appears to be P_{CO_2}, there being a marked increase in cerebral blood flow with hypercapnia above 45 torr and marked vasoconstriction with reduced cerebral blood flow in hypocapnic states. When the P_{CO_2} tension falls below 25 torr, sufficient vasoconstriction and shunting occurs within the brain that ischemic damage to nervous tissue can result [11]. When the patient is in the danger zone of the volume–pressure response curve, the additional 100% increase in cerebral blood flow produced by hypercapnia can produce a transient increase of intracranial pressure beyond systolic pressure so that cerebral perfusion fails. Cerebrovascular autoregulation does not remain intact in many pathologic states involving the CNS. When the cerebrovascular autoregulatory reflexes are lost, cerebral blood flow linearly follows cardiac output, and this important reflex protective mechanism against fluctuating cardiac output, hypoxia, or hypercapnia is lost, so that continuous monitoring of cardiopulmonary function may be necessary. It is now recognized that the cerebrovascular autoregulation is not an "all or none" phenomenon, but autoregulation may be partially impaired in various neuropathologic states [4]. The plateau wave of increased intracranial pressure may well represent a transient vasomotor paresis, causing an increase in brain blood volume. Also in brain death, with demonstrated absence of cerebral blood flow, release of intracranial pressure with restoration of blood flow is frequently followed by a state of vasomotor paresis and loss of all cerebral autoregulatory reflexes.

Due to the many deficiencies in monitoring cerebral metabolism, the clinical goal becomes that of supplying in excess the substrates necessary for aerobic cerebral metabolism. Hyperthermia is counterbalanced by cooling measures and the hypermetabolism of convulsions controlled by anticonvulsants. Glucose is administered by continuous intravenous drip, and oxygen is supplied even though the Pa_{O_2} is >100 torr. Hypocapnia below 25 torr is avoided to prevent ischemia and shunting.

When the battle to preserve cerebral metabolism is going poorly, measures can be taken to artificially reduce cerebral metabolism. Most available are hypothermic techniques, particularly useful in children and young adults, whose cardiopulmonary system readily holds up under the stress. The specialized technique of hyperbaric oxygenization works but is not readily available. On the horizon are pharmacological means of reducing cerebral metabolism, such as a continuous barbiturate anesthesia.

FUTURE MONITORING TRENDS

Efforts for neurological monitoring of the critically ill patient are destined to become increasingly popular. The advent of the computed tomogram has vastly expanded the accuracy of neurological diagnosis. Brain bulk, spinal-fluid pool, intracranial brain shifts, hydrocephalus, hematomas, neoplasms, and zones of brain edema are graphically displayed. The ability to differentiate between an infarcted brain, white matter, and gray matter is possible. The noninvasive and benign nature of this technique means that it can be repeated in order to graphically display the trends of brain response to injury or treatment. The information promised from computed tomograms, coupled with the elaborate available techniques for monitoring the cardiopulmonary system applied in neuroanesthesia, gives the neurosurgeon the opportunity to intervene with definitive surgical procedures with relative immunity from the unknowns that prevented immediate surgical intervention in the past. In the next decade, neurosurgeons will be able to operate at an earlier hour in order to hold the loss of nerve tissue in response to injury at an absolute minimum.

Summary

Neurologic monitoring of the critically ill patient involves a custom design individualized for each patient. The clinical neurologic examination of the patient by the neuroclinicians and the physicians and nurses of the intensive care unit continues to be the mainstay of neurologic monitoring. The full array of devices and techniques which have been developed for monitoring cardiopulmonary dynamics, renal function, and metabolism may be necessary for a given patient. Additionally, the simple technique of intracranial pressure monitoring can be added within any intensive care unit environment. The electroencephalogram is available, and electroencephalographic monitoring, either continuous or repeated, can be accomplished, by a willing technician. Techniques for cerebral blood flow measurement, the automated and continuous monitoring of the electroencephalographic frequency spectrum, and the specialized technique of evoking cortical potentials at present remain in the experimental realm. In the near future, the promise of high speed and high resolution computed tomographic techniques will greatly advance the art of neurologic monitoring. The role of intraventional neuropharmacology and neurosurgery is expanded by the more precise understanding of the physiologic response of the brain to injury. Neurologic monitoring occurs when the emergency-room nurse instructs the worried mother as to how to observe her son following a subconcussive head injury, and also occurs in the operating room when the skilled neuroanesthesiologist utilizes all available monitoring techniques in sheparding a high-risk patient through a critical intracranial procedure. Between these two extremes, those involved in the care of the critically ill can employ a variable range of monitoring techniques customized for each patient.

References

1. **Becker, D. P., Young, H. F., Vries, J. K.,** and **Sakalas, R.** (1974). Monitoring in patients with brain tumors. *Clin. Neurosurg. 22:*364–388.
2. **Brodkey, J. S., Claque, B. H., Lorig, R. J., Good, W., Lorek, D.,** and **Nulsen, F .E.** (1974). The role of computers in neurosurgery. *Clin. Neurosurg. 22:*432–443.
3. **Langfitt, T. W.** (1968). Increased intracranial pressure. *Clin. Neurosurg. 16:*436–471.
4. **Langfitt, T. W.** (1974). Clinical methods for monitoring intracranial pressure and measuring cerebral blood flow. *Clin. Neurosurg. 22:*302–320.
5. **Lundberg, N.** (1960). Continuous recording and control of ventricular fluid pressure in neurosurgical practice. *Acta Psychiat. Neurol. Scand. 36:*Suppl. 149.
6. **Miller, J. D.** (1974). Volume and pressure in the craniospinal axis. *Clin. Neurosurg. 22:*76–105.

7. **Obrist, W. D.** (1974). Cerebral blood flow and its regulation. *Clin. Neurosurg. 22:*106–116.
8. **Plum, F.,** and **Posner, J.** (1972). *Diagnosis of Stupor and Coma.* Philadelphia: Davis.
9. **Sundt, T. M., Sharbrough, F. W., Trautmann, C.,** and **Gronert, G. A.** (1974). Monitoring techniques for carotid endarterectomy. *Clin. Neurosurg. 22:*199–213.
10. **Vries, J. K., Becker, D. P.,** and **Young, H. F.** (1973). A subarachnoid screw for monitoring intracranial pressure (technical note). *J. Neurosurg. 39:*416–419.
11. **Wyte, S. R.** (1974). Ventilation of the neurosurgical patient. *Clin. Neurosurg. 22:*444–461.

Opportunistic Infections in Critical Care Units

PAUL F. WEHRLE, M.D.
Hastings Professor of Pediatrics, Director of Pediatrics, the Los Angeles County/University of Southern California Medical Center, Los Angeles, California

The value of intensive care units for newborn infants, medical and pediatric patients, and surgical patients both during the immediate recovery period and following trauma has been amply demonstrated. Due to the critical nature of the illness and the need for frequent and virtually continuous attention by various categories of personnel, there is increased opportunity for transfer of infection between patients and from personnel to patients as well. The type of equipment employed—with frequent use of catheters, inhalation-therapy equipment, and various monitoring devices—also offers increased opportunities for nosocomial infection to develop. To further complicate the situation for the patient, these patients are often those with impaired host defense, due both to the underlying disease and to the antimicrobial or other forms of therapy employed. Due to these multiple problems and factors, relatively small numbers of organisms of comparatively low virulence often produce disastrous opportunistic infections.

Additional factors include the degree of crowding of patients within intensive care units despite the monitoring by staff to prevent temporary overloading, and the frequency with which various emergency procedures, such as tracheostomy, cardiac resuscitation, or intravenous cut-downs, are performed. The urgency accompanying this performance combines to further increase the risk of nosocomial infection. Considerations important in the prevention of these infections include:

1. Attention to the design of these units as they are developed, with attention given to providing ample space to permit emergency care activities for each individual patient. Space should be provided for all necessary equipment such as respirators, monitors, and other technical units. Since the traffic is unduly heavy in these units, strict attention should be paid to minimize environmental contamination. Scheduled daily cleaning routines are necessary. Hospital hygiene, particularly handwashing, often deteriorates under emergency conditions, so ample provision should be made to provide appropriate facilities in the design of these units.
2. The staffing pattern for nurses, respiratory therapists, and laboratory and other technicians should permit flexibility, as it is difficult to predict the specific requirements with accuracy on a daily basis.
3. Special attention should be paid to the utilization of strict aseptic precautions during procedures such as tracheostomy, central venous catheter insertion, and similar invasive techniques.
4. Patients with infections known to present hazards to others should not be admitted to intensive care units. Such patients should receive modified intensive care support in an individual isolation unit elsewhere in the hospital.
5. While visitors are important in maintaining morale for the patients, the total number of visitors and the duration of the visit under supervision should not interfere with the efficient operation of the intensive care unit.
6. If the unit is to function effectively, the medical staff must agree as to occupancy limits of the number of patients for whom adequate care can be provided. The natural instinct of a physician to provide the best care for his patient is understandable, but strict rules must be developed and enforced if the purpose for the intensive care unit is not to be destroyed.

As indicated above, patients admitted to intensive care units, and particularly those most critically ill, often have factors that predispose to infection. Of importance are those factors which:

1. Circumvent external anatomical barriers. These factors include severe burns, the use of catheters, decubiti, and various types of extensive surgical procedures.
2. Impair granulocyte behavior and cellular immunity. Factors associated with such impairment include intensive glucocorticoid therapy, antineoplastic drug utilization, leukemia, and related problems and shock.
3. Impair immunoglobulin defenses. Underlying diseases and conditions

such as cirrhosis, acquired immunoglobulin deficiencies, and splenectomy are examples of problems in this category.

4. Adversely influence normal microbial flora. Antimicrobial drug-induced alterations in microbial flora, inoculation of unusual organisms from environmental reservoirs in contaminated equipment or medications, and failure by the medical, nursing, and technical staff to observe proper aseptic precautions.

The mechanisms responsible for these changes in susceptibility have been outlined elsewhere [4].

The organisms implicated most frequently as opportunists include any of those responsible for nosocomial infections in any other area of the hospital. In addition, those seen less frequently in other hospital areas are often of greater importance in the intensive care unit. Examples of infections seen most frequently among compromised hosts in intensive care units include the following: (a) bacteria (e.g., *Listeria, M. Tbc., Salmonella, Pseudomonas, Serratia,* and *Bacteroides*), (b) *viruses* (e.g., *Cytomegalovirus, Herpesvirus,* and *Varicella–Zoster*), (c) protozoa (e.g., *Toxoplasma*), (d) fungi (e.g., *Aspergillus, Candida, Cryptococcus, Nocardia,* and *Phycomycetes*), and (e) unclassified (e.g., *Pneumocystis carinii*).

There has been a significant relationship between specific factors associated with predisposition of infection and specific microorganisms. This relationship is sufficiently clear to assist the physician in the selection of specific diagnostic procedures and in guiding initial antimicrobial therapy, if available, based upon the clinical features of the illness and the underlying condition. For example, extensive abdominal surgery is often associated with peritonitis due to gram-negative bacilli, *Bacteroides,* and anaerobic *Streptococci* as well as *Staphylococci.* Burns and trauma interfering with skin continuity include *Pseudomonas, Serratia, Proteus, Staphylococci, Candida,* and *Mucor.* Bacteremias following cardiac surgery include *Staphylococci,* gram-negative bacilli, *Candida,* and *Diphtheroids.*

While the frequency of phlebitis associated with the use of intravenous catheters has decreased somewhat during recent years due to the use of occlusive dressings, there is increased attention to surgical technique during their insertion, and antimicrobial ointment at the point of insertion. Infections at this site are due to *Staphylococci, Pseudomonas, Candida,* and *Mimae.* Various gram-negative bacilli and *Enterococci* often follow urinary tract instrumentation.

Infections of the respiratory tract associated with tracheostomy, nebulizer utilization, and respirators includes *Pseudomonas, Klebsiella, Serratia, Staphylococci,* and *Candida. Staphylococci* are important causes of sepsis in patients with agranulocytosis and diabetes mellitus, although various gram-negative bacilli are also important. *Mucor* and *Candida* particularly infect the diabetic patient.

In individuals with various forms of neoplasms, particularly patients receiving immunosuppressive or antimetabolite therapy, virtually any bacterial infection is possible. In addition, various fungi have been reported, and some viruses such as cytomegalovirus and *Herpes Zoster* are seen. *Pneumocystis carinii* is seen almost exclusively in this type of patient.

Since potentially effective antimicrobial therapy is now available for virtually all of the usual infections, both common and rare, accurate diagnosis as promptly as possible is essential to the welfare of the patient. Gram stains of exudate and material removed from trachea, joint spaces, or abscesses often provide some guidance for initial therapy. Appropriate cultures with attention to identification of anaerobic organisms is required for definitive diagnosis and effective continued therapy. During the course of therapy, depending on the clinical response, it may be necessary to make additional efforts to identify specific infectious agents. This latter step is necessary, since in patients with impaired resistance superinfections are frequent and the original organism may be replaced or superseded by another with different requirements for effective treatment.

It should be noted that despite improved methods of recovery of organisms, therapy must be directed at times toward the most probable etiology without specific identification of the particular organism during the course of illness.

Selected Readings

Burke, J. F. (1971). Clinical determinants of host susceptibility to infection in surgical patients. In: *Proceedings of the International Conference on Nosocomial Infections.* Chicago: American Hospital Association, pp. 169–172.

Cluff, L. E. (1971). Medical determinants of nosocomial infections. In: *Proceedings of the International Conference on Nosocomial Infections.* Chicago: American Hospital Association, pp. 164–168.

Fekety, F. R., Jr., and **Murphy, J. F.** (1972). Factors responsible for the development of infections in hospitalized patients. *Surg. Clin. N. Amer. 52:*1385.

Infection Control in the Hospital. 3rd Edition, 840 North Lake Shore Drive, Chicago, Illinois 60611: American Hospital Association.

Klainer, A. S., and **Beisel, W. R.** (1969). Opportunistic infection: a review. *Am. J. Med. Sci. 258:*431.

IV

CARDIOVASCULAR CRISES

The Relationship of Pulmonary Edema to Hydrostatic and Colloid Osmotic Pressures in Man

PROTASIO L. DA LUZ, M.D.
Instituto do Coraçãs
Faculdade de Medicina da Universidade de Sao Paulo,
São Paulo, Brazil

Years ago Starling [8] demonstrated that the fluid movement between the capillaries and surrounding tissues was a function of five variables: (a) capillary permeability, (b) capillary hydrostatic pressure, (c) plasma colloid osmotic, (d) interstitial hydrostatic, and (e) interstitial colloid osmotic pressures. Subsequently, Guyton and Lindsey [3] studied specifically the relationship of intravascular forces, namely, capillary hydrostatic and plasma colloid osmotic pressures, to the development of pulmonary edema in dogs. In these experiments pulmonary edema occurred at left-atrial pressure levels of 24 mm Hg when the albumin concentration in the plasma was normal. After the albumin concentration was reduced to 47% of the control values, pulmonary edema appeared when left-atrial pressure was increased only above 11 mm Hg.

In humans, pulmonary edema has been classically assessed on the basis of pulmonary capillary pressure measurements alone. Increased pulmonary capillary pressure is characteristic of the "hemodynamic" type of pulmonary edema. However, pulmonary edema also occurs in the absence of increases in pulmonary capillary pressure. In such cases, alterations in capillary membrane permeability have been assumed to account for pulmonary edema. Although techniques for measurements of interstitial hydrostatic and colloid osmotic pressure are not yet available for clinical use, a method for clinical measurement of plasma colloid osmotic pressure was recently developed in the University of Southern California Center for the Critically Ill [10]. Since pulmonary capillary pressures can be easily obtained in the critically ill patients by the Swan–Ganz catheter, it was possible to relate pulmonary edema to changes in the plasma colloid osmotic–hydrostatic pressure gradient. Accordingly, studies were performed in 26 patients with acute myocardial infarction, 14 of whom developed pulmonary edema.

PATIENTS AND METHODS

The study included 17 men and nine women aged 40–89 (median 65) years. Pulmonary edema was more frequent in older patients (Table 1). Seven patients presented with clinical signs of shock, including clammy skin, mental confusion, reduction in intraarterial systolic blood pressure to <90 mm Hg, urine output <30 ml/hr, and arterial lactate concentration >1.4 mM/l.

Pulmonary-artery pressure measurements were obtained by means of a Swan-Ganz catheter. Colloid osmotic pressure was measured by an oncometer modified in our laboratory [10]. Cardiac output was measured by the dye-dilution technique. Portable chest x-rays were obtained within 2 hr of the hemodynamic studies and interpreted by two radiologists who had no prior knowledge of clinical status of the patients. Pulmonary circulation was analyzed according to the criteria of Turner, Lau and others [9]

TABLE 1 Clinical Data in Patients with Acute Myocardial Infarction

	PULMONARY EDEMA ABSENT (12 PATIENTS)	PULMONARY EDEMA PRESENT (14 PATIENTS)	STATISTIC *p* VALUE
Age, years	40–68 (median 53)	44–89 (median 75)	<0.001
Sex			
Male	8	9	Not significant
Female	4	5	
Location			
Anterior	4	10	Not significant
Inferior	8	4	
Outcome			
Survived	10	5	Not significant
Died	2	9	

adapted for reading supine chest x rays. In this classification, 0 = normal pulmonary vessels with orderly tapering toward the periphery; 1+ = equal perfusion of upper and lower lung zones; 2+ = minimal interstitial prominence and perivascular edema insufficient to obliterate vascular markings; 3+ = prominent interstitial markings (Kerley's B lines) and diffuse reticular pattern with obliteration of the vascular markings; and 4+ = bilateral confluent shadows of relatively uniform density but ill-defined margins. In 12 patients, chest x-rays were classified in groups 0 and 1+ and designated as uncomplicated myocardial infarction. There were two cases in category 2+ and 12 patients with more advanced stages of pulmonary edema.

Cardiac pulmonary edema with mild increases in pulmonary capillary pressure. The mean arterial pressure and heart rate were within normal range in patients with and without pulmonary edema. Although the cardiac index and stroke-work index were reduced in both groups of patients, no significant difference was observed after the onset of pulmonary edema (Table 2). However, pulmonary artery systolic, mean, diastolic, and wedge pressures were slightly but significantly higher in patients with pulmonary edema. The PAWP averaged only 15.7 ± 1.5 (SEM) mm Hg in patients with pulmonary edema and 11.0 ± 1.2 mm Hg in the absence of pulmonary edema (Table 2). Although the pulmonary capillary pressures were higher among patients with pulmonary edema, it is unlikely that this mild increase alone would explain the presence of pulmonary edema. Since these measurements were obtained during the course of pulmonary edema rather than preceding it, it is possible that higher levels of pulmonary pressures occurred earlier. Most reports [2,5] have shown a good correlation between the level of pulmonary capillary pressure and the presence or absence of pulmonary edema in patients with acute myocardial infarction. Exceptions, however, are not uncommon and an adequate explanation for pulmonary edema associated with low capillary pressure has not been given.

Plasma colloid osmotic pressure and pulmonary edema. In the absence of pulmonary edema, mean colloid osmotic pressure was 20.8 ± 1.0 mm Hg but it was reduced to 16.9 ± 1.1 mm Hg in patients with pulmonary edema. Although this difference is statistically significant ($p < 0.02$), a considerable overlap between the two groups is observed (Fig. 1). Since colloid osmotic pressure was measured after appearance of pulmonary edema, it is possible that reduction in colloid osmotic pressure was the result rather than the cause of pulmonary edema. Circulatory failure was more common among patients with pulmonary edema. Circulatory failure alone may increase alveolar capillary membrane permeability, and this could alter interstitial and hydrostatic and colloid osmotic pressures. Since these variables were not measured in this study, their role remains speculative. Thus, a cause–effect relationship between reductions in plasma colloid osmotic

TABLE 2 Hemodynamic Measurements

	HR (BEATS/ MIN)	AP (MM HG)	CI (L/MIN· M^2)	SWI (g· M/M^2)	PASP	PAP	PADP (MM HG)	PAWP	COP
AMI	90	83	2.1	24	27	17.6	13.2	11.0	20.8
Uncomplicated	±6.5	±4.3	±0.2	±3.1	±2.7	±1.7	±1.5	±1.2	±1.0
AMI	89	73	1.9	18.8	34.9	23.8	17.8	15.7	16.9
Pulmonary edema	±4.7	±4.6	±0.2	±3.5	±1.9	±1.5	±1.4	±1.5	±1.1
p value	ns	ns	ns	ns	<0.05	<0.02	<0.05	<0.05	<0.02

Legend:
AMI—Acute myocardial infarction
AP—Mean arterial pressure
CI—Cardiac index
COP—Colloid osmotic pressure (plasma)
HR—Heart rate
PADP—Diastolic pulmonary artery pressure
PAP—Mean pulmonary artery pressure
PASP—Systolic pulmonary artery pressure
PAWP—Wedge pulmonary artery pressure
SWI—Stroke work index (left ventricular)

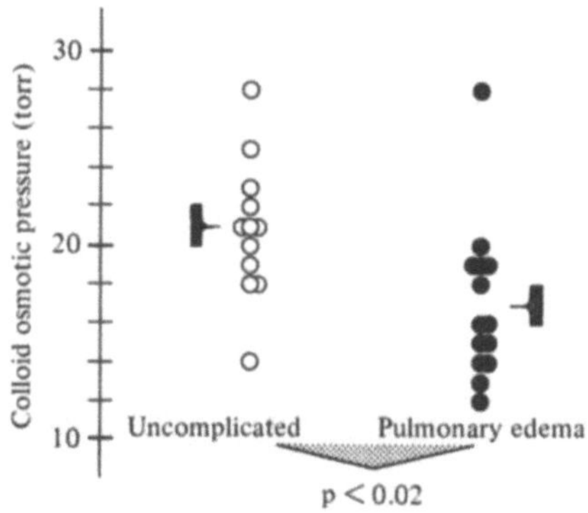

FIGURE 1 Plasma colloid osmotic pressure in patients with and without pulmonary edema (uncomplicated) following acute myocardial infarction; O indicate the mean value. Published by permission of the American Heart Association, from da Luz *et al. Circulation 51*:350, 1975.

pressure and the appearance of pulmonary edema is not demonstrated. Nevertheless, a decrease in plasma colloid osmotic pressure alone would, regardless of cause, facilitate water transudation into the lungs at a relatively low pulmonary capillary pressure.

The plasma colloid osmotic–PAWP gradient. When the gradient between plasma colloid osmotic pressure and PAWP was calculated for estimation of the net balance between the intravascular and extravascular forces governing fluid movement at the capillary level, highly significant differences were demonstrated. In 13 normal supine individuals previously studied in this laboratory, the plasma colloid osmotic pressure averaged 20.6 ± 3.9 (standard deviation) mm Hg. The PAWP range is normally 4–12 mm Hg. Based on these values, a gradient of 9–17 mm Hg normally favors fluid retention within the intravascular compartment. Among the patients without pulmonary edema, the colloid osmotic hydrostatic pressure gradient averaged 9.7 ± 1.7 mm Hg, a low-normal value. In 14 patients with pulmonary edema, however, the gradient was reduced to 1.2 ± 1.3 mm Hg, and it exceeded 3.0 mm Hg in only three cases (Fig. 2). Thus a reduction in the colloid osmotic–hydrostatic pressure gradient correlated better with the presence of radiographic signs of pulmonary edema than either increases in pulmonary capillary pressure or reduction in plasma colloid osmotic pressure alone.

EFFECTS OF THERAPY

Changes in colloid osmotic pressure and PAWP following treatment with Digoxin and furosemide were also assessed. In three patients in whom pulmonary edema was reversed, the plasma colloid osmotic pressure re-

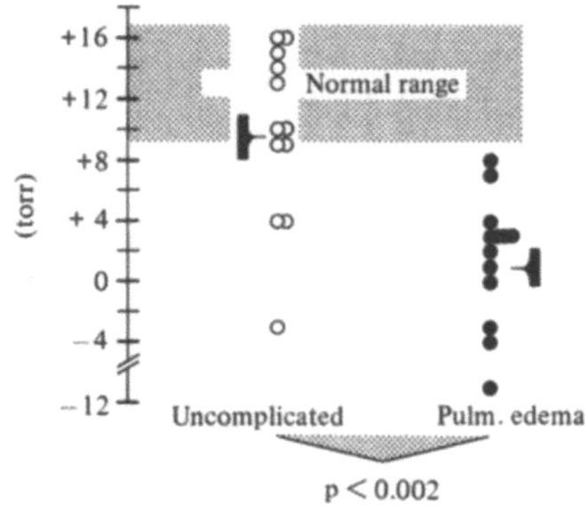

FIGURE 2 The gradient between plasma colloid osmotic pressure and PAWP in 26 patients. Uncomplicated cases are those without pulmonary edema. ■ indicate the mean value. Published by permission of the American Heart Association, from da Luz *et al. Circulation 51*:350, 1975.

mained in the normal range or increased. A concomitant decline in PAWP was also observed (Fig. 3). In six cases in which treatment failed to reverse pulmonary edema, plasma colloid osmotic pressure was either unchanged or further reduced. The effects on PAWP were variable. Changes in the colloid osmotic hydrostatic pressure gradient more consistently reflected the course of pulmonary edema (Fig. 4). In each of the patients in whom

FIGURE 3 Changes in PAWP (left) and plasma colloid osmotic pressure (right) during conventional treatment of pulmonary edema in nine patients. Published by permission of the American Heart Association, from da Luz *et al. Circulation 51*:350, 1975.

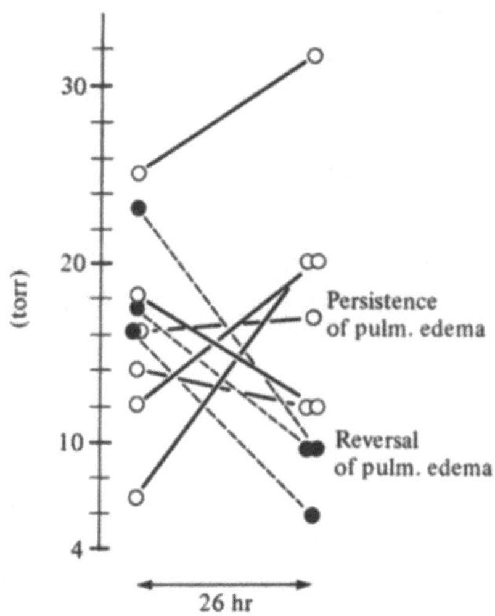

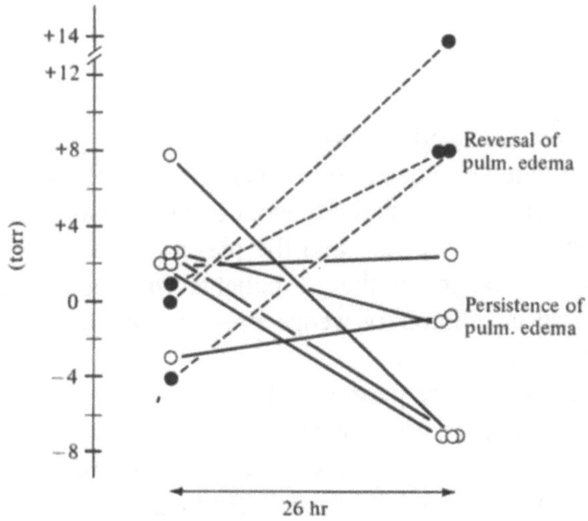

FIGURE 4 Changes in the gradient colloid osmotic–PAWP in relation to treatment in 9 patients. Note consistent directional changes when both reversal or persistence of pulmonary edema occurred with conventional measures including O_2, digitalis, and diuretics administration. Published by permission of the American Heart Association, from da Luz *et al. Circulation 51:*350, 1975.

pulmonary edema was reversed, the gradient increased. In all six patients in whom treatment failed, this gradient remained <4 mm Hg or was further reduced. Thus, it is apparent that the combined effects of changes in pulmonary capillary and plasma colloid osmotic pressures correlate with reversal or persistence of pulmonary edema.

Pathophysiologic and therapeutic implications. The present data should be cautiously interpreted in relation to the mechanism of pulmonary edema. Left ventricular failure and increases in pulmonary capillary pressure are primary and probably the initial factors accounting for pulmonary edema after acute myocardial infarction. The study does indicate though, that after acute myocardial infarction, pulmonary edema occurs in close relationship to simultaneous changes in both plasma colloid osmotic and pulmonary capillary pressures.

The therapeutic implication relates to the control of fluid administration in critically ill patients. Volume loading is an effectve means to reverse circulatory failure in select groups of patients [1]. Pulmonary artery wedge pressure measurements serve as the guide for fluid infusion. Levels of ⩽18 mm Hg have been suggested as safe [6]. On the basis of present data, we regard simultaneous measurements of colloid osmotic pressure and PAWP as a more reliable basis for guiding fluid administration. Optimally, the colloid osmotic PAWP gradient should be calculated throughout fluid administration. As this gradient decreases below 9 mm Hg, the risk of pulmonary edema increases.

Summary

Plasma colloid osmotic and pulmonary artery wedge pressures and their relationship to pulmonary edema were investigated in 26 patients with acute myocardial infarction. In 12 patients without pulmonary edema, both the pulmonary artery wedge pressure and the plasma colloid osmotic pressure were in the normal range; in the 14 patients with pulmonary edema, a moderate increase in pulmonary wedge pressure and reduction in plasma colloid pressure were observed.

The gradient between the plasma colloid osmotic pressure and the pulmonary artery wedge pressure emerged as a sensitive index to separate the patients with and without pulmonary edema. In the absence of pulmonary edema, this gradient averaged 9.7 (±1.7 SEM) mm Hg; it was reduced to 1.2 (±1.3) mm Hg, following appearance of pulmonary edema. During therapy with Digoxin and furosemide, the course of pulmonary edema was closely related to concomitant changes in the colloid osmotic-hydrostatic pressure gradient. These data indicate that both increases in pulmonary capillary pressure and decreases in colloid osmotic pressure may follow the onset of pulmonary edema. The reduction in the colloid osmotic–hydrostatic capillary pressure gradient may favor transudation of fluid into the lungs.

References

1. **da Luz, P. L., Weil, M. H., Liu, V. Y.,** and **Shubin, H.** (1974). Plasma volume prior to and following volume loading during shock complicating acute myocardial infarction. *Circ. 49:*98.
2. **Forrester, J. S., Diamond, G., McHugh, T. J.,** and **Swan, H. J. C.** (1971). Filling pressures in the right and left sides of the heart in acute myocardial infarction. A reappraisal of central venous pressure monitoring. *New Engl. J. Med. 285:*190.
3. **Guyton, A.,** and **Lindsey, A. W.** (1959). Effect of elevated left atrial pressure and decreased plasma protein concentration on the development of pulmonary edema. *Circ. Res. 7:*649.
4. **Hamosh, P.,** and **Cohn, J. M.** (1971). Left ventricular function in acute myocardial infarction. *J. Clin. Invest. 50:*523.
5. **Lassers, B. W., George, M., Anderton, J. L., Higgins, M. R.,** and **Philip, T.** (1970). Left ventricular failure in acute myocardial infarction. *Am. J. Cardiol. 25:*511.
6. **McHugh T. J., Forrester, J. S., Adler, L., Zion, D.,** and **Swan, H. J. C.** (1972). Pulmonary congestion in acute myocardial infarction: Hemodynamic and radiologic correlations. *Ann. Intern. Med. 76:*29.
7. **Nixon, P. G. F.** (1968). Pulmonary edema with low left ventricular diastolic pressure in acute myocardial infarction. *Lancet 2:*146.

8. **Starling, E. H.** (1896). On the absorption of fluids from the connective tissue spaces. *J. Physiol. 19:*312.
9. **Turner, A. F., Lau, F. V., and Jacobson, G.** (1972). A method for the estimation of pulmonary venous and arterial pressure from the routine chest roentgenogram. *Amer. J. Roentgenol. 116:*97.
10. **Weil, M. H., Morissette, M., Michaels, S., Boycks, E., Shubin, H.,** and **Jacobson, E.** (1974). Method for routine measurement of plasma colloid osmotic pressure. *Crit. Care Med. 2:*229.

Indications for and Use of Flow-directed Catheters for Diagnosis and Treatment

WILLIAM GANZ, M.D., C.SC. and H. J. C. SWAN, M.D., PH.D.
Department of Cardiology, Cedars-Sinai Medical Center and the Department of Medicine, University of California at Los Angeles, Los Angeles, California

Balloon-tipped flow-directed catheters allow the measurement of pressures in the right-heart chambers and pulmonary artery at the bedside of critically ill patients [5]. The pulmonary capillary wedge pressure (PCWP) is one of the most useful single parameters from the standpoint of patient management. It is recorded when the inflated balloon impacts into a pulmonary vessel slightly smaller in diameter than the inflated balloon and interrupts the flow to the vessel; pressure is then transmitted backward from the left atrium and pulmonary veins.

A larger version of the balloon-tipped flow-directed catheter [2] also allows the determination of cardiac output and the simultaneous measurement of the right atrial and pulmonary artery or PCWP. The cardiac output is estimated by the thermodilution technique [3], which does not require withdrawal of blood for measurement and calibration and allows about two measurements per minute. In connection with simple bedside computers, the estimates of cardiac output are immediately available and are highly reproducible (±3.5% with 10 ml of cold solution and ±4.7% with a room-temperature solution).

ASSESSMENT OF CARDIAC PERFORMANCE IN CRITICALLY ILL PATIENTS

The initial application of balloon-flotation catheters was in the management of acutely ill patients with acute myocardial infarction. The assessment of circulatory function in the preoperative, intraoperative, and postoperative periods is of particular interest to the practicing surgeon and anesthesiologist. In addition, the application of such techniques in the management of critically ill patients suffering from other disease is self-evident, particularly in cases of pulmonary or renal disease and disturbance of intra- and extravascular volumes.

In the critically ill, performance of the left ventricle must be closely observed. While the level of CVP is occasionally valuable in the assessment of the blood volume, imbalances between the complex and the interrelated functions of right and left ventricles in disease require a knowledge of left-ventricular filling pressure reflected with reasonable accuracy by the PCWP. The mean PCWP is a direct determinant of the degree of pulmonary congestion and of fluid transfer at the pulmonary capillary level and relates closely with x-ray changes in the lungs [4]. In patients with myocardial infarction, the PCWP relates closely to left-atrial pressure and, in the absence of mitral valve disease, to left ventricular diastolic pressure and can therefore be used for the assessment of left ventricular performance on the basis of the Frank-Starling mechanism.

A knowledge of cardiac output as a basic component of cardiovascular function has always been accepted as important by the cardiovascular physiologist. With an ability now to measure this variable without particular difficulty or increased hazard to the patient, the significance of such measurements in clinical practice is becoming recognized more widely. Several definable states of cardiovascular function can now be identified in pathophysiological terms and specific therapies can be indicated on hemodynamic basis.

Normal cardiac output. A normal output associated with a normal left-ventricular filling pressure does not require specific cardiovascular therapy and indicates that abnormal symptoms or signs suggestive of cardiovascular dysfunction may have another basis. The observation of normal hemodynamic data in the early portion of an illness is valuable as changes may occur with the passage of time. Left ventricular filling pressure of 8–12 mm Hg, right-ventricular filling pressures of 0–5 mm Hg, and cardiac index of $\geqslant 2.5$ $l/min/m^2$ characterize a normal cardiovascular state in a patient confined to bed in a hospital.

Pulmonary congestion with adequate cardiac output. Many patients with acute myocardial infarction of small or moderate size have pulmonary congestion and dyspnea, yet the cardiac output is found to exceed

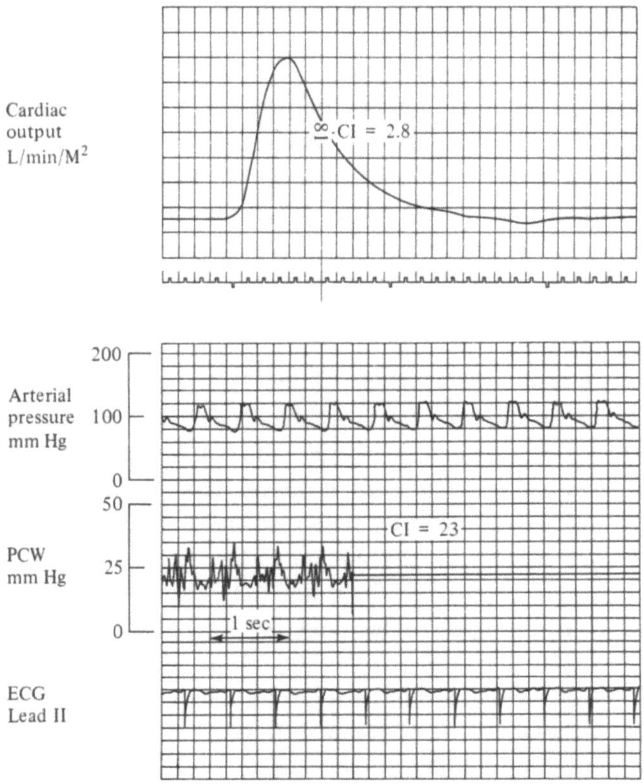

FIGURE 1 Tracing from a patient with acute myocardial infarction. The cardiac output and systemic arterial pressure are within normal limits; the pulmonary capillary wedge pressure indicates pulmonary congestion.

2.5 $l/min/m^2$. However, PCWP may be elevated—exceeding 18 mm Hg and perhaps as high as 25 mm Hg. In this instance, cardiac performance is usually adequate and therapy should not be directed to its alteration (Fig. 1).

Reduced cardiac index. In the presence of more severe degrees of heart failure, particularly in association with extensive acute myocardial infarction or cardiomyopathy, the cardiac index may be depressed to levels below 2.2 $l/min/m^2$ (Fig. 2). Pressure levels above 18 mm Hg are associated with increasing degrees of pulmonary congestion, dyspnea, and pulmonary edema, resulting in increases of both cardiac and respiratory work. In these instances, the effects of impedance reduction [1] to facilitate left ventricular emptying have proven to be of immense significance in management of severe power failure of the heart. If the reduction in cardiac index is due to

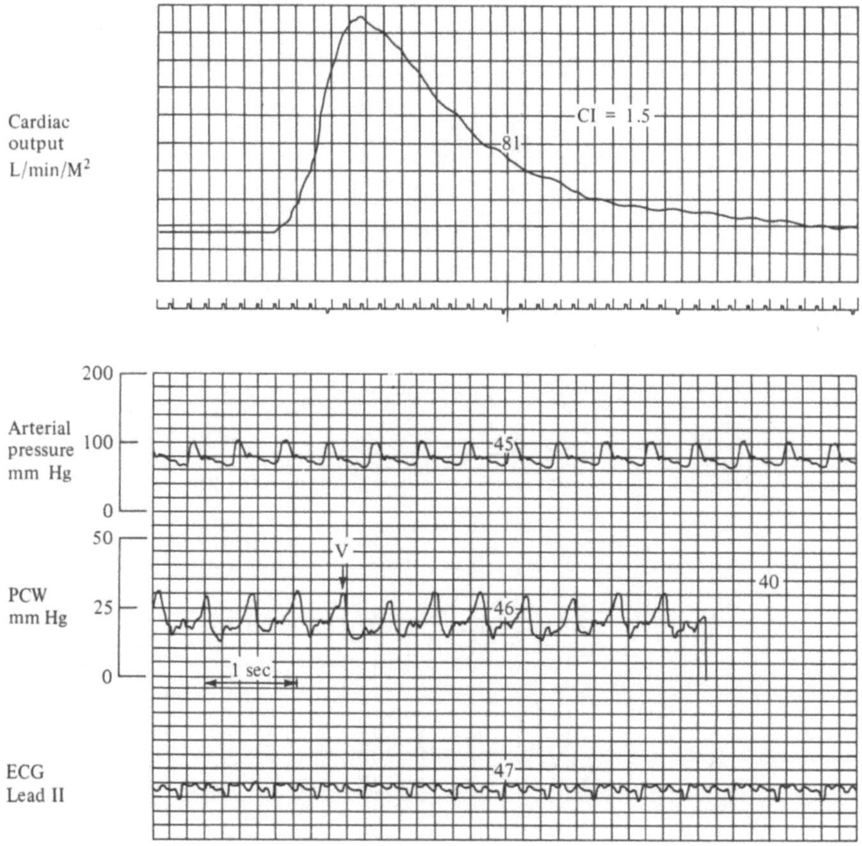

FIGURE 2 Tracing from a patient with acute myocardial infarction and clinical signs of shock. The cardiac output is low. The pulmonary capillary wedge pressure is high, indicating that myocardial depression is the main cause of the low cardiac output and shock.

hypovolemia, a filling pressure of 6 mm Hg or less may be seen (Fig. 3). If the filling pressure is severely depressed (0–4 mm Hg), such patients will respond promptly to fluid loading by increases in cardiac index and arterial blood pressure. If the filling pressure is 9–12 mm Hg, it is our practice to elevate filling pressures to approximately 18 mm Hg. Beneficial effects on cardiac index are not seen in patients in whom left ventricular filling pressures are already elevated above these levels.

Changes in cardiac performance associated with slow heart rate. These may be accurately measured by use of the multipurpose catheter incorporating atrial and ventricular pacing electrodes, and, if necessary, optimal heart rate may be established by selective pacing (Fig. 4).

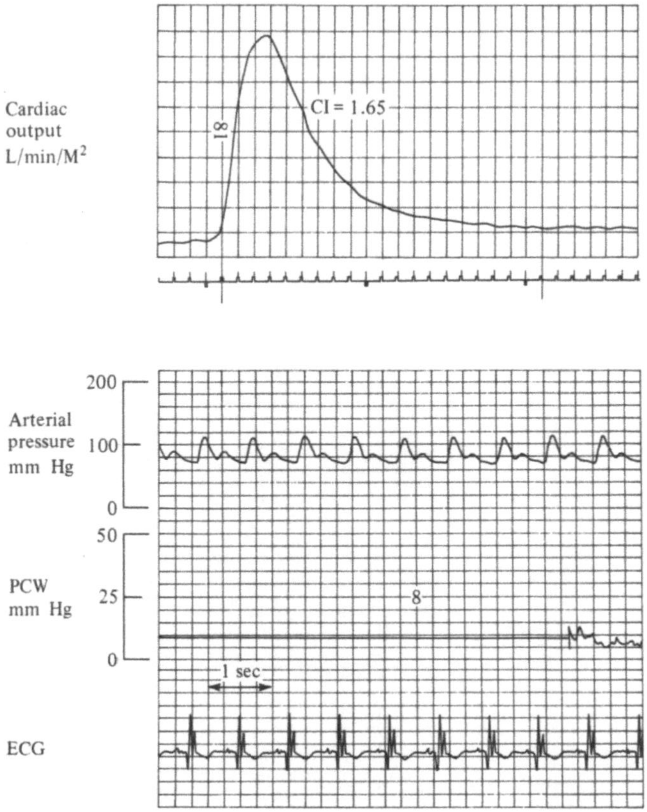

FIGURE 3 Tracing from a patient with acute myocardial infarction and clinical signs of shock. The cardiac index is low. The mean pulmonary capillary wedge pressure is not elevated, implicating hypovolemia as the main cause of the low cardiac output.

DIFFERENTIAL DIAGNOSIS OF CIRCULATORY SYNDROMES

Balloon-flotation catheterization has been used to establish a precise diagnosis in more complex situations in the acutely ill. These include identification of mitral regurgitation as evidenced by a tall peaked V wave in the wedge postion (Fig. 5), ventricular septal defect due to ruptured ventricular septum (Fig. 6), significant pulmonary hypertension, and an increase in the oxygen saturation of the blood in the pulmonary artery over and above that of blood in the right atrium or in the cavae. Chronic pulmonary disease is associated with a differential between diastolic pulmonary artery pressure and a mean or average PCWP in excess of 10 mm Hg. Cardiac tamponade [6] may be suspected by equivalency of pressures in the right atrium and in

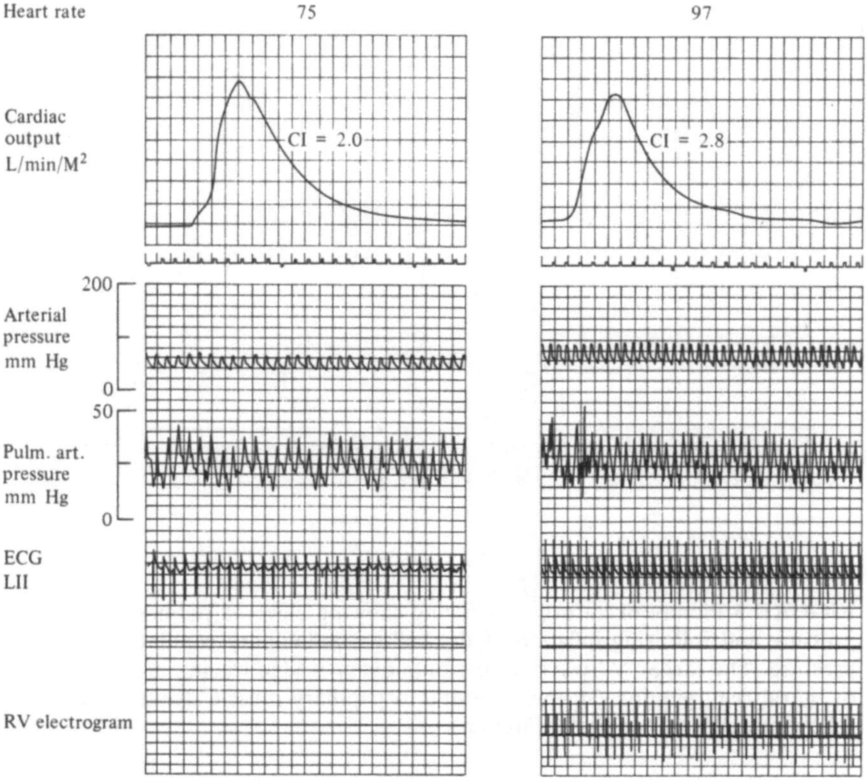

FIGURE 4 Patient hospitalized with an acute myocardial infarction and severe hypotension (systolic pressure in radial artery ~60 mm Hg). A multipurpose flow-directed catheter inserted into the pulmonary artery showed a low cardiac index (2.0 l/min/m²) at a relatively low heart rate of 75 beats/min (left-hand panel). It was therefore decided to gradually raise the heart rate by atrial pacing, using the multipurpose catheter. The right-hand panel illustrates the dramatic effect of elevated heart rate (≤97/min) on cardiac index (2–2.8 l/min/m²) and arterial pressure (systolic value 60–95 mm Hg).

the pulmonary capillary wedge position. In cardiac tamponade, the difference between these pressures is small in contrast to a minimal difference of 7 mm Hg in normal subjects.

The diagnosis of cardiac arrhythmias. The multipurpose catheter incorporating sensing electrodes in the ventricle and atrium allows for a differentiation of a number of complex cardiac arrhythmias (Fig. 7). The clear identification of ventricular activation, atrial activation, and their interrelationship allows for the recognition of a large number of important and specific arrhythmias. The quality of these signals is such as to facilitate

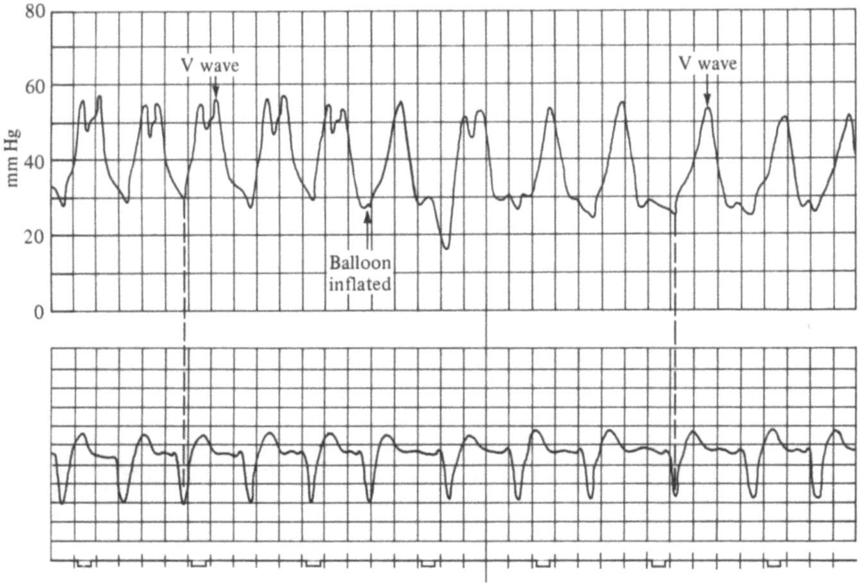

FIGURE 5 Picture of an original tracing showing elevated pulmonary artery pressure and following inflation of the balloon pulmonary capillary wedge pressure. The large "V" waves in the pulmonary wedge tracing are indicative of mitral regurgitation (in this case due to papillary muscle dysfunction following acute myocardial infarction).

FIGURE 6 Pulmonary artery hypertension and higher hemoglobin O_2 saturation in the pulmonary artery (PA—93%) than in the right atrium (RA—71%) in a patient with ruptured interventricular septum following acute myocardial infarction.

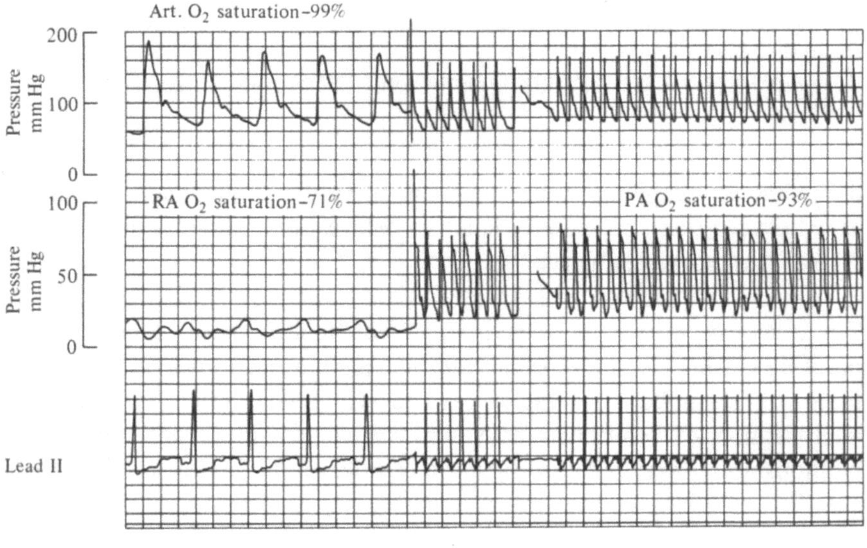

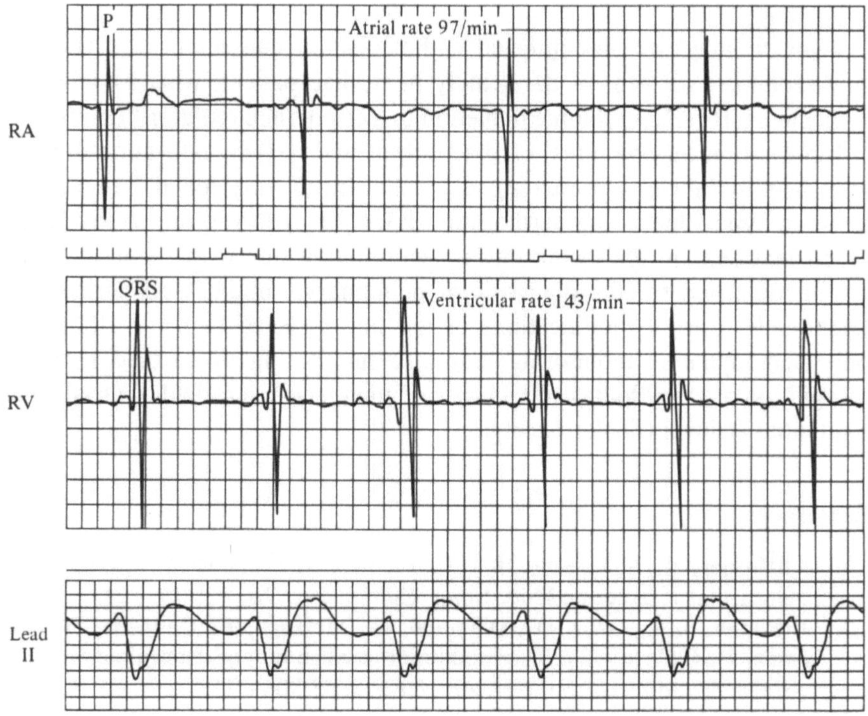

FIGURE 7 Diagnosis of ventricular tachycardia by means of a flow-directed multipurpose catheter. The surface electrocardiogram (Lead II) shows wide QRS complexes appearing at a rate of 143/min with no clearly identifiable atrial complexes. In the right atrial (RA) intracavity ECG atrial complexes appear at a regular rate of 97/min, lower than the rate of ventricular complexes in the right ventricular (RV) intracavity ECG, indicating atrioventricular dissociation.

automatic data processing applied to the recognition of dysrhythmias, their categorization, and the frequency of their occurrence.

In addition, the effectiveness of conventional antiarrhythmic agents may be assessed with great objectivity and hard data end-points by use of such signals that may be categorized and tabulated by automated detecting equipment.

Summary

Flow-directed balloon tipped catheters allow the catheterization of the pulmonary artery without fluoroscopic control, with relative safety and without the special skill required by the use of semirigid catheters. In addition, to right heart and pulmonary artery pressures, pulmonary capillary wedge pressure can be determined by inflating the balloon and floating it into wedged position. The same catheter will also supply on-line information on cardiac output in connection with a single purpose thermodilution computer.

Data obtained by flow-directed catheterization can serve as a reliable guide for the treatment of the acutely ill cardiac patient, whether afflicted by acute heart failure, volume depletion or peripheral circulatory failure.

Information on pressures, cardiac output and oxygen saturation can be very helpful in cases presenting diagnostic problems, for differentiation between hypovolemic and cardiogenic shock, between rupture of the interventricular septum and acute mitral regurgitation due to papillary muscle dysfunction, and for the diagnosis of pulmonary embolus and pericardial tamponade. Recent modifications of the flow-directed catheter allow not only hemodynamic monitoring, but also monitoring of cardiac rhythm, recognition of arrhythmias and, in case of emergency, ventricular, atrial, and sequential atrioventricular pacing.

References

1. **Chatterjee, K.**, and **Swan, H. J. C.** (1974). Vasodilator therapy in acute myocardial infarction. *Mod. Conc. Cardiovasc. Dis. 43:*119–124.
2. **Forrester, J. S., Ganz, W., Diamond, G., McHugh, T., Chonette, D.** and **Swan, H. J. C.** (1972). Thermodilution cardiac output determination with a single flow-directed catheter. *Am. Heart J. 83:*306–311.
3. **Ganz, W.**, and **Swan, H. J. C.** (1972). Measurement of blood flow by thermodilution. *Am. J. Cardiol. 29:*241–245.
4. **McHugh, T., Forrester, J. S., Adler, L., Zion, D.**, and **Swan, H. J. C.** (1972). Pulmonary vascular congestion in acute myocardial infarction: Hemodynamic and radiologic correlations. *Ann. Int. Med. 76:*29–33.
5. **Swan, H. J. C., Ganz, W., Forrester, J. S., Marcus, H., Diamond, G.,** and **Chonette, D.** (1970). Catheterization of the heart in man with use of a flow-directed balloon-tipped catheter. *New Engl. J. Med. 283:*447–451.
6. **Weeks, K., Chatterjee, K., Block, S., Matloff, J. M.**, and **Swan, H. J. C.** (in press). Bedside hemodynamic monitoring—its value in the diagnosis of tamponade complicating cardiac surgery. *New Engl. J. Med.*

Indications for the Treatment of Myocardial Infarction with Corticosteroids

JOHN K. VYDEN, M.D.
Medical Director, Vascular Diagnostic Laboratory,
Cedars-Sinai Medical Center, Associate Professor of Medicine,
University of California at Los Angeles School of Medicine,
Los Angeles, California

TERUO TAKANO, M.D.
Research Fellow, Department of Cardiology,
Cedars-Sinai Medical Center, Los Angeles, California

For over 20 years, only sporadic attention has been given to the use of corticosteroids in the treatment of acute myocardial infarction and its various complications. There is now considerable interest as to whether this agent or any other type of therapeutic intervention can limit the size of an acute myocardial infarction. Laboratory experimentation indicates that this may apply, to humans as well as animals, and if so, it would be reasonable to assume that the use of corticosteroids will become far more widespread.

HISTORICAL PERSPECTIVE

In 1952 Chapman and his colleagues [2] found that corticosteroids given to dogs with experimentally induced myocardial infarction did not deleteriously affect the size of the infarction or the rate of quality of myocardial healing.

One year later, Johnson [9] and his colleagues found that corticosteroids appeared to reduce the average size of an infarct. However, part of this work was disputed by Opdyke and his colleagues [15]. Although randomly controlled trials with low-dosage methylprednisolone in acute myocardial infarction showed no beneficial effects [16,19], a further trial was reported by Dall wherein only severe cases of myocardial infarction were selected which showed improved survival [4,18]. Later Dall and his colleagues organized a double-blind trial of hydrocortisone in cases of acute myocardial infarction, the results of which showed no difference in mortality between treated and controlled patients. In retrospect, it seems unfortunate that this study used mortality as its only end point as we now know that heart-attack sufferers are not a homogeneous group and that it may be quite incorrect to expect that all patients would benefit equally from corticosteroid treatment during the acute and convalescent phases of illness. Weil, Dietzman, and Lillehei [5,23] later suggested that the use of large doses of corticosteroids were more efficacious than the small dosages used previously. In various publications these workers suggested dosages as large as 30 mg/kg of methylprednisolone.

POSSIBLE INDICATIONS FOR THE USE OF CORTICOSTEROIDS IN ACUTE MYOCARDIAL INFARCTION

At the present time, it would appear that there are six areas in which corticosteroids may be of some benefit in the management of acute myocardial infarction and/or its complications: (a) treatment of high-degree heart block, (b) as adjunct to surgical management of acute myocardial infarction, (c) treatment of Dressler's syndrome, (d) treatment of septic shock complicating acute myocardial infarction, (e) treatment of cardiogenic shock secondary to acute myocardial infarction, and (f) reduction of myocardial infarct size.

High-degree Heart Block

Prinzmetal and Kennamer [17] showed that cortisone could abolish heart block, which led to its extensive use for this complication of acute myocardial infarction until it was superseded by the advent of the electrical pacemaker. With the use of the modern temporary pacemaker, which can be placed on an emergency basis, corticosteroids are virtually no longer used for this complication.

Adjunctive Therapy in Cardiac Surgery

In the therapy of acute myocardial infarction, there have been operative attempts to improve coronary and systemic hemodynamics, particularly in the presence of such conditions as shock, aneurysm, septal rupture, and mitral-valve dysfunction. It has become standard in some groups undertaking these procedures to use corticosteroids, often in the pump, as adjunctive therapy, particularly if people are chronic smokers or have a history of chronic lung disease and also if long bypass time is anticipated in surgery. The rationale for steroids in this situation is that: (a) they can protect the lung against the development of "shock lung" and (b) it has been demonstrated that steroids appear to improve pulmonary capillary blood flow [24].

Dressler's Syndrome

This postmyocardial syndrome, as emphasized by Dressler, occurs in a small percentage of patients. This condition may be treated with corticosteroids, aspirin, and indomethacin. However, prolonged use of corticosteroids in the management of this complication is probably contraindicated since it may give rise to delayed healing and poor scar formation.

Septic Shock Complicating Acute Myocardial Infarction

When hemodynamic deterioration occurs in a patient with acute myocardial infarction, it is essential that the attending physician rule out causes of shock other than that of true "cardiogenic shock" resulting from badly damaged myocardial tissue. Thus, if an elderly patient with myocardial infarction needs bladder catheterization and develops the shock syndrome on the second or third day of illness, it is quite possible that this may be due to a gram-negative bacteremia rather than to myocardial infarction per se. Since urinary-tract instrumentation in the elderly is associated with a high incidence of bacteremia, precipitation of bacteremic shock in acute myocardial infarction is probably more common than is recognized. While the indication for large doses of corticosteroids is somewhat controversial, if this agent given early in combination with specific antimicrobial therapy, it is likely to be of benefit in overcoming bacteremic shock [20].

Another form of shock complicating acute myocardial infarction more commonly than bacteremic shock is hypovolemic shock. Corticosteroids are contraindicated in this situation because their peripheral vasodilatory action could worsen the shock state.

True Cardiogenic Shock Secondary to Acute Myocardial Infarction

Corticosteriods have been used with varying degrees of enthusiasm and sporadically by clinicians treating the development of true cardiogenic shock and power failure in acute myocardial infarction. It is recognized that if the stroke-work index is <20 g-m/beat/m^2 associated with a left-ventricular filling pressure of >15 mm Hg, the mortality rate exceeds 95%. Recently 100 shock patients were examined in relation to clinical profile and hemodynamic studies undertaken. This study showed that patients with profoundly depressed hemodynamics are not a homogenous entity but constitute three different clinical subsets [6,21].

Subset 1 resembles experimental coronary artery occlusion and patients present with rapidly developing shock with minimal enlargement of the heart. Necropsy reveals slightly increased heart size and a recent complete occlusion or subtotal obstruction of diffuse disease in the left coronary artery in all patients. Since such lesions result in massive blockage of the main blood flow to the left ventricle and, hence, cause massive infarction, corticosteroid therapy is unlikely to reverse the underlying anatomic mechanism of the lesion.

Subset 2, gross hemodynamic depression, usually follows rupture of the ventricular septum or infarction of the mitral-valve apparatus. Corticosteroids again appear unlikely to be of benefit since they cannot repair the anatomic defect.

Subset 3 is characterized by severe hemodynamic depression superimposed on end-stage heart disease. Nearly all patients have a previous history of myocardial infarction, while 60% are in heart failure before admission. At necropsy replacement of heart muscle by fibrous scar resulting from previous infarcts is encountered. Again, while corticosteroids may benefit a borderline patient, they cannot be expected to overcome the basic anatomic defect.

Unfortunately, the treatment of pump failure and terminal shock after acute myocardial infarction may not expose the possible usefulness of these agents. However, in patients with less severe myocardial infarction, corticosteroids may be of value if they reduce infarct size.

Reduction of Infarct Size

In 1965 Ebdid and his colleagues [7] found that corticosteriods given intravenously in large doses caused regression of the ST segment elevation in both experimental myocardial infarction in dogs and (human) myocardial infarction patients. More recently, Libby and his colleagues [11] studied the effects of large doses of intravenously administered hydrocortisone on the size of experimental infarction. On the basis of ECG, enzymatic, and histological criteria, they found that corticosteriods prevented myocardial cells from undergoing extreme necrosis and that the magnitude of myocardial ischemic injury was markedly reduced. They also found that pharmacological doses of corticosteroids helped prevent subsequent necrosis when given even as late as 6 hr after the experimental coronary arterial occlusion. Vyden and his colleagues [22] have shown that the use of corticosteroids in acute myocardial infarction can produce marked increases in cardiac, stroke, and stroke-work indexes and coronary arterial blood flow with a narrowing of the arterio-venous oxygen difference. In addition, cardiac efficiency, defined as stroke-work index divided by myocardial oxygen consumption, was markedly improved after treatment with corticosteroids. This work has been confirmed by Masters and his colleagues [14], who showed that large doses of corticosteroids improved collateral blood flow into the infarcted area with a significant improvement in metabolism. There may also be a direct beneficial metabolic effect on carbohydrate metabolism by the steroid. Maley and his colleagues [12] recently published data to suggest that the use of methylprednisolone succinate in human acute myocardial infarction tends to limit the size of infarct as measured by a CPK isoenzyme technique.

In addition to corticosteroids, nitrites, glucose-insulin-potassium, hyaluronidase, beta blocking agents, and certain forms of circulatory assistance have experimentally proven to be of value in reducing the size of the infarct after acute myocardial infarction [1,13].

OTHER PROPERTIES

Methylprednisolone possess other properties of value in treating acute myocardinal infarction. It is known that release of the myocardial depressant factor from the ischemic pancreas caused by splanchnic hypoperfusion in acute myocardial infarction is reduced after administration of corticosteroids [3]. Corticosteroids may also attentuate the changes in ventricular compliance that occur after acute myocardial infarction [8] and prevent the disruption of cellular lysosomes and subsequent release of destructive proteases into the bloodstream [10].

Summary

Experimental and clinical evidence on the effects of corticosteroids on the course of acute myocardial infarction are described. Corticosteroids in pharmacological doses may reduce infarct size. Yet, the exact role of corticosteroids for treatment of myocardial infarction remains to be determined.

References

1. **Braunwald, E., Maroko, P. R.,** and **Libby, P.** (1974). Reduction of infarct size following coronary occlusion. *Circ. Res. 34/35:*III–192.
2. **Chapman, D. W., Skaggs, R. H., Thomas, J. R., and Greene, J. A.** (1952). The effect of cortisone in experimental myocardial infarction. *Am. J. Med. Sci. 223:*41.
3. **Crampton, R. S., Wangensteen, S. L.,** and **Lovett, W. L.** (1972). Production of myocardial depressant in shock following acute myocardial depressant in shock following acute myocardial infarction: Preliminary evaluation of treatment with methylprednisolone. *Am. J. Cardiol. 29:*257.
4. **Dall, J. L. C.,** and **Peel, A. A. F.** (1963). A trial of hydrocortisone in acute myocardial infarction. *Lancet 2:*1098.

5. **Dietzman, R. H.,** and **Lillehei, R. C.** (1968). The treatment of cardiogenic shock. V. The use of corticosteroids in the treatment of cardiogenic shock. *Am. Heart J. 75:*274.
6. **DonMichael, T. A., Forrester, J. S., Allen, H. N.,** and **Swan, H. J. C.** (1972). Identification of clinical subset in cardiogenic shock. *Am. J. Cardiol. 29:*280.
7. **Ebdid, M., Caramell, Z., Netos, S. M., Dossantos, M. I. R., Tranchesi, J., Barbato, E., Pilleggi, F.,** and **Decourt, L. V.** (1965). The effects of large intravenous dose of hydrocortisone or hyaluronidase on the electrocardiographic pattern of acute myocardial infarction. *Arch. Inst. Cardiol. Mex. 35:*3.
8. **Jewitt, D. E., Skelton, C. L.,** and **Sonnenblick, E. H.** (1972). Salutary effect of methylprednisolone (MP) on the viability of heart muscle exposed to anoxia (abstr.). *Circulation 45/46:*II–121.
9. **Johnson, A. S., Scheinberger, S. R., Gerish, R. A.,** and **Saltzstein, H. C.** (1953). The effect of cortisone on the size of experimentally produced myocardial infarcts. *Circulation 7:*224.
10. **Lefer, A. M.,** and **Martin, J.** (1969). Mechanism of the protective effect of corticosteroids in hemorrhagic shock. *Am. J. Physiol. 216:*314.
11. **Libby, P., Maroko, P. R.,** and **Bloor, C. M.** (1973). Reduction of experimental myocardial infarct size by corticosteroid administration. *J. Clin. Invest. 52:*599.
12. **Maley, T., Gulotta, S.,** and **Morrison, T.** (1974). Effect of methylprednisolone on predicted myocardial infarct size in man. *Clin. Res. 22:*288A.
13. **Maroko, P. R., Kjekshus, J. K., Sobel, B. E., Watanabe, T., Covell, J. W.,** and **Ross, J., Jr.** (1971). Factors in influencing infarct size following experimental coronary artery occlusions. *Circulation 43:*67.
14. **Masters, T. M., Harbold, N. B.,** and **Hall, D. G.** (1974). Beneficial effects of methylprednisolone sodium succinate (MPSS) with acute myocardial infarction. *Circulation 50:*III–119.
15. **Opdyke, D. A., Lambert, A., Stoerk, H. C., Zanetti, M. E.,** and **Kuna, S.** (1953). Failure to reduce the size of experimentally produced myocardial infarcts by cortisone treatment. *Circulation 8:*544.
16. **Peel, A. A. F.** (1962). Steroid therapy in acute myocardial infarct. Proceedings of World Congress of Cardiology, Mexico City.
17. **Prinzmetal, M.,** and **Kennamer, R.** (1954). Emergency treatment of cardiac arrhythmias. *J. Am. Med. Assoc. 154:*13.
18. **Semphe, T.,** and **Dall, J. L. C.** (1965). Steroids in myocardial infarction. *Am. Heart J. 70:*716.
19. **Sieves, J., Johansen, T.,** and **Prednine, L. N.** (1962). Treatment of myocardial infarction. Proceeding of World Congress of Cardiolcgy, Mexico City.
20. *Steroids and Shock.* Baltimore: Thomas M. Glenn, University Park Press, 1974.
21. **Swan, H. J. C.** (1972). Power failure of the heart in acute myocardial infarction. In: Likoff, W., Segal, B. L., Insull, W., and Moyer, J. H. (eds.), *Atherosclerosis and Coronary Heart Disease,* New York: Grune and Stratton, pp. 453–467.
22. **Vyden, J. K., Nagasawa, K., Rabinowitz, B., Parmley, W. W., Tomoda, H.,**

Corday, E., and **Swan, H. J. C.** (1974). Effects of methylprednisolone administration in acute myocardial infarction. *Am. J. Cardiol. 34:*677.

23. **Weil, M. H.**, and **Whigham, H.** (1965). Corticosteroids for reversal of hemorrhagic shock in rats. *Am. J. Physiol. 209:*815.
24. **Wilson, J. W.** (1972). Treatment or prevention of pulmonary cellular damage with pharmacologic doses of corticosteroids. *Surg. Gynec. Obstet. 134:*675.

Avoiding Emergencies in the Pregnant Patient with Heart Disease

PHIL R. MANNING, M.D.
Professor of Medicine and Associate Dean,
Post Graduate Division
University of Southern California School of Medicine
Los Angeles, California

CHANGES IN NORMAL PREGNANCY THAT MAY SIMULATE HEART DISEASE

Physiologic changes that occur in normal pregnancy may cause signs and symptoms that will simulate heart disease even though no heart disease is present. To begin with, the normal pregnant patient tends to hyperventilate. This happens relatively early in pregnancy, and is believed to be related to elevated progesterone levels [4]. Most patients do not react to the hyperventilation, but some will be concerned and bothered. There are several ausculatory findings in the normal pregnant state that could lead a physician to suspect heart disease when, in fact, no heart disease is present.

First, functional murmurs, frequently present in young women, are more common and usually louder in the pregnant state. These are usually systolic ejection murmurs heard over the second interspace to the left of the sternum, but occasionally may be heard in the aortic and mitral areas as well. A third heart sound is more apt to be heard during pregnancy than in the nonpregnant state. Hurst has described two extra-cardiac murmurs that occasionally occur and may confuse the clinician [3]. The first is a systolic murmur due to increased blood flow in the internal mammary artery. A continuous murmur, which may suggest a patent ductus arteriosus, is occasionally heard due to the increased flow of blood in the veins of the breast.

Palpation of the chest may disclose misleading signs. A systolic pulsation at the lower left sternal border over the area of the outflow tract of the right ventricle is often palpated in the pregnant state. This may be confused with the pathologic lift at the lower left sternal border that is associated with right-ventricular hypertrophy. Usually, the systolic pulsation felt in pregnancy will be of shorter duration and of less magnitude than that associated with right-ventricular hypertrophy.

Pulmonary-closure taps are common in the pregnant state and should not immediately suggest pulmonary hypertension. Pulmonary blood flow is increased in pregnancy, but pulmonary blood pressure remains normal. Pretibial edema is, of course, very common in pregnancy and, most frequently, totally unrelated to heart failure.

There is some controversy in the literature concerning changes of the heart shadow and vascular markings. Recently, Turner has reviewed films on pregnant patients, and has concluded that the same criteria for cardiac size and degree of pulmonary vascularity may be used in both nonpregnant and pregnant states [7]. He did not consider there to be significant increase in either cardiac size or pulmonary vascular markings during pregnancy.

Circulatory Changes During Pregnancy

In the normal pregnant state, the heart rate increases about 10–15 beats/min, particularly in the last trimester [1]. Cardiac output increases almost to maximum by the 20th week ([2]. When the measurement of cardiac output is made with the patient supine, there is a significant drop in cardiac output toward term. Lees and others have indicated that the drop in the cardiac output toward term does not occur with the patient lying on her side [5]. Ueland's work shows that there is a decrease in cardiac output toward term in all positions, but significant only in supine position [8].

The mechanism for the drop of cardiac output appears to be related to the pressure of the uterus and products of conception on the pelvic veins, causing a decreased venous return to the right side of the heart and, consequently, a decrease in cardiac output.

MITRAL STENOSIS IN PREGNANCY

Because of the increased blood volume and cardiac output and the slight increase in heart rate, which shortens the diastolic filling time, mitral stenosis and pregnancy are a dangerous combination. In a previously asymptomatic patient with mitral stenosis, congestive failure may occur for the first time during pregnancy, delivery, or during the postpartum period. The main difficulty appears to be related to the mechanical problem of the increased blood volume crossing the narrow valve orifice with a shortened diastolic filling time due to the increased heart rate.

Despite the intrinsic dangers of mitral stenosis and pregnancy, cautious modern management will usually allow a pregnancy to proceed with safety. There are four general therapeutic goals in management of the pregnant patient with mitral stenosis: (a) prevention of congestive failure, (b) prevention of acute rheumatic fever, (c) prevention of infective endocarditis, and (d) early treatment of congestive failure.

In most cases, congestive failure should be preventable, even during pregnancy. The patient should be schooled in the principles that may prevent heart failure. She should be carefully supervised on a 2-g sodium diet and instructed to contact her physician in event of infection or fever, to avoid strenuous exercise, and to report to her physician any unusual palpitation or cardiac irregularities.

In our clinic, we prefer to have patients with mitral stenosis admitted 7–10 days prior to the estimated date of delivery. This allows the attending physician the opportunity of having the patient in the optimal state of compensation and avoids the hasty automobile ride across town during labor. As in the nonpregnant state, it is wise to give regular antibiotics to patients with rheumatic heart disease in order to prevent a recurrent episode of rheumatic fever. The American Heart Association's recommendation of 1.2 million units of intramuscularly administered bicillin monthly would seem to be the best approach to this problem for patients not sensitive to penicillin.

Infective endocarditis rarely follows delivery, but the consequences are so great that in most centers antibiotics are used at the time of delivery and during the first 2–3 days of the postpartum period. We are currently using 2.4 million units of penicillin per day for 3 days, beginning with the onset of labor. Streptomycin 1 g twice daily is also used for a 3-day period. To avoid possible injury to the infant's ears, we usually begin the streptomycin immediately following the clamping of the cord. However, there is no evidence that 1 g of streptomycin given during labor would pose a risk to the fetus.

If congestive failure cannot be avoided, it must be treated as early as possible. It is, therefore, necesary to develop a monitoring system that facilitates detection of early signs of congestive failure. It is important that these patients be seen weekly and that significant data be recorded on a flow sheet. The development of a flow sheet avoids the possibility of omitting a significant observation and displays the information in a convenient fashion. In our clinic, we weekly observe and record information on the following monitoring points: (a) weight, (b) blood pressure, (c) pulse, (d) urine protein, and glucose, (e) respirations per minute, (f) neck veins, (g) rales, (h) liver, (i) edema, (j) dyspnea, (k) orthopnea, (l) hemoptysis, (m) cough, and (n) chest pain. This almost always allows us to detect and treat congestive failure in the very early stages.

If the early signs of congestive failure appear, the patient is hospitalized and maintained on bed rest. Treatment includes more stringent dietary salt restriction and diuretics. If atrial fibrillation is present, digitalis is given or increased to slow the heart rate. If the patient is in regular sinus rhythm, we have not been impressed that digitalis is helpful in treating patients with mitral stenosis.

These simple measures are almost always successful. Cardiac surgery is rarely necessary during the pregnancy. While it is usually unnecessary to perform cardiac surgery during pregnancy, it can be performed with little or no increase in risk to the mother. Open heart surgery apparently does increase the risk to the fetus; in a combined study, fetal mortality was 33% [10].

From the standpoint of individuals interested in critical care, it is appropriate to remember that congestive failure may occur in patients with mitral stenosis previously asymptomatic for the first time in the postpartum period.

Several hemodynamic changes contribute to this potential risk. Significant volumes of fluid may be mobilized from the legs in the postpartum period. Probably more important is the injudicious use of intravenous fluids. Finally, it is now accepted that oxytocins have an antidiuretic effect [6,9]. Since most obstetricians utilize oxytocins to avoid the risk of uterine hemorrhage, their use may contribute to heart failure. However, with careful observations for early signs of failure and restriction of fluids, oxytocins do not seem to be unduly dangerous. Nevertheless, it is sensible for all patients with mitral stenosis to be followed in a well-equipped recovery room or, better, an intensive care unit where appropriate monitoring can take place for at least 12–16 hr postpartum. Heart rate, respiration, basal rales, and fluid intake/output should be carefully monitored.

Summary

With the current state of development in critical care, patients with mitral stenosis in pregnancy can almost always be carried through a normal and safe pregnancy, delivery, and postpartum period. This, however, should not obscure the fact that patients with mitral stenosis in the pregnant state and postpartum period, even those who have been totally asymptomatic, may develop severe and life threatening pulmonary edema.

References

1. **Burwell, C. S.,** and **Metcalfe, J.** (1958). *Heart Disease in Pregnancy. Physiology and Management.* London: Churchill, pp. 11–12.
2. **Hamilton, H. F. H.** (1949). The cardiac output in normal pregnancy as determined by the Cournand right heart catheterization technique. *J. Obstet. Gynaec. Brit. Emp. 56*:548.
3. **Hurst, J. W., Staton, J.,** and **Hubbard, D.** (1958). Precordial murmurs during pregnancy and lactation. *New Engl. J. Med 259*:515.

4. **Hytten, F. E.,** and **Leitch, I.** (1964). *The Physiology Of Human Pregnancy*. Oxford: Blackwell, p. 102.
5. **Lees, M. M., Scott, D. B., Kerr, M. G.,** and **Taylor, S. H.** (1967). The circulatory effects of recumbent postural change in late pregnancy. *Clin. Sci. 32:*453.
6. **Potter, R. R.** (1964). Water retention due to oxytocin. *Obstet. Gynec. 23.*
7. **Turner, A. F.** (in press). The chest radiograph in pregnancy. *Clin. Obstet. Gynec.*
8. **Ueland, K., Novy, M. J., Peterson, E. N.,** and **Metcalfe.** (1969). Maternal cardiovascular dynamics. IV. The influence of gestational age on the maternal cardiovascular response to posture and exercise. *Am. J. Obstet. Gynec. 104:*856.
9. **Whalley, P. J.,** and **Pritchard, J. A.** (1963). Oxytocin and water intoxication. *J. Am. Med. Assoc. 186.*
10. **Zitnik, R. S., Brandenburg, R. O., Sheldon, R.,** and **Wallace, R. B.** (1969). Pregnancy and open-heart surgery. *Cardiovasc. Surg.* 1968; Suppl. I, *Circulation 39/40.*

Sudden Death and Acute Myocardial Infarction – What Are We Talking About?

WILLIAM J. GRACE, M.D.*
Department of Medicine, St. Vincent's Hospital and Medical Center of New York, and Professor of Clinical Medicine, New York University School of Medicine, New York, New York

Sudden death outside the hospital is very common in our country. Vital statistics indicate as many as one-half million people die in this way every year. However, vital statistics record that the bulk of such deaths is due to an acute myocardial infarction. Despite this rather well-entrenched tradition, there is some question about whether such is the truth. For example, in an autopsy study of sudden death by Kuller in Baltimore, 61% of the patients had only arteriosclerostic heart disease; 14% had alcoholism and fatty liver, and the rest of the deaths were due to a variety of causes. Fifty percent of the patients with sudden deaths had extensive, severe coronary artery disease. In this particular study of sudden death, only 13% of patients had an acute myocardial infarction. Therefore, to say that sudden death is due to acute myocardial infarction is far from accurate.

Roberts has recently reviewed the problem. He made a meticulous dissection of coronary arteries in patients who died within a few hours of the onset of symptoms. Neither coronary thrombosis nor acute myocardial infarction was present in any significant number of the patients. In this

***Unfortunately, Dr. Grace's untimely death precluded preparation of the bibliography for his contribution to this volume.**

regard there is a special experience reported by Cobb (Seattle, Washington), who treated a number of patients in ventricular fibrillation outside of the hospital. These patients were promptly defibrillated and 20% survived to leave the hospital in good condition. In this particular report very few of these patients had ECG evidence of acute myocardial infarction. Nagel (Miami, Florida) reports similar findings in patients outside the hospital. It is therefore important to realize that the patient dying suddenly outside of the medical care system did not die of an overwhelming and irreversible myocardial necrosis, but in all probability of cardiac arrhythmia. The types of arrhythmia seen here and in coronary care units are predominantly ventricular fibrillation, ventricular tachycardia, and occasional bradycardiac arrhythmias with hypotension. Inasmuch as these arrhythmias are treatable, we must give considerable thought to instituting systems in our community for arrhythmia control and cardiopulmonary resuscitation A study by Pantridge indicates that those patients with acute myocardial infarction and ventricular fibrillation had as smooth a post-hospital course as those who did not have ventricular fibrillation. A 1-year follow-up study indicated no disadvantage to the patient who had been successfully resuscitated from ventricular fibrillation.

Of particular note is ambulance service throughout the world. Reports which have been summarized by Lambrew indicate that in such places as Baltimore, Belfast, Charlottesville, Maryland, North London and Rochester, a percentage of patients have cardiac arrest in the ambulance; this percentage is not insignificant and varies from 8.7% reported from Montgomery County, Maryland, to as high as 17% (Virginia) and 21.7% (North London). It is presumed that these deaths are likewise due to arrhythmia. This is an additionally sad event, for here the patient is under some kind of a medical care system which is seemingly unable or unauthorized to deal with ventricular fibrillation. Lambrew has transmitted electrocardiograms on all patients transported to the hospital by the rescue squad in Suffolk County, New York. A surprisingly large number of life-threatening arrhythmias occur in the patients who seemingly have called the ambulance solely because of trauma or automobile accident. In the chest-pain patients, cardiac arrhythmia was recorded in 22%. Eight percent had ventricular fibrillation as the initial rhythm. For example, in 2744 patients for whom the ambulance responded because of a call of trauma, 4.2 % had a significant cardiac arrhythmia recorded. The initial arrhythmia was ventricular fibrillation in 0.1%, and ventricular standstill in 0.2%. Cardiac arrest occurred in transit in this ambulance study—in patients with chest pain (1% of 1728 patients) and trauma (0.3% of 2744). Although the percentage of arrhythmic deaths in the trauma patient is statistically small, it is an extremely important observation. Arrhythmia control and cardiopulmonary resuscitation are necessary for the ambulance teams, even when approaching a patient whose only problem presumably is trauma. Hence, it is advantageous for practicing physicians to be aware that sudden death is associated with lethal cardiac arrhythmias and that, importantly, this may occur in the setting of trauma, as well as in the setting of symptomatic coronary artery disease. Physicians should be concerned about out-of-hospital deaths, and should be actively engaged in community organization to solve this therapeutic problem. Reports from Pantridge in Ireland, Grace in New York City, Cobb and Rose in the far West, and Warren in Ohio all indicate that out-of-hospital rescue squads are effective in salvaging patients from ventricular fibrillation. Reports from our own experience (Grace and Chadbourn) indicate that beginning coronary care outside of the hospital lowers the hospital mortality rate.

Potentially Fatal Ventricular Arrhythmias

MILFORD G. WYMAN, M.D.
Clinical Professor of Medicine
Director Coronary Care Unit
San Pedro Community Hospital
San Pedro, California

Ventricular arrhythmias are potentially fatal depending on the setting in which they occur. It has long been recognized that a single premature ventricular beat may initiate ventricular fibrillation in the presence of an acute myocardial infarction or an acute ischemic episode. Such depolarization will initiate ventricular fibrillation most often if it occurs on the apex of the T wave (the vulnerable zone), but in the presence of an acute infarction the single ectopic ventricular beat can initiate ventricular fibrillation during any portion of the cardiac cycle. Evidence has accumulated to document the increased hazard of: (a) two consecutive ventricular beats, (b) "R on T" ventricular beats, and (c) multifocal or multiform ventricular beats. The number of ventricular beats per minute (or preferably per 100 beats) may be a factor in predicting fibrillation, but data are not available to define what that number is. Data on the duration of the vulnerable period following acute infarction are also lacking. After the acute infarction there is an exponential decrease in the prevelance of ventricular fibrillation with time, but vulnerability to ectopic ventricular beats may continue for as long as 3–6 months. It is the purpose of this chapter to classify the types of ectopic ventricular beats and to suggest an approach to their treatment, and most importantly, to define a rational approach to the prevention of these potentially lethal ventricular rhythms in the setting of an acute ischemic episode or infarction.

Our classification of the ectopic ventricular rhythms is as follows: (a) automatic ventricular rhythm; (i) "protected" rhythm, with parasystole and (ii) "nonprotected" rhythm, with "escape" and accelerated idioventricular rhythm and (b) re-entry ventricular rhythm.

PARASYSTOLE

An automatic ventricular rhythm is one that originates in the Purkinje cells and has its own independent rate. When a discharge from the sinus node does not disturb the rhythm of the automatic ventricular pacemaker, that pacemaker is said to be "protected." This single electrophysiologic property differentiates a parasystolic ventricular rhythm from an accelerated idioventricular rhythm. Since the automatic focus of a parasystolic rhythm has an independent rate, it will have no fixed relation to the preceding sinus beat.* The ventricular impulse becomes manifest depending both on the presence of an exit block and the refractory period of the ventricle at the time of parasystolic discharge. Since the parasystolic impulse has a fixed rate despite the degree of exit block or refractory period of the ventricle, the rate can easily be calculated by determining the lowest common denominator between the ectopic ventricular complexes. Figure 1 is an example of parasystolic ventricular tachycardia.

NONPROTECTED AUTOMATIC VENTRICULAR RHYTHMS

Nonprotected ventricular rhythms are a frequent event in an acute myocardial infarction and are recognized by: (a) a variable coupling interval (as in parasystole) and (b) ability of the sinus impulse to penetrate the region of the automatic focus, thereby discharging it and upsetting its regularity (unlike parasystole). When the automatic ventricular focus occurs as a manifestation of slowing of the sinus node, it is termed an "escape ventricular rhythm." If the ventricular pacemaker reaches threshold prior to or at the same time (fusion beat) as the next expected sinus beat and continues to function as the dominant pacemaker, it is known as an "accelerated idioventricular rhythm" (Fig. 2).

The decision as to whether these ventricular rhythms should be treated depends on the following criteria: (a) sinus rate, (b) rate of the automatic ventricular pacemaker and its acceleration, (c) presence of additional

*Accordingly the coupling interval is not constant. At times, the sinus impulse and the impulse from the ventricular parasystolic focus fuse. Such fusion beats combine the characteristics of the sinus and parasystolic complexes and they are commonly observed in patients with parasystolic rhythms.

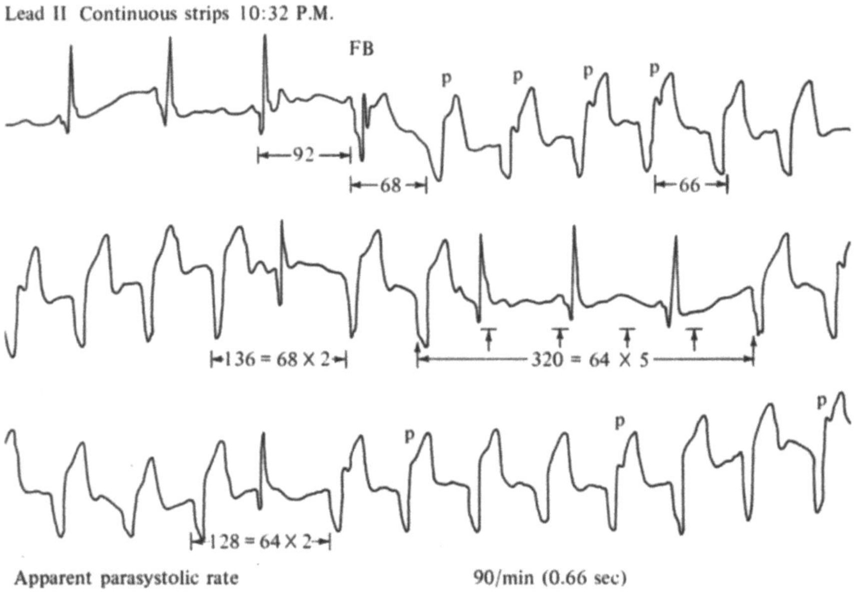

FIGURE 1 Parasystolic ventricular tachycardia, demonstrating protection, variable coupling, and a fusion beat (FB).

ectopic ventricular beats from different foci, and (d) effect of the ventricular rhythm on arterial blood pressure. If the escape or accelerated ventricular rhythm occurs in the presence of sinus bradycardia, the automatic ventricular rhythm may be abolished by accelerating the sinus pacemaker with atropine. When its discharge is increased with atropine, the sinus node becomes the dominant pacemaker and the ventricular pacemaker becomes latent. It is frequently stated that accelerated idioventricular rhythms are benign. Nevertheless, idioventricular rhythms may accelerate or the rhythm may be further complicated by the simultaneous appearance of other ectopic ventricular pacemakers. When this occurs in the presence of sinus rates that exceed 80 beats/min, lidocaine may be the drug of choice (Fig. 3). If sinus bradycardia is present and the above conditions exist, both atropine and lidocaine may be used. We have observed accelerated idioventricular rhythms to be less responsive to intravenous lidocaine or procainamide than the second major subgroup of ventricular arrhythmias, re-entry or extrasystolic ventricular tachycardia.

RE-ENTRY VENTRICULAR RHYTHMS

The clinical diagnosis of re-entry ventricular beats depends on the demonstration of fixed coupling, that is, a constant interval between the sinus beat and the premature ventricular beat. This assumes that the ectopic beat is

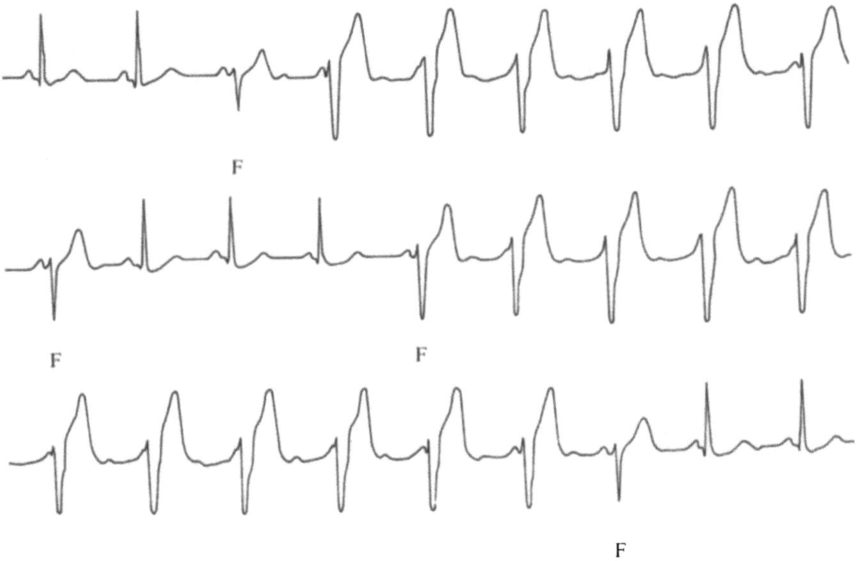

FIGURE 2 Accelerated idioventricular beginning and ending with a fusion beat (F). This could be treated with atropine.

dependent on the preceding normal sinus beat requiring a conduction block that is unidirectional. When this occurs in the ventricle a single premature ventricular depolarization results or ventricular tachycardia occurs from a continuous circulation of impulses within the circuit (Fig. 4). This type of ectopic ventricular rhythm in an acute myocardial infarction is frequently rapid and provides the fragmentation and disorganization of the

FIGURE 3 Accelerated ventricular tachycardia (continuous strip) with acceleration of ventricular rate and a sinus rate of 84; best treated with lidocaine.

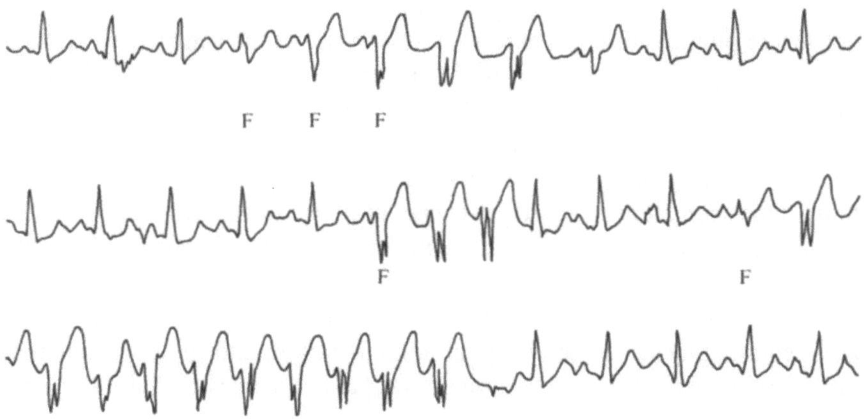

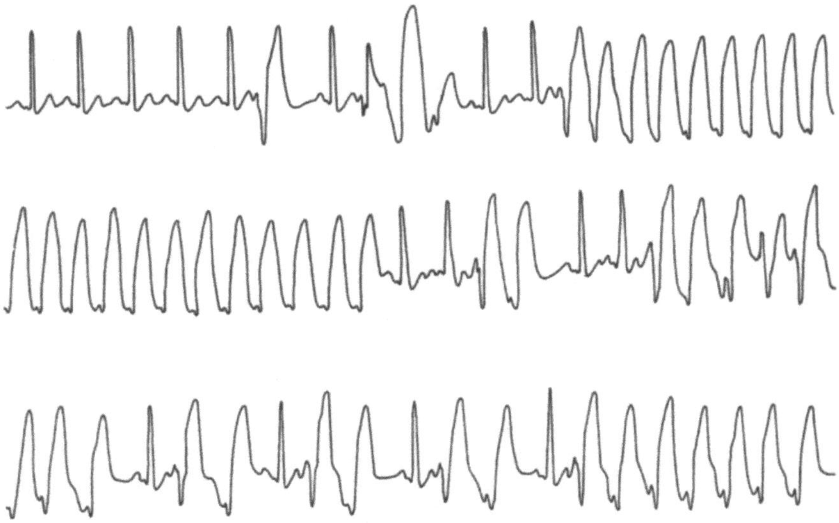

FIGURE 4 Re-entry ventricular tachycardia with demonstration of fixed coupling preceding the runs of tachycardia.

impulse necessary for ventricular fibrillation. Re-entry ventricular rhythms respond to lidocaine and procainamide but the approach to both prevention and treatment demands a coordinated system, a protocol that we shall now outline.

PREVENTION AND TREATMENT OF VENTRICULAR ARRHYTHMIAS

The goal in treatment of ectopic ventricular rhythms is the prevention of primary ventricular fibrillation. Primary ventricular fibrillation is defined as fibrillation in the absence of pulmonary edema or shock. If the patient without severe pump failure has exhibited none or all of the ventricular rhythms defined above, then develops ventricular fibrillation and expires, his death can be attributed to arrhythmia. Primary ventricular fibrillation should be prevented, but data from muliple centers document the continued prevalence of primary ventricular fibrillation and an excessive associated mortality. One such study suggests an excess of 50,000 lives lost each year due to arrhythmias in patients with acute myocardial infarction *within the hospital*. The system required to prevent such deaths begins in the emergency room and continues until hospital discharge. A protocol approved by all attending physicians, the hospital administration, and the department of nursing must be set into action when the patient arrives at the emergency room. The training of personnel includes clerks, nurses, and physicians. The protocol, the set of standing orders, clearly defines the responsibility of each member of the staff and requires a specific response of each individual involved.

Emergency room. The method herein outlined has now been used in excess of 800 myocardial infarctions. The first step is the injection of a 75 mg bolus of lidocaine followed by a pump-controlled 2-mg/min infusion to every patient with suspected myocardial infarction on hospital admission. It is mandatory that treatment of the patient with chest discomfort take precedence of the emergency room. Sudden death from an acute ischemic episode or myocardial infarction decreases exponentially with time. The patient must, therefore, be treated immediately after hospital admission. In our study of 800 infarctions in the emergency room, primary ventricular fibrillation was prevented with this method in all patients who received lidocaine. Four patients developed fibrillation before the intravenous needle could be inserted.

Transport of the patient. The control of arrhythmias is continued as the patient is transported to the coronary care unit. A portable monitor–defibrillator and infusion pump accompanies each patient into the elevator, the corridors, and the coronary care unit.

Treatment within the critical care unit. The control of ectopic ventricular beats requires specialized knowledge of the pharmacology of all drugs used, particularly lidocaine and procainamide. A protocol that allows the nurse to give multiple 50-mg boluses of lidocaine every 5 min, not exceeding 250 mg, is a safe procedure if the patient is not in severe pump failure. With each additional bolus the infusion rate is increased to a maximum of 4 mg/min. However, it must be appreciated that the increase in the infusion rate will not reach a plateau for hours after it is adjusted. Hence the bolus is used for the treatment of the ectopic ventricular beats occurring at that precise moment; increments in the infusion rate slowly increase the blood level of lidocaine to prevent ventricular arrhythmias that may occur hours later.

The time for addition of a second drug, procainamide, must be clearly delineated in the protocol. When the lidocaine boluses and infusion of $\leqslant 4$ mg/min have been ineffective, the nurse will use multiple 100-mg boluses of procainamide over a 3-min period. Procainamide given in excess of five separate 100-mg boluses at 5-min intervals is rarely necessary to control the ectopic ventricular beats, but up to one gram procainamide is tolerable. A constant infusion of procainamide (2–6 mg/min) controlled by a pump is then used to achieve a stable effective blood level. The dosage of these drugs depends on the degree of heart, kidney, or liver failure. There are remarkably few side effects when the drugs are used carefully. Within the coronary care unit, primary ventricular fibrillation has been almost completely eliminated. In our study, primary ventricular fibrillation occurred in less than 0.5% in the last 800 myocardial infarctions with no deaths. Death in our coronary care unit has been due only to severe pump failure.

Arrhythmia deaths on the medical floor. The problem of arrhythmia deaths in the patient after discharge from the unit has received very little attention. One study reported that 23% of the deaths after discharge from the critical care unit were due to arrhythmia. Monitoring by telemetry is a necessity until hospital discharge. We utilize telemetry after the patient is discharged from the coronary care unit to determine: (a) incidence of ventricular arrhythmias (number of ectopic ventricular beats, bursts, "R on T," and ventricular tachycardia), both at rest and in the presence of pain, (b) effect of exercise on rate, rhythm, and conduction, and (c) effect of drug therapy on ventricular arrhythmias and conduction. A new episode of sustained chest pain unresponsive to nitroglycerine is treated as a possible extension of either an old or new infarction. Hence the patient again receives prophylactic lidocaine. The incidence of sudden death after discharge from the critical care unit has been reduced to less than 1%.

Summary

Ectopic ventricular beats may be fatal depending on the setting in which they occur. An "R on T" ectopic ventricular beat in the normal heart will be harmless; in an acute myocardial infarction it may be fatal. A plan for treatment of ventricular rhythms should begin with an understanding of their mechanism and of the pharmacology of the drugs necessary for their control.

The treatment of ventricular rhythms cannot be left to those physicians with little or no experience in this specialized area of critical care medicine. It requires the organization of a comprehensive plan that begins in the emergency room and continues to time of discharge. It requires the cooperation of administration, the entire attending physician staff, and the nursing department.

The plan or protocol is set in motion when the patient is brought to the emergency room by the paramedics or presents himself to the clerk at the emergency room desk complaining of chest pain. Every suspected myocardial infarction is treated. Such a plan demands the recognition of ventricular rhythms by the nursing personnel with a precise approach to treatment. In each instance when treatment is not successful an alternate plan must be available to the nurse to avoid the unnecessary time delay of contacting a physician. The use of a comprehensive plan with a complete protocol that can be utilized by the nurse has resulted in the complete prevention of primary ventricular fibrillation in the emergency room in over 800 infarctions. In the CCU there have been 3 cases of primary ventricular fibrillation (all resuscitated) in 800 myocardial infarctions. On the medical floor sudden death occurred in five cases in 945 infarctions. Potentially fatal ventricular arrhythmias can both be successfully treated and prevented.

Techniques for Establishing Appropriate Dose Regimens of Digitalis

ROGER W. JELLIFFE, M.D.
Associate Professor of Medicine
University of Southern California, School of Medicine,
Los Angeles, California

ABSORPTION AND BIOAVAILABILITY OF DIGITOXIN AND DIGOXIN

Much recent attention has been directed to the problem of bioavailability. While oral digitoxin appears to be essentially completely absorbed [28], the bioavailability of oral digoxin appears to be somewhere between 85% [3–5] and 50% [7]. Other digoxin preparations may be even less well absorbed. Because of this, parenteral doses of digoxin probably should be reduced to 50–85% of the corresponding oral dose when using oral digoxin of good bioavailability, while little or no such reduction appears necessary for digitoxin.

Strict FDA regulations have been developed to improve the bioavailability of digoxin [8]. Even here, however, the goal has been only to achieve about 70% dissolution of the tablet as judged by a standard method. It is likely, however, that more complete dissolution may yield even greater reproducibility of pharmacologic effect [23], possibly without any significant increase in toxicity from the higher transient serum levels that may occur. Generally, then, the data suggest the bioavailability of oral digitoxin to be essentially complete and that of oral digoxin incomplete and often poor. Better formulations may well improve this.

METABOLISM AND EXCRETION

Digitoxin is extensively metabolized in the body. Its renal losses are small [9,14]. When renal function is normal, 30% of the total daily loss of digitoxin takes place by urinary excretion of unchanged digitoxin. Approximately 62% of the total daily loss of digitoxin is nonurinary, the digitoxin being converted to inactive metabolites [14]. About 8% of the total daily loss of digitoxin is due to is hydroxylation by the liver to digoxin [14]. The kinetic behavior of this digitoxin–digoxin system in patients is only modestly altered by impaired renal function [9,14]. The daily percentage loss of digitoxin from the body can be calculated from the formula:

$$D = 7.7 + 0.035\ \mathrm{CCr}, \qquad (1)$$

where D represents the daily percentage loss; and CCr, the patient's endogenous creatinine clearance in ml/min/1.73 m^2 of body-surface area [16].

In contrast, a much larger proportion of digoxin is eliminated by the kidney, and a much smaller amount is catabolized. When renal function is normal, approximately 60% of the total daily loss of digoxin is renal and 40% is nonurinary, resulting from metabolic degradation to essentially inactive products. The kinetic behavior of digoxin in patients is greatly altered by impaired renal function [9].

The daily percentage loss of digoxin from the body can be calculated from the formula:

$$D = 14 + 0.2\ \mathrm{CCr}, \qquad (2)$$

where D and CCr are defined as before [10].

Evaluation of Renal Function

Evaluation of renal function is an integral part of planning rational cardiac glycoside therapy. Measurement of CCr is far superior to that of the level of blood-urea nitrogen or serum creatinine alone. Measurement of CCr by standard techniques, however, involves very careful collection of a timed urine specimen. All too often this simply cannot be done. A reasonable estimate of CCr is often a helpful alternative. Such an estimate has been made by a computer program [18] that takes into account the patient's age, sex, height, weight, and the constancy of serum creatinine concentration.

Renal function falls progressively with age. This is not revealed to us by mere inspection of serum creatinine levels. Failure to recognize reduced

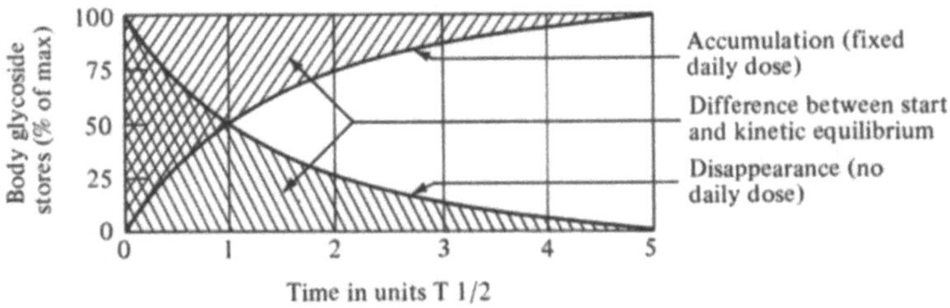

FIGURE 1 Accumulation of glycoside on a fixed daily dose compared with its disappearance after dosage is stopped. Time is expressed in units of drug half-times. (See text for discussion.)

renal function in elderly patients is a pitfall in planning cardiac glycoside therapy, which has led to a high incidence of digitalis toxicity in the past [12].

Kinetics of Cumulation

Most drugs disappear from the body in a logarithmic manner and have an apparent half-life or $T_{1/2}$. After five half-lives, 31/32 of the original drug has disappeared from the body.

On the other hand, as shown in Fig. 1, if a loading dose is omitted and the patient is simply started on a fixed maintenance dose, the drug cumulates in the body by the mirror image of the decay curve. After five half-lives on such a dosage regimen, the total amount of drug in the body will have cumulated to 31/32 of the maximum that it will ever achieve in the body, other factors remaining unchanged. The basic aspects of such kinetic behavior of cardiac glycosides have been reviewed elsewhere [1,9,14]. Because of this, the full clinical response to a change in either a patient's renal function or his daily maintenance dosage will not be seen for at least five drug half-lives. As shown in Table 1, these half-lives range from about 1.6 to 4.4 days for digoxin and from about 5.8 to about 8.7 days for digitoxin.

INTUITIVE CARDIAC GLYCOSIDE THERAPY

It has been traditional to attempt to individualize cardiac glycoside therapy very carefully by following a process of clinical titration. This has generally been accomplished by careful clinical assessment of the patient for evidence of either under- or overdosage, followed by appropriate adjustment of dosage when the manifestations are encountered. Other more recent approaches, such as measurement of serum glycoside levels or salivary electrolytes, have been widely used to monitor patients and to attempt to detect incipient toxicity.

TABLE 1 Digitoxin and Digoxin Half-Lives ($T_{1/2}$) at Different Creatinine Clearance Rates (CCr)

DRUG	CCr	$T_{1/2}$ (DAYS)	FIVE $\times$ $T_{1/2}$ (DAYS)
Digitoxin	100	5.8	29
	75	6.6	33
	50	7.3	37
	25	8.0	40
	0	8.7	44
Digoxin	100	1.6	8
	75	2.0	10
	50	2.4	12
	25	3.0	15
	0	4.4	22

The traditional intuitive approach to therapy suffers from being entirely retrospective with respect to the patient. Furthermore, it fails to employ the wealth of data gathered by many investigators concerning the kinetic behavior of cardiac glycosides in patients and has resulted in a considerable incidence of adverse reactions, ranging from 20% of hospitalized patients [25], to 29% of consecutive hospital admissions [2], to 35% of a group of patients with a higher than usual incidence of renal disease [12]

Digitalis intoxication carries a high mortality. For example, in one clinical report it was felt to be a direct cause of death in six of 148 toxic patients, a 4% incidence. Five of the six patients were autopsied and no anatomic cause of death could be found [26].

Digitalis toxicity is also an important contributing cause of death. Mortality was 17% in nontoxic hospitalized patients receiving cardiac glycosides but 41% in toxic patients, a significant difference [2]. In that study, an arrhythmia was required for a patient to be included in the "toxic" group. In another study, two patients' deaths were related to toxicity among 32 adverse reactions, an overall mortality of 6% [12]. Of these 32 episodes, 13 were instances of major sustained arrhythmias. The two deaths were both noted in this group, an incidence of 15%.

In summary, completely retrospective intuitive therapy has been accompanied by a high incidence of toxicity and a significant mortality.

Advance Planning of Dosage Regimens

It seems reasonable to adjust glycoside dosage to a patient's body weight and renal function. If this is done, the total amount of drug in the body—and therefore serum [12,22,24,27] and myocardial [20] levels—can be better kept within reasonable bounds.

In general, for patients with normal sinus rhythm, a total body concentration of about 10 μg/kg will result in a reasonable therapeutic effect and a low incidence of toxicity [12,22]. Greater amounts ($\sim$13–15 μg/kg) are usually required for adequate control of ventricular rate in patients with atrial fibrillation.

It is useful to divide the total loading dose into two or three parts at 6-hr intervals to allow adequate time to observe the effect of each previous part. This approach permits a gentle touch and yet usually completes the loading dose in 12–18 hr. So-called loading doses, which are given over more than 1 day, are actually combinations of loading and maintenance doses.

It seems best to use this approach even in an apparently elective clinical situation. This forces a gentle examination of the patient's ability to tolerate the selected body concentration when everyone is more alert to the possibility of toxicity. In contrast, if the loading dose is omitted and cumulation is allowed to occur in a prolonged manner, at least five glycoside half-lives are required before it is safe to assume that the patient can tolerate the regimen. A degree of control is lost. The problems associated with such uncontrolled cumulation and with the sudden appearance of an adverse reaction have been previously discussed [11].

If the patient tolerates the total loading dose, given in the above gradual increments, there is strong evidence he may well continue to tolerate it, other things being equal. When the loading and maintenance doses are both given by the same route, one can plan the maintenance dose by the following formula:

$$\text{M} = \text{LD} \times \text{daily percentage loss,} \tag{3}$$

where M = maintenance dose and LD = loading dose.

The daily percentage loss of digitoxin or digoxin can be found from formulas 1 and 2 given earlier.

Computer-Assisted Glycoside Therapy

Development of proper dosage regimens becomes more difficult when renal function or previous glycoside dosage has been changing, thereby requiring repetitive serial calculations of past total-body glycoside concentrations.

A general-purpose computer program [15] was developed to perform these functions rapidly and practically for patients receiving any possible combination of digitalis leaf, digitoxin, digoxin, or cedilanid-D (deslanoside). The computer program has been designed for use by community hospitals and by medically underserved areas as well as by urban centers. The program employs remote time-sharing terminals connected to the computer by an ordinary telephone line. Thus one can run the program simply by telephoning the computer and placing the telephone in the box or coupler, thereby linking the terminal to the computer. This program has been in active clinical use since 1967.

Use of this program has significantly reduced the incidence of digitalis toxicity [12]. Figure 2 shows that the incidence of digitalis toxicity was reduced from 36% to 12% in a retrospective study (Computer Group A versus Intuitive Therapy Group). Renal function in these patients ranged from normal to anuric. Many were hospitalized and placed in intensive care units. Computed total-body glycoside concentrations averaged 18.4 and 14.6 μg/kg in the intuitively treated group and the computer-assisted group, respectively. Similarly, in a *prospective* study of otherwise comparable

FIGURE 2 Frequency of adverse reactions to digitalis in the intuitive therapy group and in computer groups A (middle) and B (right). (See text for discussion.) Column 1 (large dots) indicates all manifestations of adverse reactions; Column 2 (clear bar), arrhythmias due to digitalis toxicity; and Column 3 (small dots), major sustained toxic arrhythmias.

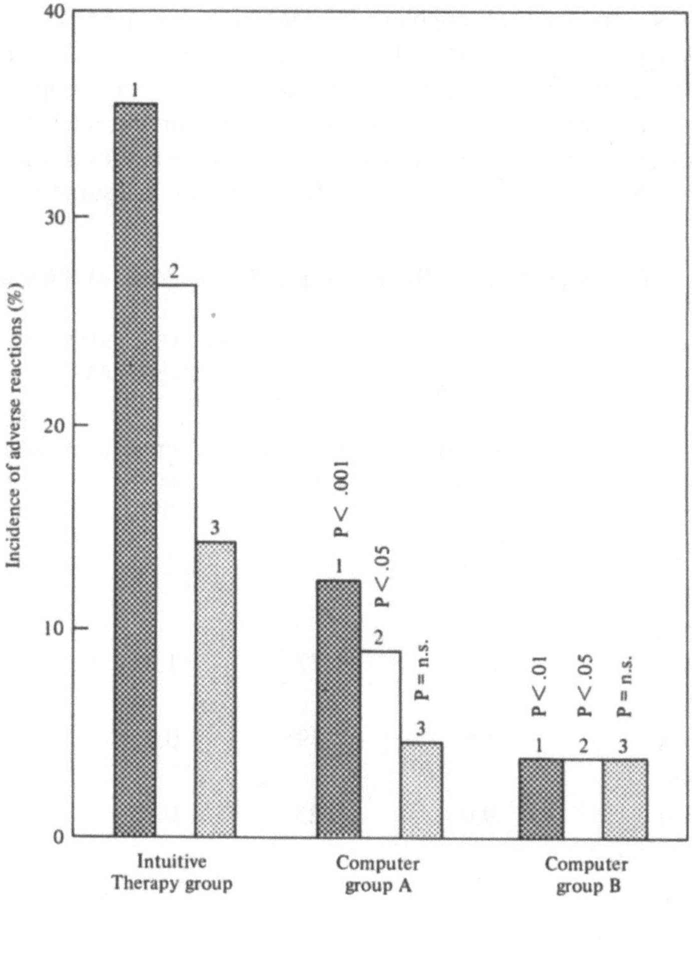

patients with a similar full range of renal function from normal to anephric (Computer Group B in Fig. 2), an average body glycoside concentration of 9.9 μg/kg was achieved, and a 4% incidence of toxicity was found, also a significant reduction [12].

It is interesting to examine this incidence in relation to the period of time the patients were receiving these various regimens. As shown in Table 2, in the retrospective study, 1.8 adverse reactions were noted per patient-year of therapy with the intuitive regimens, but only 0.5 adverse reactions were found with computer assistance (Computer Group A), a significant difference. In the prospective study (Computer Group B), the incidence was only 0.25 adverse reactions per patient-year, also a significant difference. It is noteworthy that the above reduction of adverse reactions was achieved between 1967 and 1969, without a single measurement of serum glycoside level being performed.

Use of serum glycoside assays. Because of the kinetics of cumulation and the five half-lives required to reach a new steady state following a change, the changes in serum levels are blunted by the kinetic properties of the drug itself. Changes in serum levels will therefore inevitably lag behind changes in renal function. Monitoring renal function, coupled with proper adjustment of dosage when such changes occur, allows for the maintenance of total-body glycoside concentrations (and therefore serum levels) at the desired value. Serum levels can then be advantageously measured to test the

TABLE 2 Observed Adverse Reactions per Patient-Year of Therapy

	AVERAGE BODY GLYCOSIDE LEVEL	ADVERSE REACTIONS PER PATIENT-YEAR		
		ALL MANIFESTATIONS	ARRHYTHMIAS	MAJOR ARRHYTHMIAS
	μg/kg body weight			
Intuitive therapy group	18.4	1.77	1.33	0.72
Computer group A	14.6	0.49^{a}	0.35^{a}	0.26^{b}
Computer group B	9.9	0.25^{c}	0.25^{b}	0.25^{b}

^{a} $p < 0.001$.
^{b} $p =$ not significant.
^{c} $p < 0.05$.

effectiveness of this plan. Waiting for serum levels to change, however, inevitably means that dosage adjustment will be after the fact, and invites a greater risk to the patient. The combination of kinetically oriented advance planning and careful clinical observation and monitoring of serum levels uses each tool to its own best advantage.

Digitoxin versus Digoxin

Of the two glycosides, digoxin is more rapidly excreted and is thus also more rapidly cumulative, usually in about 8 days (five half-times) when renal function is normal. The clinical response to a change in the maintenance dose of digitoxin is much more difficult to observe, however, as five of its half-times take place more slowly, usually over about 1 month. The kinetics of digitoxin are much less affected by renal function than those of digoxin. The bioavailability of digitoxin is generally greater and thus probably digitoxin is more reproducible than digoxin in its effect.

One of the main reasons advocated for using digoxin is its relatively rapid excretion, using the rationale that when toxicity occurs, one can reverse it more rapidly than with digitoxin. This is presumed to be an advantage. One certainly cannot argue against the general case that rapid excretion is useful when toxicity is present.

Toxicity, however, represents a failure of advance planning of the dosage regimen by any method. Reduction of the mortality associated with digitalis toxicity is best accomplished by prevention and by adjusting dosage to changes in renal function.

Let us now consider what appear to be the relative penalties of failing to do this, first for a patient receiving digoxin, then for one receiving digitoxin. Let us set up a hypothetical "worst case," where a patient is on a long-term maintenance dosage and his CCr is 100 ml/min per 1.73 m^2. Let us assume that he suddenly becomes totally anuric but that his dosage continues unchanged.

As shown in Figure 3, the patient receiving digoxin will cumulate to 83% above his previous control level after 1 week without dosage adjustment and to 137% above control (more than doubling) when the steady state is approached in about 22 days. The patient receiving digitoxin, however, will cumulate only to 19% above his previous control level after 1 week and to only 46% above control at the steady state, which will require about 44 days to be closely approached. Thus the cumulation of digoxin at 1 week is 83/19 more than that of digitoxin, a factor of 4.3, and in the steady state is 137/46 more than that of digitoxin, a factor of 3.0.

It is therefore most important that transient changes of a patient's renal function, following myocardial infarction or surgery, be closely watched and dosage properly adjusted. If this is not done, the risk of digitalis toxicity appears to be considerably greater for the patient receiving digoxin than digitoxin.

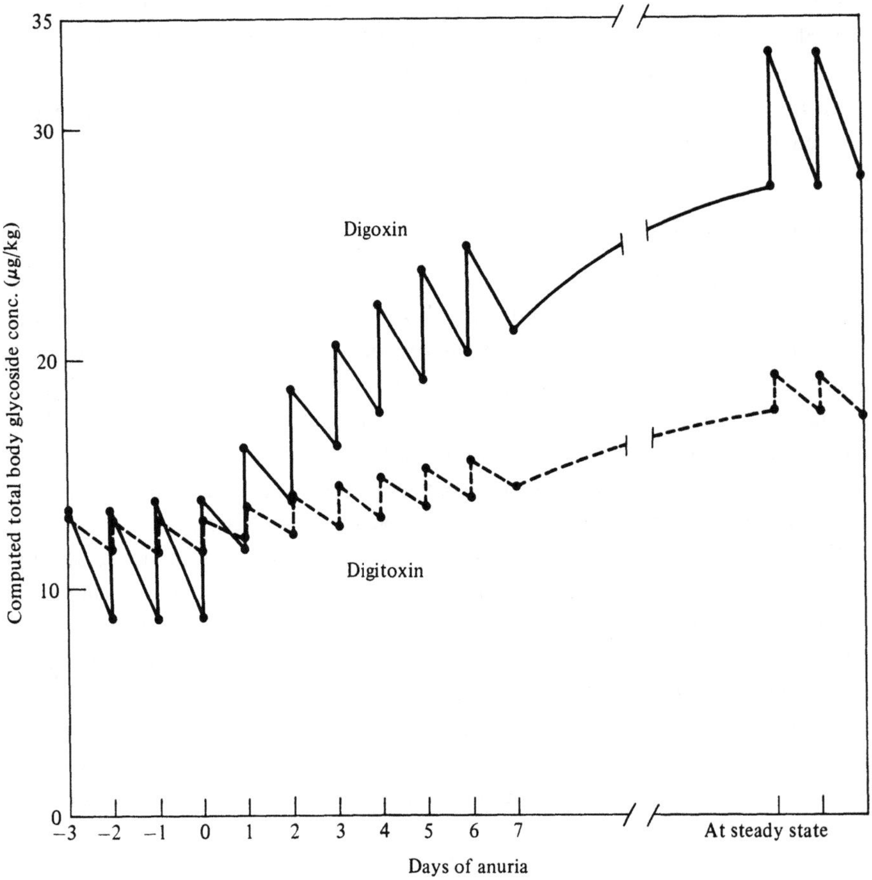

FIGURE 3 Cumulation of digitoxin and digoxin during a hypothetical sudden change from a normal creatinine clearance rate (CCr = 100 ml/min) to a 1 week period of total anuria (CCr = 0 ml/min). Digitoxin kinetics are much less disturbed by a sudden change in renal function without dosage adjustment. In addition, prolonged anuria without adjustment of dosage ("at steady state," right) is also associated with a much smaller total cumulation of digitoxin than digoxin.

Summary

Purified digitalis glycosides such as digitoxin or digoxin are preferred for precision in therapy over preparations such as digitalis leaf or gitalin. Measurement of serum levels is useful but provides only retrospective data.

The lesser renal excretion of digitoxin and its longer half-life provide a degree of stability that may well make it preferable to digoxin in patients with changing renal function where such changes cannot readily be monitored and dosage adjusted.

Retrospective evaluation is always the final arbiter of the success or failure of a dosage regimen. Application of the known kinetic behavior of drugs to plan such dosage regimens has led to the formulas described herein, and to a conversational computer program for community hospital use [12]. For digitalis glycosides, such programs have significantly reduced the incidence of adverse reactions [12] and have controlled serum glycoside levels within reasonable limits [22].

Similar programs are also available to plan infusion regimens of lidocaine [17] and procainamide [6] and of kanamycin [21] gentamicin [19], and streptomycin [13], as well as programs for processing data from the cardiac catheter laboratory, the pulmonary function laboratory, from echocardiograms, and from systolic time intervals.[1]

References

1. **Augsberger, A.** (1954). Quantitatives zur therapie mit herzglycosiden. *Klin. Wschr., 32:*945.
2. **Beller, G. A., Smith, T. W.,** and **Abelmann, W. H.** (1971). Digitalis intoxication. A prospective clinical study with serum level correlations. *New Engl. J. Med. 284:*989–997.
3. **Doherty, J. E., Flanigan, W. J.,** and **Murphy, M. L.** (1970). Tritiated digoxin. XIV. Enterohepatic circulation, absorption, and excretion studies in human volunteers. *Circulation 42:*867–874.
4. **Doherty, J. E.,** and **Perkins, W. H.** (1962). Studies with tritiated digoxin in human subjects after intravenous administration. *Am. Heart J. 63:*528–536.
5. **Doherty, J. E., Perkins, W. H.,** and **Mitchell, G. K.** (1961). Tritiated digoxin studies in human subjects. *Arch. Int. Med. 108:*531–539.
6. **Goicoechea, F. J., Haywood, J., deGuzman, M., Jelliffe, R. W., Gallardo, C.,** and **Rodman, J.** (1974). Kinetics of procainamide after single and multiple oral doses. *Circulation 49/50:*Suppl.: III–228.
7. **Greenblatt, D. J., Duhme, D. W., Koch-Weser, J.,** and **Smith, T. W.** (1973). Evaluation of digoxin bioavailability in single-dose studies. *New Engl. J. Med 289:*651–654.
8. **Harter, J. G., Shelly, J. P.,** and **Steers, A. W.** (1974). Digoxin—The regulatory viewpoint. *Circulation 49:*395–398.
9. **Jelliffe, R. W.** (1967). A mathematical analysis of digitalis kinetics in patients with normal and reduced renal function. *Math Biosci. 1:*305–325.
10. **Jelliffe, R. W.** (1969). Therapeutic guidelines. Administration of digoxin. *Dis. Chest 56:*56–60.
11. **Jelliffe, R. W.** (1971). Factors to consider in planning digoxin therapy *J. Chron. Dis. 24:*407–416.
12. **Jelliffe, R. W., Buell, J.,** and **Kalaba, R.** (1972). Reduction of digitalis toxicity by computer-assisted glycoside dosage regimens. *Ann. Int. Med. 77:*291–906.

[1] Available over the international time-sharing network maintained by Network Software Services, General Electric Information System, 401 North Washington Street, Rockville, Maryland 20850, (213)385-9411. Also available over the network of Comshare, Inc., Los Angeles Office, 700 South Flower Street, Suite 1218, Los Angeles, California 90017, (213)629-5551.

13. **Jelliffe, R. W., Buell, J., Kalaba, R.,** and **Ivler, D.** (1972). A computer program for streptomycin dosage. *Fed. Proc. 31:*576.
14. **Jelliffe, R. W., Buell, J., Kalaba, R., Sridhar, R.,** and **Rockwell, R.** (1970). A mathematical study of the metabolic conversion of digitoxin to digoxin in man. *Math. Biosci. 6:*387–403.
15. **Jelliffe, R. W., Buell, J., Kalaba, R. Sridhar, R.,** and **Rockwell, R.** (1970). A computer program for digitalis dosage regimens. *Math. Biosci. 9:*179–193.
16. **Jelliffe, R. W., Buell, J., Kalaba, R., Sridhar, R., Rockell, R. W.,** and **Wagner, J. G.** (1970). An improved method of digitoxin therapy. *Ann. Int. Med. 72:*453–464.
17. **Jelliffe, R. W., Goicoechea, F. J., Tuey, D., Wyman, M. G., Rodman, J.,** and **Goldreyer, B.** (1975). An improved computer program for lidocaine infusion regimens. Paper presented at the Western Society for Clinical Research, February 7, Carmel, California.
18. **Jelliffe, R. W., and Jelliffe, S. M.** (1972). A computer program for estimation of creatinine clearance from unstable serum creatinine levels, age, sex, and weight. *Math Biosci. 14:*17–24.
19. **Jelliffe, R. W., Knight, R., Buell, J., Kalaba, R.,** and **Rockwell, R.** (1970). Computer assistance for gentamicin therapy. *Clin. Res. 18:*441.
20. **Jelliffe, R. W.,** and **Stephenson, R. G.** (1969). A fluorometric determination of myocardial digoxin at autopsy. *Am. J. Clin. Path. 51:*347–357.
21. **Knight, R., Buell, J., Kalaba, R., Rockwell, R.,** and **Jelliffe, R. W.** (1970). Computer-assisted kanamycin dose programs. *Clin. Res. 18:*137.
22. **Kolendorf, K., Christiansen, N. J. B., Siersbaek-Nielsen, K.,** and **Moholm Hansen, J.** (1972). Serum digoxin after dosage regimen based on body weight and renal function. *Lancet 2:*326.
23. **Levy, G.,** and **Gibaldi, M.** (1974). Bioavailability of drugs. *Circulation 49:*391–394.
24. **Ogilvie, R. L.,** and **Ruedy, J.** (1972). An educational program in digitalis therapy. *J. Am. Med. Assoc. 222:*50–55.
25. **Rodensky, P. L.,** and **Wasserman, F.** (1961). Observations on digitalis intoxication. *Arch. Int. Med. 108:*61–78.
26. **von Capeller, D., Copeland, G. D.,** and **Stern, T. N.** (1959). Digitalis intoxication: A clinical report of 148 cases. *Ann. Int. Med. 50:*869–878.
27. **Wang, S. P.,** and **Chiang, B. N.** (1973). An appraisal of Jelliffe's method, in digoxin therapy. Symposium, Republic of China Society of Cardiology, September 30.
28. **Weissler, A. M., Snyder, J. R., Schoenfeld, C. D.,** and **Cohen, S.** (1966). Assay of digitalis glycosides in man. *Am. J. Cardiol. 17:*768–780.

Tissue Blood Flow and Oxygen Transport in Critically Ill Patients

CHRISTOPHER W. BRYAN-BROWN, M.D.
Departments of Anesthesiology and Surgery, Mount Sinai School of Medicine, City University of New York, New York

"Anoxaemia not only stops the machine but wrecks the machinery."
J. S. Haldane

The expectation that oxygen might improve the ailing patient is nearly as old as the discovery of oxygen itself. The belief that his newly found "dephlogisticated air" would be of medical benefit was recorded by Joseph Priestly after the meager trial of being sampled by two mice and himself [35]. John Hunter proposed its use for resusciation in 1776 [21]. Since then, the desire to get more oxygen into patients has been pursued with great vigor, even though its pulmonary toxicity had been noted in the literature (albeit in mice) by 1796 [4]. Since then, the methodology, understanding, and limitations of getting more oxygen to the tissues have been, in large part, worked out. Now the problems of oxygen delivery have become so seemingly trivial that they are prematurely being treated with indifference by those who fund research programs. This will continue unless something dramatic is offered, such as extracorporeal oxygenation.

The purpose of this chapter is to outline the limits of oxygen transport and to show how present knowledge and practice may be extending the adaptations of circulatory physiology to meet the needs of the tissues in hypoxic and low-flow states.

HYPOXIA

The term "hypoxia" lacks a good definition. The common description "lower arterial oxygen tension that should be expected from the inspired oxygen concentration" is more a commentary on the performance of a patient's lungs than on an insufficient oxygen supply. Joseph Barcroft tried to face this problem when giving his famous address on anoxemia to the British Association for the Advancement of Science in 1920 [3]. In this he proposed the well-known classification of oxygen deficiencies: (a) anoxic—when blood was not filled with oxygen in the lungs due to pulmonary insufficiency or reduced inspired oxygen tension, (b) anemic—when the oxygen carrying capacity of the blood was reduced by anemia or conversion of hemoglobin to methemoglobin, and (c) stagnant—when various or all tissues become short of oxygen due to diminished blood flow.

In this paper, Barcroft pointed out that in anoxemia it was not possible to produce a predictable permanent deficit of function unless the subjects were pushed to "within a measurable distance of death" or were "elderly or unsound persons."

Later, the hypoxic quartet was completed by Peters and Van Slyke with histotoxic anoxemia [33]. This condition was considered to be of secondary importance. The oxygen delivered to the cell was in sufficient quantity to meet metabolic needs, but the cell could not use the oxygen—the sort of condition that might be due to cyanide poisoning. In the field of shock, this had now become the most grave of the hypoxic states, and when severe, has the very worst prognosis.

The study of oxygen transport to the tissues is fraught with the problem of estimating whether delivery is adequate. Oxygen transport (the product of arterial-blood oxygen content and cardiac output) was used by Nunn [31] to restate Barcroft's classification in therapeutic terms. Venous oxygen tensions and saturations can be measured as a reflection of tissue oxygenation. It is still questionable whether it is better to measure central venous or mixed venous blood. The former has the advantage that it is more easily obtained, and most of the blood comes from a region of fairly constant oxygen uptake. Mixed venous oxygen may reflect the contributions of various organ systems (e.g., splanchnic and renal) that have very differing venous oxygen tensions.

The value of oxygen tension over saturation has been demonstrated by such observations as the state of consciousness being related to tension [14] and not saturation [22] during inadequate cerebral oxygen delivery. The absolute oxygen utilization (uptake) can be used as a measure of oxygen delivery, and the efficiency of the system measured in the utilization coefficient [19] or extraction (the ratio of the oxygen used by the body to the amount of oxygen delivered). The more basic arteriovenous content difference has also been established as a reasonable prognostic and therapeutic indicator [38]. Regarding the assessment of oxygen transport in terms of anaerobic metabolism, the lactate level can readily be used to follow progress and prognosis [9,12]. Chronically maintained low-flow states, hypoxemia or anemia can be diagnosed and followed by measuring the affinity of red cells for oxygen. When the two in vivo oxyhemoglobin-dissociation curve is right shifted, oxygen delivery at the tissue level is at a higher tension, allowing for greater extraction without injurious levels of hypoxia. This compensatory mechanism can be used as an index of oxygen shortage [40]. The clinical assessment of the patient is still one of the most reliable indicators of the adequacy oxygen transport. Alterations in CNS function, cardiac arrythmias, and renal failure can all be picked up at the bedside. Although this type of monitoring can be difficult to quantitate, it often warns that hypoxia has become significantly deleterious.

The quantitation of hypoxia can be severely questioned when applied to the whole body measurement. A local, severe shortage of oxygen may be masked by the compensatory mechanisms that allow the body to tolerate elsewhere a diminished oxygen transport [23]. The normal response to a shortage of oxygen in any part of the body is an automatic or autoregulatory controlled increase in blood flow. When this is limited in low-flow states, other mechanisms come into play to conserve the cardiac output for vital organs most in need. Thus blood is diverted from skin, resting muscle, and the splanchnic region, by increased sympathetic tone, and to the brain and heart, respectively, with an elevated carbon dioxide and lowered oxygen tension. Acidosis develops in the severely hypoxic tissues, reducing the affinity of hemoglobin for oxygen (Bohr effect), thus allowing for a reduced blood flow to deliver more oxygen at a higher tension. Eventually the erythrocytes start to manufacture and accumulate more 2-3 diphosphoglycerate (2-3 DPG) and the oxyhemoglobin-dissociation curve becomes permanently shifted to the right. These mechanisms have been reviewed more fully elsewhere [9,16,40].

OXYGEN THERAPY AND CARDIOPULMONARY FAILURE

The foremost therapy for the treatment of the hypoxic state is the elevation of the inspired oxygen tension. Although this simple maneuver may cure the condition, it is surprising how many physicians avoid giving high concentrations for fear of toxicity.

The patient with combined cardiopulmonary disease may well have inadequate oxygen delivery to the tissues through both incomplete filling of the blood oxygen capacity in the lung and low cardiac output. Some of the myocardial insufficiency may be secondary to the lowered oxygen content of the blood flowing through the coronary circulation. The possible benefit of increasing the arterial oxygen content has been recorded by Ayres and colleagues [1]. Under normal circumstances, arterial blood at Pa_{O_2} of 80 torr would contain about 19.5 ml of oxygen per 100 ml. Increasing the P_{O_2} to 400 torr would increase the oxygen content to 21.4 ml per 100 ml. About half of this increase would be due to the saturation of hemoglobin, and the rest to dissolved oxygen. This would allow the same oxygen delivery to be made with about 15–20% less cardiac output or, more importantly, would allow 15–20% more oxygen to be extracted by tissues at a safe oxygen tension when blood flow is limited. In combined cardiopulmonary disease, increasing the inspired oxygen tension can increase oxygen delivery, more by increasing cardiac output than by increasing blood oxygen content [1]. In patients with established coronary artery disease, myocardial performance and oxygenation can be improved, with an increase in myocardial lactate extraction [18]. It has also been demonstrated that hyperbaric oxygenation can provide sufficient extra oxygen to improve a failing cardiorespiratory system until function is restored sufficiently for survival [7,24,32]. It is also possible that the addition of more oxygen to the system may improve oxygenation still further by a reduction of pulmonary vascular resistance.

Pulmonary insufficiency is often the limiting factor in oxygen delivery. Assessment of the major areas of acute respiratory failure is beyond the scope of this chapter [11,34]. The maintenance of an adequately expanded lung with minimal decrease in the cardiac output will optimize oxygen delivery [39].

CARDIAC OUTPUT

When cardiac output becomes limited, physiologic mechanisms come into play, reducing the blood flow to tissues that normally have a low oxygen consumption (e.g., skin, resting muscle, and kidneys). This is mainly achieved by an overall increase in sympathetic tone. Tissues that have a demand for more oxygen will then get a relative increase in blood flow by an autoregulatory loss of tone in resistance blood vessels. This is mediated either directly by tissue hypoxia or by acidosis [20]. The determinants of cardiac output are the filling pressure (preload) of the ventricles, the contractility of the myocardium, and the pressure it has to generate to push the blood into the circulation (afterload). Under conditions of normothermia, the most oxygen delivery for the least energy expenditure is achieved when the hematocrit is 40–44 percent [20]. In hypothermic states, probably because of decreased viscosity, hemodilution has been found to optimize oxygen transport.

In the post-traumatic and surgical shock patient, hypovolemia causes a marked reduction of oxygen delivery [2]. Restoration of blood volume can markedly reduce systemic and pulmonary vascular resistance and increase cardiac output. The real problem of cardiac output occurs when the circulation is impaired by inadequate myocardial performance, particularly if myocardial ischemia is present. The heart is the organ with the least margin for impaired oxygen delivery. Under normal circumstances, the myocardium extracts 60% of the oxygen presented to it in the coronary circulation. When the coronary sinus oxygen tension falls to around 20 torr, hypoxia is demonstrated by the heart, having converted from a net consumer to a producer of lactate. Coronary sinus blood normally has an oxygen tension of 23–29 torr [29]. When oxygen delivery to the myocardium is critical, the performance of the heart may be reduced to cut the oxygen requirement, and may make consumption match transport [5,6]. This can be done by reducing afterload with vasodilators such as sodium nitroprusside or alpha-adrenergic blockade [13,17,37]. When systemic oxygen delivery is being considered, alpha-blockade has the possible disadvantage that skin and resting muscle will receive a greater portion of any increase in cardiac output, whereas a universal vasodilator such as sodium nitroprusside will alter the distribution less. Myocardial contractility can be reduced with beta-blockade. The benefit of this has been clearly demonstrated by Mueller and colleagues [30], who have maintained the oxygenation of ischemic myocardium with propranalol.

OXYHEMOGLOBIN DISSOCIATION

The reduction of the affinity of hemoglobin for oxygen is a well-recognized mechanism that will allow for more oxygen to be delivered to a tissue with a fixed blood flow without a reduction of oxygen tension. A right shift of the oxyhemoglobin-dissociation curve due to acidosis or hypercarbia can be accounted for with fair accuracy. In the study of shock and low-flow states, other factors that alter this aspect of oxygen delivery may have been missed because of methodology. A typical example of this was picked up in a review of some unpublished data on blood flow and oxygen delivery to a limb. The workers found that when a large bolus dose of methylprednisolone was given to a patient, the blood flow did not change but the femoral venous oxygen tension rose about 6 torr. This was interpreted, from *derived* saturation values, as an increase in saturation from 69% to 77% (Fig. 1: x — y) or a reduction of oxygen uptake by nearly a quarter. As can be seen, if the midpoint (P_{50}) of the oxyhemoglobin dissociation curve had been right-shifted by 4 torr, then the actual saturation would not have changed (Fig. 1: x —x'). This is the order of change that can occur with this strategy [10, 26]. The data could be taken to show that the oxygen needs of the leg were being met at a higher oxygen tension. Thus, it is now usual to measure content or saturation as well as tension.

It is very difficult to demonstrate that shifts in the oxyhemoglobin dis-

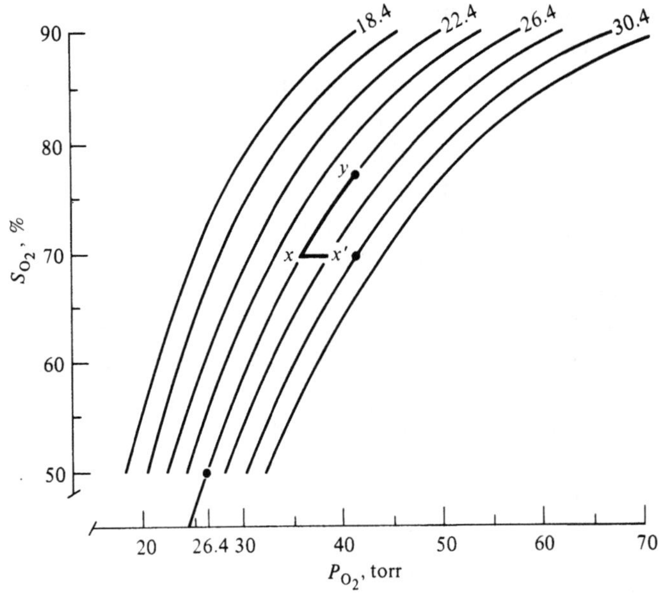

FIGURE 1 Normal oxyhemoglobin-dissociation curves plotted at P_{50} intervals of 2 torr: $x - y$ shows the change in saturation if the oxygen tension rises 6 torr; $x - x'$ shows that the same change in oxygen tension could mean no change in saturation if the curve is right-shifted from a P_{50} of 26.4 to 30.4.

sociation curve significantly affect the progress or prognosis of the patient in the shock or low-flow state, especially if the total economy of the body is examined.

Figure 2 shows the relationship of the standard oxyhemoglobin-dissociation curve ($P_{50} = 26.4$ torr) to the cardiac output that would be required to deliver oxygen at the same normal tension to the tissues. It can be seen that if the P_{50} is 19.1 torr, the cardiac output would have to be more than doubled to prevent reduction of tissue oxygen tension. This is the order of Bohr shift that would be produced if the pH of the patient suddenly rose from 7.4 to 7.7 (e.g., the change that may be seen after cardiopulmonary resuscitation when the patient has been given overgenerous doses of sodium bicarbonate). The recent presentation of da Luz and colleagues [15] showed that an 18% increase of oxygen uptake by patients with fixed low cardiac indexes could be accounted for by a spontaneous increase in P_{50} of 4.6 torr, which occurred in cardiogenic shock patients in the days after infarction. The rate of this change was probably too slow to significantly affect the prognosis of these patients.

Other compensations and alterations of the oxygen-transport system are able to mask a lethal deficit in one organ. When a tissue with a high oxygen-extraction ratio is embarrassed with a limited blood supply, this mechanism

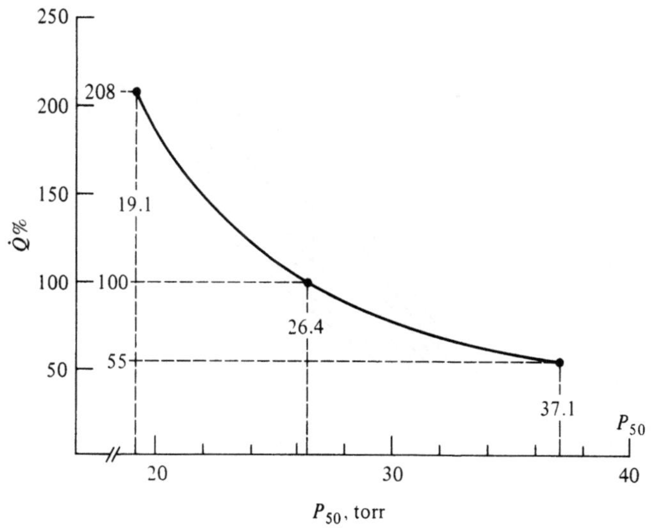

FIGURE 2 Cardiac output plotted against P_{50} to show how increased cardiac output is needed to maintain tissue oxygenation when P_{50} falls.

could be life-saving [23]. Such a region is the ischemic area that surrounds a myocardial infarction.

When the venous oxygen tension falls below 20 torr, the needs of the body probably exceed the capacity of the delivery system. It is therefore reasonable to consider any oxygen available below this tension as obtainable only at the price of deleterious hypoxia, and not actually available for consumption. [8]. The *consumable* oxygen can equally be considered as that available above 20 torr. The saturation point on the oxyhemoglobin-dissociation curve at a tension of 20 torr (S_{20}) then becomes the determinant of the adequacy of the transport system when blood flow, hemoglobin, or oxygen tension are low. In Figure 3, the lower portions of eight oxyhemoglobin-dissociation curves have been plotted with P_{50} intervals of 2 torr. These curves cover the range of in vivo P_{50} values seen in the mixed venous blood of most critically ill patients. The saturation at a tension (P_{O_2}) of 20 torr is marked on each curve. For easier reference, the curve position, as defined by the P_{50}, has been plotted against these points (S_{20}) in Figure 4. A change in the P_{50} from 20.4 to 24.4 torr could potentially increase *consumable* oxygen by over 20%, but further down the curve, the changes would be relatively less. This is the range of curve shift that has been reported in vivo from the use of pharmacologic doses of methylprednisolone [8,10,26].

Much benefit has been described by the early use of steroids in pharmacologic doses for acute myocardial infarction. The preservation of ischemic myocardium [5], with reduction of infarct size [27,36], improved oxygena-

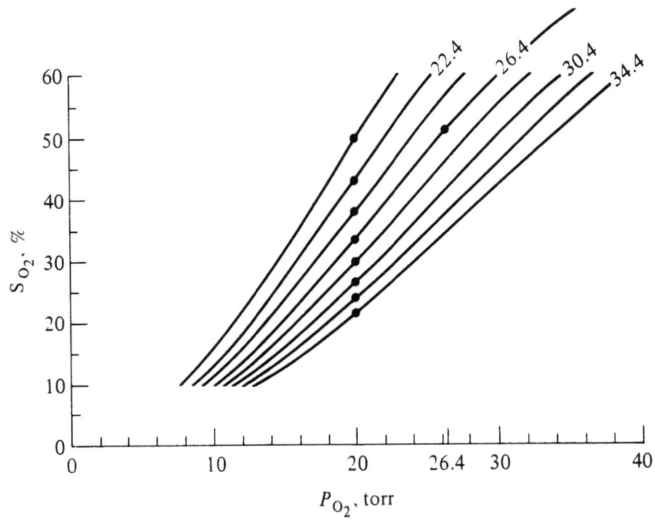

FIGURE 3 Normal oxyhemoglobin-dissociation curves plotted at intervals of 2 torr at the P_{50} value. The points of saturation at an oxygen tension of 20 torr (S_{20}) are marked. Oxygen above these points can be termed *consumable*, whereas below this it may only be available at deleterious hypoxic cost.

tion [5,17], and improved performance [41] have all been demonstrated. One of the benefits of this therapy might easily be the increase in oxygen delivery to the ischemic myocardium due to a decreased affinity with hemoglobin. Propranalol which shifts the oxyhemoglobin-dissociation curve to

FIGURE 4 Points of S_{20} shown in Fig. 3 plotted against P_{50} of respective curves. A curve shift of 20.4 to 24.4 could increase *consumable* oxygen by over 20% by a drop of saturation at a tension of 20 torr from 48% to 37%.

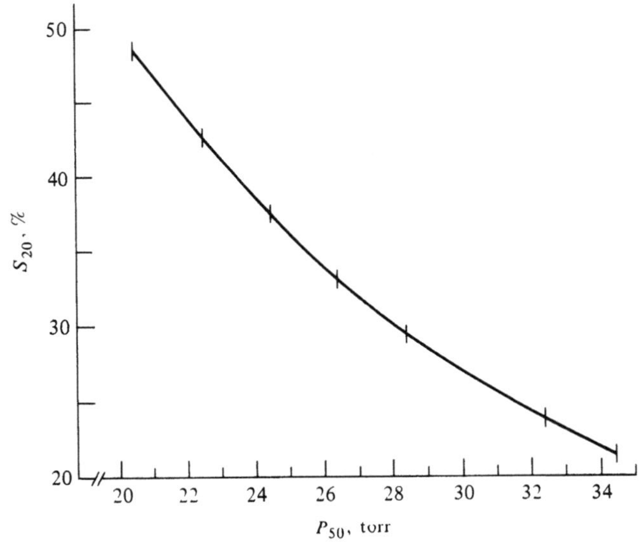

the right, but to a lesser extent, may also be of help in this regard. It may well be that these data have already been obtained and are in need only of analysis [28].

Summary

The theoretical and practical solutions to the problems of increasing oxygen transport are now well understood. Unfortunately, the quantitation of hypoxia, both as an absolute deficit and as a precise indicator of prognosis, is not yet available. In part, it is the effect of regional hypoxia in vital tissue which is not detected in the measurement of mixed venous blood.

Oxygen delivery may be increased during low-flow states by redistribution of cardiac output, reduction of oxygen uptake of tissues, by reducing the work load of an organ (especially the heart), by increasing the oxygen capacity and physical oxygen content of blood, or by decreasing the affinity of hemoglobin for oxygen. The decrease in affinity of hemoglobin for oxygen with increases of P_{50} induced by pharmacologic doses of methylprednisolone may be therapeutically useful.

References

1. **Ayres, S. M., Gianelli, S.,** and **Mueller, H.** (1974). *Care of the Critically Ill.* New York: Appleton-Century-Crofts.
2. **Baek, S.-M., Makabali, G. G., Bryan-Brown, C. W., Kusek, J.,** and **Shoemaker, W. C.** (1973). Inadequacy of high CVP as a guide to volume therapy. *Surg. Forum 24:*14–16.
3. **Barcroft, J.** (1920). On anoxaemia. *Lancet 2:*485–489.
4. **Beddoes, J.,** and **Watt, J.** (1796). Considerations on the medicinal use of factitious airs. Bristol: Johnson.
5. **Braunwald, E.,** and **Maroko, P. R.** (1973). Investigations on the protection of the ischemic myocardium. *Trans. Am. Clin. Climatol. Assoc. 84:* 80–115.
6. **Braunwald, E.,** and **Maroko, P. R.** (May 1973). Protection of the ischemic myocardium. *Hosp. Pract.* 61–74.
7. **Bryan-Brown, C. W.** (1973). Respiratory intensive care: a review with possible indications for membrane oxygenator support. *Mt. Sinai J. Med. 40:*181.
8. **Bryan-Brown, C. W., Baek, S.-M., Makabali, G., Shoemaker, W. C.** (1973). Consumable oxygen: Study of oxygen availability in relation to oxy-hemoglobin dissociation. *Crit. Care Med. 1:*26–31.
9. **Bryan-Brown, C. W.** (in press). Oxygen transport and the oxy-hemoglobin dissociation curve in the critically ill patient. In: Berk, J. L. *et al.* (eds.), *Manual of Critical Care Medicine*, Boston: Little Brown, Ch. 17.
10. **Bryan-Brown, C. W., Baek, S.-M., Makabali, G.,** and **Shoemaker, W. C.** (1974). Hemodynamic responses on oxygen delivery after methylprednisolone sodium succinate. In: Glenn, T. (ed.), *Steroids and Shock*, Baltimore: University Park Press.

11. **Bryan-Brown, C. W.**, and **Shoemaker, W. C.** (1973). Acute respiratory failure after trauma and surgery. *Semin. Drug Treat. 3:*269.
12. **Cady, L. D., Weil, M. H., Afifi, A. A., Michaels, S. F., Liu, V. Y., Shubin, H.** (1973). Quantitation of severity of critical illness with special reference to lactate. *Crit. Care Med. 1:*75–80.
13. **Chatterjee, K., Parmley, W. W., Ganz, W., Forrester, J., Walinsky, T., Crexells, C.**, and **Swan, H. J. C.** (1974). Hemodynamic and metabolic responses to vasodilator therapy in acute myocardial infarction. *Circulation 48:*1183–1193.
14. **Cohen, P. J., Alexander, S. C., Smith, T. C., Reivich, M.**, and **Wollman, H.** (1967). Effects of hypoxia and normocarbia on cerebral blood flow and metabolism in conscious man. *J. Appl. Physiol. 23:*183–189.
15. **da Luz, P., Weil, M. H., Cavanilles, J.**, and **Michaels, S.** (1975). Oxygen delivery, anoxic metabolism and P_{50} in acute myocardial infarction and shock. *Am. J. Cardiol. 36:*2, 148–154.
16. **Finch, C. A.**, and **Lenfant, C.** (1972). Oxygen transport in man. *New Engl. J. Med. 286:*407.
17. **Franciosa, J. A., Guiha, N. H., Limas, C. J., Rodriguera, E.**, and **Cohn, J. N.** (1972). Improved left ventricular function during nitroprusside infusion in acute myocardial infarction. *Lancet 1:*650.
18. **Ganz, W., Donoso, R., Marcus, H.**, and **Swan, H. J. C.** (1972). Coronary hemodynamics and myocardial oxygen metabolism. *Circulation 45:* 763.
19. **Grenvik, A.** (1966). Respiratory, circulatory and metabolic effects of respirator treatment: a clinical study in postoperative thoracic surgical patients. *Acta Anaesthesiol. Scand. (Suppl.)* XIX.
20. **Guyton, A. C., Jones, C. E.**, and **Coleman, T. G.** (1973). *Circulatory Physiology: Cardiac Output and its Regulation.* Philadelphia: Saunders.
21. **Hunter, J.** (1776). Proposals for the recovery of people apparently drowned. *Phil. Trans. Roy. Soc.* (Lond.) *66:*412.
22. **Larson, C. P., Jr., Ehrenfeld, W. K., Wade, J. G.**, and **Wylie, E. J.** (1967). Jugular venous oxygen saturation as an index of adequacy of cerebral oxygenation. *Surg. 62:*31–39.
23. **Laver, M. B.** (1974). The arthurian legend. *Anesthesiol.* 40:523–524.
24. **Lipton, B., Toth, A.**, and **Jacobson, J. H.** (1973). The hyperbaric changer and pulmonary oxygen toxicity: a clinical and pathological study. *Mt. Sinai J. Med. 40:*7.
25. **Masters, T. N., Harbol, N. B.**, and **Hall, D. G.** (1974). Beneficial effects of methylprednisolone sodium succinate (MPSS) with acute myocardial infarction (abstr.). *Circulation 49/50:*Suppl. III–119.
26. **McConn, R.**, and **Del Guercio, L. R. M.** (1970). Respiratory function of blood in the acutely ill patient and the effect of steroids. *Ann. Surg. 174:*436–450.
27. **Morrison, J., Maley, T., Reduto, L., Victa, C., Pyros, I., Brandow, J.**, and **Gulota S.** (1975). Effect of methylprednisolone on predicted myocardial infarction size in man. *Crit. Care Med. 3:*94–102.
28. **Mueller, H. S.** (1975). Personal communication.
29. **Mueller, H., Ayres, S. M., Gregory, J. J., Gianelli, S.**, and **Grace, W. J.** (1970). Hemodynamics, coronary blood flow and myocardial metabo-

lism in coronary shock: Response to 1-norepinephrine and isoproterenol. *J. Clin. Invest. 49:*1885.

30. **Mueller, H. S., Ayres, S. M., Religa, A.,** and **Evans, R. G.** (1974). Propranalol in the treatment of acute myocardial infarction. *Circulation 49:* 1078–1087.
31. **Nunn, J. F.,** and **Freeman, J.** (1964). Problems of oxygenation and oxygen transport during haemorrhage. *Anaesthesia 19:*206–216.
32. **Peirce, E. C., Bryan-Brown, C. W., Lukban, S. B., Jacobson, J. H.,** and **Rothschild, J. J.** (1973). The use of hyperbaric oxygenation in conjunction with membrane perfusion for respiratory insufficiency. *Mt. Sinai J. Med. 40:*228.
33. **Peters, J. P.,** and **Van Slyke, D. D.** (1932). *Quantitative Clinical Chemistry.* Vol. II, Baltimore: Williams and Wilkins, 1932.
34. **Pontopiddan, H., Geffin, B.,** and **Lowenstein, E.** (1972). Acute respiratory *failure in the adult. New Engl. J. Med. 287:*690, 743, and 799.
35. **Priestly, J.** (1777). Experiments and observations on different kinds of air. London.
36. **Shatney, C. H.,** and **Lillehei, R. C.** (1974). Effects of methylprednisolone on myocardial infarct volume (abstr.) *Circulation 49/50:* Suppl. III–205.
37. **Shell, W. E., Eshani, A. A.,** and **Sobel, B. E.** (1973). Reduction of infarct size in hypertensive patients with acute myocardial infarction. *J. Clin. Invest. 52:*76a.
38. **Siegel, J. H., Farrell, E. J., Goldwyn, R. M.,** and **Friedman, H. P.** (1972). Myocardial function in human septic shock states. In: Forscher, B. K., Lillehei, R. C., and Stubbs, S. S. (eds.), *Shock in Low and High-Flow States.* Amsterdam: Excerpta Medica, pp. 250–262.
39. **Suter, P. M., Fairley, H. B.,** and **Isenberg, M. D.** (1975). Optimum end-respiratory airway pressure in patients with acute pulmonary failure. *New Engl. J. Med 292:*284.
40. **Valeri, C. R., Zaroulis, C. G.,** and **Fontier, N. L.** (1972). Peripheral red cells as a functional biopsy to determine tissue oxygen tension. In Rorth, M., and Astrup, P. (eds.), *Symposium IV.* New York: Academic, p. 650.
41. **Vyden, J. K., Nagasawa, K., Rabinowitz, B., Parmley, W. W., Tomada, H., Corday, E.,** and **Swan, H. J. C.** (1974). Effects of methylprednisolone administration in acute myocardial infarction. *Am. J. Cardiol. 34:*677–686.

Influence of Pharmacologic Agents on Tissue Metabolism in Circulatory Shock

WILLIAM SCHUMER, M.D.
Professor and Chairman, Department of Surgery, University of Health Sciences/The Chicago Medical School, Chicago, Illinois

Our research activities have been oriented to the effect of pharmacologic agents on tissue metabolism in the low-flow state, or circulatory shock. Specifically, we have been most interested in the effect of glucocorticoids on cellular metabolism because these agents exert a reproducible protective effect during septic and endotoxic shock in rats and monkeys. Further, we have studied the differences between untreated animals in shock and those treated with pharmacologic agents in an attempt to determine which cellular metabolic changes are critical to survival. This chapter presents our studies and those of other laboratories, which have defined the effects on tissue metabolism of groups of pharmacologic agents: (a) those that stimulate cyclic adenosine monophosphate (AMP) (viz., epinephrine, norepinephrine, glucagon, and prostaglandin) and (b) those that do not stimulate AMP (viz., the glucocorticoids).

CYCLIC AMP STIMULATORS

Studies of hemorrhagic shock in dogs and rabbits show a progressive decline in hepatic cyclic AMP [18,19]. Evidence for this decrease was also found in an investigation of liver slices, which revealed a 30% decrease in epinephrine responses during advanced hypovolemic shock. Bitensky [1] studied glucagon's activation of hepatic adenylate cyclase in rabbits. He found that during hemorrhagic shock the basal cyclic AMP level was depressed, as was the response to glucagon. The in vitro exposure of the preparation of hepatic adenylate cyclase to glucagon resulted in a 50% reduction of the production of cyclic AMP compared with controls.

If the activation of cyclic AMP were depressed, then the effects of the alpha-adrenergic drugs would diminish. This may, therefore, indicate the need to reinforce the dosages of such drugs to ensure their important metabolic effect.

Epinephrine and Norepinephrine

Epinephrine is one of the first hormones of the adrenal medulla to be released during shock. Its metabolic effect can be described in terms of two processes: (a) glycogenolysis and (b) lipolysis.

Epinephrine is one of the primary stimulators of the adenyl cyclase system which increases cyclic AMP. Cyclic AMP then activates a protein kinase that changes phosphorylase A, an inactive form, to phosphorylase B. The phosphorylases are the catabolic enzymes that cause the degradation of glycogen to glucose units.

Epinephrine has a marked effect on lipolysis that rapidly increases the levels of both fatty acids and glycerol. Apparently, epinephrine is another of the hormones that aid in the release of substrates from the peripheral tissues for hepatic gluconeogensis. A high level of epinephrine may partially account for the depression of insulin secretion. Epinephrine in the shock state has the following functions: (a) provision of fatty acids for gluconeogenesis, (b) mobilization of glucose by increased glycogenolysis and gluconeogenesis, and (c) reduction of insulin secretion and the consequent depression of glucose utilization in the peripheral tissues, which preserves glucose for vital organ function.

Epinephrine usually stimulates alpha- and beta-adrenergic receptors in the tissues. Fatty-acid mobilization and glycogenolysis are beta-type metabolic reactions, since they can be simulated by beta-adrenergic drugs such as isoproterenol. *The beta effects are associated with increases in cyclic AMP, while the alpha effects are associated with decreases in cyclic AMP.* Since epinephrine can stimulate either adrenergic response, its effect on tissue metabolism depends upon the quantity and sensitivity of the receptors—either alpha or beta. For example, the pancreas has mainly an alpha-adrenergic response to epinephrine; therefore, insulin secretion is inhibited. But in the presence of an alpha-blocking agent such as phentolamine, the beta response predominates; therefore, the production of cyclic AMP and the release of insulin are both enhanced.

Hansen and co-workers [5] studied human volunteers in whom hemorrhage was limited to 15% of the total volume. They showed that norepinephrine also significantly raised the levels of blood sugar and fatty acids but produced no change in the level of lactate. In studies of dogs and rats with 30% of their volume bled, the administration of norepinephrine markedly increased the production of lactate and markedly decreased redox potential and pH [20]. Whether these changes occurred as a primary metabolic effect or as a result of vasoconstriction is not yet clear. Certainly, the increased rates of glycogenolysis and glycolytic cycling could increase the lactate level, and the depression of peripheral microcirculatory perfusion could produce ischemia and, consequently, cause an increase in lactate.

Glucagon

The effect of glucagon appears to be mediated by adenyl-cyclase stimulation. In a liver perfusion system, glucagon increases cyclic AMP; and, as described with epinephrine, it increases the hepatic level of phosphorylase, accelerates glycogenolysis, and augments the hepatic output of glucose. Glucagon is also a potent gluconeogenic stimulator, which utilizes lactate, amino acids, and perhaps fatty acids. All of these substrates are converted to glucose in the liver. The lipolytic effect of glucagon appears to be more pronounced in the liver, while that of epinephrine is more active in the peripheral tissue.

Studies in our laboratory have indicated that glucagon may have a salutary effect for the monkey in hypovolemic shock. We were able to show that, in addition to its microcirculatory effects, glucagon decreased the levels of serum lactate, amino acids, and fatty acids and increased the pH [22]. Whether the improved hemodynamics noted by Siegel and associates [27] is a product of an increased supply of nutritive substrates to the cell or is purely an effect of microcirculatory perfusion is not yet known. In our study, however, with the in vitro liver perfusion maintained at a constant rate, glucagon increased lactate extraction.

Prostaglandin

Prostaglandin is another ubiquitous hormone. It is derived from prostanoic acid and the dietary linoleic acid and stimulates the cyclic AMP system in cardiac muscle, adipose tissue, thyroid, corpus luteum, kidney, pituitary, ovary, thymus, brain, liver, lung, adrenal, and platelets.

Kessler and associates [9] reported the presence of a prostaglandin A_1 type of substance in endotoxified dogs, which had a vasodilatory activity that potentiated the vasopressin action of the renal tubules. This effect inhibited water reabsorption and resulted in both a decrease in urine osmolality and the appearance of free water at a low rate of solute clearance. We studied the effect of prostaglandin A (PGA) in endotoxemia and found that in 10-μg doses PGA was lethal to adrenalectomized rats and was not protective to intact rats. The effect of prostaglandin E (PGE) in hemorrhagic shock was reported by Hissen and co-workers [6], who found decreased platelet aggregation induced by adenosine diphosphate. This would have a beneficial effect on the endotoxified animal by preventing the further release of histamine or serotonin. In normal, anesthetized dogs, PGE_1 has been shown to increase both cardiac output and myocardial contractile force and to decrease total peripheral resistance. Machiedo and associates [13] showed that PGE_1 significantly protected dogs in hemorrhagic shock. They ascribed this salutary effect to a decreased plasma level of cathepsin and improved arterial pH and oxygen consumption and found no statistical difference in hemodynamics between the PGE_1-treated dogs and controls. Thus, the use of prostaglandin remains experimental at this time. Many more basic studies in animals are necessary before its role for treatment of clinical shock may be competently assessed.

GLUCOCORTICOIDS

During injury, the neuroendocrine system stimulates the production of emergency energy to maintain vital organ function. The adrenal cortex produces glucocorticoids that activate gluconeogenesis. These hormones influence various steps in the glucose pathway, including the conversion of the amino acid, alanine, to pyruvate. Further, they stimulate other amino acids to enter the tricarboxylic acid cycle, in which glucose is catabolized to water, carbon dioxide, and energy. Fatty acids enter the glucose pathways through the oxidation of long-chain fatty acids to shortened three- or four-carbon fragments and through the entrance of glycerol into the glucose breakdown scheme.

The breakdown of fatty acids can be stimulated by either epinephrine or a glucocorticoid acting on the enzyme that allow more glucose to enter the bloodstream for energy production in the peripheral tissues [11,15]. Oji and Shreeve [17] described the effects of corticoids on the cellular metabolic pathways and found that corticoid administration increased fivefold the radioactivity of free glucose produced from labeled lactate and malate. In our experiments with corticoids in shocked rats, radioactive labeling decreased in lactate and increased in pyruvate and the citric acid intermediates, particularly malate. The malate radioactivity may have been due to the entrance of ^{14}C-glucose into the dicarboxylic shunt [21,24]. The dicarboxylic shunt may allow the metabolism of energy production to bypass the anoxic block in the pyruvate to acetyl coenzyme-A reactions. After corticoid administration, Oji and Shreeve [17] found an increase in labeled carbon dioxide, which was attributed to a general increase in respiration.

Studying adrenalectomized rats, Feigelson and associates [2] reported that anoxia caused the hepatic level of adenosine triphosphate (ATP) to decrease, an effect which was reversed after corticoid administration. In Fleck's human studies [4], the decrease in serum inorganic phosphates after corticoid therapy indicated the increased incorporation of phosphate into ATP. Thus, corticoids may indirectly stimulate ATP formation.

Williamson [28] found that endotoxin in an isolated liver perfusion system produced a defect in the formation of new sugar from fat and protein stores. LaNoue [10] had postulated this gluconeogenic block in animals in gram-negative sepsis. Since it has been well documented that glucocorticoids confer protection in endotoxemia [16], we attempted to determine whether this effect is partially attributable to the steroids' enhancement of gluconeogenesis; specifically, we studied the effect of endotoxin on gluconeogenesis in the intact rat and the modification of this effect by glucocorticoids.

Fasted Simonsen rats, weighing 180–220 g, received intravenous injections as follows: (a) endotoxin-treated group, 20 mg/kg of *Escherichia coli* lipopolysaccharide (LPS), (b) glucocorticoid-endotoxin-treated group, 10 mg/kg of dexamethasone phosphate (DMP) simultaneously with 20 mg/kg of endotoxin, and (c) control group, saline. Five hours after injection, the animals were lightly anesthetized with ether. Blood for the glucose determination was obtained by retro-orbital puncture. The abdomen was then opened and liver samples obtained by the freeze-clamp method. Glycolytic intermediates were determined spectrophotometrically by enzymatic procedures after perchlorate extraction.

Table 1 shows that, 5 hr after endotoxin challenge, the levels of glycogen, glucose-6-phosphate (G6P), and phosphoenolpyruvate (PEP) were significantly reduced in comparison with the control levels. Concentrations of fructose diphosphate (FDP), pyruvate, and lactate were significantly elevated. Administration of DMP to rats with endotoxic shock resulted in levels of FDP and PEP similar to control levels, glycogen and glucose concentrations rose, and lactate, which accumulated in untreated endotoxemia, decreased significantly.

Endotoxin caused striking alterations in carbohydrate metabolism. The elevated level of FDP and the depressed level of PEP reflected an inhibition of gluconeogenesis. For maximal gluconeogenesis, the activities of phosphofructokinase and pyruvate kinase must be depressed. For some reason, possibly a dysfunction of mitochondria, the FDP level increased during endotoxemia. This in turn activated pyruvate kinase, which may have decreased the PEP level and elevated the pyruvate level. The high-energy phosphate stores were depleted during endotoxemia. Increased levels of adenosine monophosphate may have activated phosphofructokinase and inhibited fructose diphosphatase and depressed the activity of pyruvate carboxylase. The net result was a decrease in gluconeogenesis.

The treatment of endotoxic shock with DMP increased glucose produc-

TABLE 1 Levels of Carbohydrate Metabolites in Livers of Rats[a]

METABOLITE	CONTROL ($N = 10$)	TREATMENT LPS ($N = 10$)	DMP + LPS ($N = 10$)
G6P	329.5 ± 17.5	98.4 ± 21.1[b]	255.0 ± 12.5[b]
FDP	28.6 ± 3.1	42.7 ± 8.1[b]	32.0 ± 4.4
PEP	120.0 ± 14.9	57.9 ± 6.7[b]	104.9 ± 14.4
Pyruvate	68.7 ± 5.5	99.3 ± 4.4[b]	117.0 ± 7.0[b]
Lactate	1357.0 ± 113.0	3621.0 ± 196.0[b]	2241.0 ± 229.0[b]
Glycogen (mg/g wet wt)	10.0 ± 1.3	4.2 ± 1.5[b]	6.4 ± 0.6[b]
Serum glucose (mg/100 ml)	112.2 ± 3.6	96.1 ± 8.4	139.7 ± 5.7[b]

[a] Mean concentration ± SE (nmole/g liver wet weight).
[b] $p < 0.01$ (compared with control group).

tion and resulted in levels of FDP and PEP that were comparable to the control levels. It has been shown that the short-term administration of glucocorticoids induces the important gluconeogenic enzymes, glucose-6-phosphatase, and fructose-1, 6-diphosphatase. Moreover, glucocorticoids mobilize lipids and induce protein breakdown, providing energy and substrate precursors.

Steroids stimulate liver gluconeogenesis, which uses lactic, amino, and fatty acids in the production of new sugar. The utilization of these acidic anaerobic metabolites in shock decreased the concentration of hydrogen ion and consequently decreased the metabolic acidosis of shock. In 25 patients in septic shock and 25 in oligemic shock, we found a significant decrease in lactate levels after the administration of pharmacologic doses of corticoids [24]. To facilitate the analysis of these results, we used a biochemical index—the totaled means of pH, arterial carbon dioxide, and oxygen pressure. When the biochemical index and the hemodynamic measurements were plotted against time, we found that the control patients' biochemical parameters returned to normal levels 54 min earlier than their hemodynamic parameters. There was significant correlation between hemodynamic parameters and the biochemical index notably between the venous pressure and the biochemical index ($r = 0.9058$). The relationship between the pulse rates and the metabolic parameters was not significant ($r = 0.5095$). Hemodynamic changes correlated directly with the gas index, corroborating reports by other investigators [12].

In the comparative results between corticosteroid-treated and control patients, all showed increased concentrations of serum lactic acid, amino acids, and inorganic phosphates and decreased pH, arterial carbon dioxide, and oxygen pressure. The log of the biochemical index was calculated and plotted. In the control patients who survived, the biochemical indices reverted gradually to normal levels. In those who received corticosteroids, however, the biochemical indices decreased precipitously 75 min earlier than the controls.

There was a direct relationship between the biochemical index and the death rate. There was an inverse relationship between the death rate and the gas index; a high gas index was associated with a low mortality rate. The survival rate was 80% in the corticosteroid-treated group and 60% in the control group.

Protein Metabolism

Glucocorticoids stimulate the breakdown of proteins to amino acids. They also stimulate transaminating and deaminating enzymes to facilitate the entrance of amino acids into the energy pathways. Eventually, protein catabolism may be detrimental to the organism by causing severe weight loss; however, the body's priorities during stress tend to favor the degradation of proteins to carbon skeletons, which are necessary for energy production. This should add fixed acids, such as sulfates and phosphates, to the plasma. Thus, the administration of pharmacologic doses of corticoids to a shock patient, who is already undergoing protein catabolism, may increase the weight loss and compound the metabolic acidosis. Clinical experience, however, has shown no significant decrease in pH.

Fat Metabolism

Lipolysis, the breakdown of fat tissue, is initiated by the catecholamines and the glucocorticoids. Epinephrine and norepinephrine release fatty acids and glycerol to enter the glycolytic cycle. At the pyruvate to acetyl coenzyme-A step, these molecules are converted to energy cycle intermediates and ATP.

The rapid mobilization of fats during stress is vitally important to the patient, since the calorific value of fat is much greater than that of glucose or protein. Fats approach a theoretical yield of 9 cal/g, while carbohydrates and proteins produce only 4 cal/g. The use of fatty acids for ATP production, however, has the inherent danger of acidosis. The metabolic degradation of fats during stress yields considerable quantities of acetone and ketone bodies, acetoacetic acid, and beta-hydroxybutyric acid. Recent studies by Clowes and associates showed that the septic patient utilizes fatty acids preferentially to produce energy [1A].

Membrane Function

Studies by Shires and associates [25] suggested that a shift of water from the extracellular compartment to the intracellular compartment occurs during shock. Glucocorticoids reportedly reverse this shift, especially in intracellular cerebral edema. The precise role of glucocorticoids in the restoration of water homeostasis, however, has not been established. Corticoids also reportedly stabilize plasma membranes, especially in vascular and endothelial cells. Theoretically, this would reverse endothelial permeability in the anoxic state of shock [25,26].

Ultramicroscopic studies of the cell in endotoxic shock have shown disruption of the endoplasmic reticulum and the protoplasm, the presence of mitochondrial edema, and evidence of cell lysis. This may be due to lysosomal rupture. The lysosomes contain lytic enzymes, and since the lysosomal membrane is sensitive to pH changes, marked intracellular acidosis disrupts the membrane. As the lytic enzymes are secreted, necrosis and autolysis may ensue [7,14]. Recent observation by Janoff, Weissmann, and associates [8] have focused attention on the possibility that part of the glucocorticoids' effect on tissues may be due to their ability to stabilize lysosomal membranes. The lysosomal lipoprotein membrane may be disrupted in various ways, including ischemia, hypervitaminosis A, ultraviolet irradiation, and exposure to endotoxin or streptolysin. Corticoids appear to prevent the rupture of membranes and thereby suppress acid hydrolase release, an effect that has been noted in several tissues including bone, gastrointestinal mucosa, cartilage, and liver.

Fine and associates [3] have supported the therapeutic use of glucocorticoid with their ultramicroscopic studies. Their work specifically concentrated on the morphologic nature of the vascular lesion and on the effect of corticoids on this lesion. After developing a technique to visualize vascular smooth muscle with the electron microscope, these investigators identified a severe disorder of the myofibrils during prolonged shock states in all vascular muscles except the myocardium. This lesion, which could explain the progressive pooling of blood in the periphery, was shown to be reversible by a single massive dose of corticoids. Recovery in the experimental animals was sustained only if broad-spectrum antibiotic therapy was initiated [3].

We have made ultramicroscopic studies of the effect of corticoids on hepatocellular changes during shock [23]. As shock progressed the rough endoplasmic reticulum became disorganized, probably reflecting impaired protein synthesis in the liver. The hyperplastic smooth endoplastic reticulum, which appeared in the liver at the reversible stages, could be attributed to the enhanced hepatic capacities to metabolize glycogen and to detoxify drugs. In the irreversible stages, progressive hepatocellular autophagia appeared. Corticoids, however, prevented the appearance of the irreversible ultramicroscopic changes. These findings reinforced the contention that corticoids protect the integrity of the cellular membrane in an unknown fashion.

Summary

The metabolic effects of pharmacologic agents which may be beneficial for treatment of shock are reviewed. Epinephrine, like norepinephrine, increases glycogenolysis and lipolysis. It acts as one of the primary stimulators for production of cyclic AMP by its beta-adrenergic action and decreases insulin secretion by its alpha-adrenergic action. Glucagon increases cyclic AMP and accelerates glycogenolysis and lypolysis, as does epinephrine. Prostaglandins also stimulate cyclic AMP production. Glucocorticoids activate gluconeogenesis and stimulate the entry of amino acids with the tricarboxylic acid cycle. Decreases in hepatic adenosine triphosphate (ATP) due to anoxia are reversed after glucocorticoid administration and also reverses the apparent hepatic gluconeogenic block induced by endotoxins from gram negative bacilli.

References

1. **Bitensky, M. W., Gorman, R. E.,** and **Thomas, L.** (1971). Selective stimulation of epinephrine-responsive adenyl cyclase in mice by endotoxin. *Proc. Soc. Exp. Biol. Med. 138*:773.

1A. **Clowes G. H. A., Jr., Vucinic, M.,** and **Weidner, M. G.** (1966). Circulatory and metabolic alterations associated with survival or death in peritonitis. *Ann. Surg. 163*:866.

2. **Feigelson, P.,** and **Feigelson, M.** (1964). Studies on the mechanism of cortisone actions. In: Litweck, G., and Kritchewsky, D. (eds.). *Actions of Hormones on Molecular Processes*. New York: Wiley.

3. **Fine, J.** (1970). The effect on vascular smooth muscle in shock. In: Schumer, W., and Nyhus, L. M. (eds.). *Corticosteroids in the Treatment of Shock*. Urbana: University of Illinois Press.

4. **Fleck, A.,** and **Munro, H. N.** (1963). Protein metabolism after injury. *Metabol. 12*:783.

5. **Hanson, E. L., Brennan, M. F., O'Connell, R. C.,** and **Moore, F. D.** (1973). Response of glucose, insulin, free fatty acid, and human growth hormone to norepinephrine and hemorrhage in normal man. *Ann. Surg. 177*:453.

6. **Hissen, W., Fleming, J. S., Bierwagen, M. E.,** and **Pindell, M. H.** (1969). Effect of prostaglandin E_1 on platelet aggregation *in vitro* and in hemorrhagic shock. *Microvasc. Res. 1*:374.

7. **Holden, W. D., DePalma, R. G., Drucker, W. R.,** and **McKalen, A.** (1965). Ultrastructural changes in hemorrhagic shock: Electron microscopic study of liver, kidney and striated muscle cells in rats. *Ann. Surg. 162*:517.

8. **Janoff, A., Weissmann, G., Zweifach, B. W.,** and **Thomas, L.** (1962).

Pathogenesis of experimental shock. IV. Studies on lysosomes in normal and tolerant animals subjected to lethal trauma and endotoxemia. *J. Exp. Med. 116:*451.

9. **Kessler, E., Hughes, R. C., Bennett, E. N.,** and **Nadela, S. M.** (1973). Evidence for the presence of prostaglandin-like material in the plasma of dogs with endotoxin shock. *J. Lab. Clin. Med. 81:*85.
10. **LaNoue, K. F., Mason, A. D., Jr.,** and **Daniels, J. P.** (1968). The impairment of glucogenesis by gram negative infection. *Metabol. 17:*606.
11. **Levenson, S. M., Eiheber, A.,** and **Malm, O. J.** (1961). Nutritional and metabolic aspects of shock. In: Seeley, S. F., and Weisiger, J. R. (eds.), *Proceedings of a Conference on Recent Progress and Present Problems in the Field of Shock. Fed. Proc. 20:*99.
12. **Lowery, B. D., Cloutier, C. T.,** and **Carey, L. C.** (1969). Blood gas determinations in the severely wounded in hemorrhagic shock. *Arch. Surg. 99:*330.
13. **Machiedo, G. W., Brown, C. S., Lavigne, J. E.,** and **Rush, B. F., Jr.** (1973). Prostaglandin E_1 as a therapeutic agent in hemorrhagic shock. *Surg. Forum 24:*12.
14. **Martin, A. M.,** and **Hackel, D. B.** (1966). An electron microscopic study of the progression of myocardial lesions in the dog after hemorrhagic shock. *Lab. Invest. 15:*243.
15. **Migone, L.** (1962). Metabolic aspects of shock. In: Bock, K. D. (ed.). *Pathogenesis and Therapy: An International Symposium.* New York: Academic.
16. **Mills, L. C.** (1971). Corticosteroids in endotoxin shock. *Proc. Soc. Exp. Biol. Med 138:*507.
17. **Oji, N.,** and **Shreeve, W. W.** (1966). Gluconeogenesis from ^{14}C- and 3H-labeled substrates in normal and cortisone-treated rats. *Endocrinol. 78:*765.
18. **Rutenburg, A. M.** (1973). Adenosine 3′,5′-monophosphate in experimental hemorrhagic shock. In: Kahn, R. H., and Lands, W. E. M. (eds.), *Prostaglandins and Cyclic AMP. Biological Actions and Clinical Applications.* New York: Academic.
19. **Rutenburg, A. M., Bell, M. L., Butcher, R. W., Polgar, P., Dorn, B. D.,** and **Egdahl, R. H.** (1971). Adenosine 3′,5′-monophosphate levels in hemorrhagic shock. *Ann. Surg. 174:*461.
20. **Schumer, W.** (1963). Study of the effects of norepinephrine on the microcirculation of the dog omentum in oligemic shock. *Surg. Forum 14:*19.
21. **Schumer, W.** (1968). Localization of the energy pathway block in shock. *Surg. 64:*55.
22. **Schumer, W., Miller, B., Nichols, R. L., McDonald, G. E.,** and **Nyhus, L. M.** (1973). Metabolic and microcirculatory effects of glucagon in hypovolemic shock. *Arch. Surg. 107:*176.
23. **Schumer, W.,** and **Nyhus, L. M.** (1969). The role of corticoids in the management of shock. *Surg. Clin. N. Am. 49:*147.
24. **Schumer, W.,** and **Nyhus, L. M.** (1970). Corticosteroid effect on biochemical parameters of human oligemic shock. *Arch. Surg. 100:*405.
25. **Shires, T.,** and **Carrico, C. J.** (1966). Current status of the shock problems. In: *Current Problems in Surgery.* Chicago: Year Book.

26. **Shires, T., Colin, D., Carrico, J.,** and **Lightfoot, S.** (1964). Fluid therapy in hemorrhagic shock. *Arch. Surg. 88*:688.
27. **Siegel, J. H., Levine, M. J., McConn, R.,** and **Del Guercio, L. R. M.** (1970). The effect of glucagon infusion on cardiovascular function in the critically ill. *Surg. Gynecol. Obstet. 131*:505.
28. **Williamson, J. R., Refino, C.,** and **LaNoue, K.** (1970). Effects of *E. coli* lipopolysaccharid B treatment of rats on gluconeogenesis. In: Porter, R., and Knight, J. (eds.). *Energy Metabolism in Trauma.* A Ciba Symposium. London: Churchill.

Cardiopulmonary Emergencies in the Newborn

ARNOLD C. G. PLATZKER, M.D.
Director, Neonatal-Respiratory Diseases Division

ANGELA RAMOS, M.D.
Associate Neonatologist, Children's Hospital of Los Angeles, Los Angeles, California

With the first breath after delivery, the newborn infant makes major cardiopulmonary adjustments to his new environment. A failure to make all of the adjustments will lead to respiratory insufficiency within the first few hours after birth. Although the prematurely born infant is at greatest risk for respiratory failure at birth, these disorders are the leading causes of morbidity and mortality in the newborn infant. In this chapter we discuss the cardiopulmonary adjustments at birth, the pathophysiology of neonatal respiratory insufficiency, and the differential diagnosis of neonatal respiratory distress, and outline the approach to diagnosis and treatment of these disorders.

CARDIOPULMONARY ADJUSTMENTS AT BIRTH

Circulatory Changes

In the first moments after birth, the infant makes a very vigorous inspiratory effort, which clears his airways of fluid and inflates his lungs with air. The flow of air into the terminal airspaces inflates the alveoli distending the pulmonary capillary bed, initiating a fall in pulmonary vascular resistance (PVR) and resulting in a 3–10-fold increase in pulmonary blood flow. Airflow into the lungs also raises alveolar and, thus, pulmonary arteriolar tension causing a further lowering of PVR. This fall in PVR is thought to be potentiated by the release of bradykinin, a vasoactive peptide, into the circulation. This peptide might augment the dilatation of the pulmonary vascular bed and paradoxically cause constriction of the umbilical arteries and the ductus arteriosus. However, the release of bradykinin into the circulation is dependent on an adequate arterial oxygen tension. The increased blood flowing through the lungs empties into the left atrium, raising the left atrial pressure above that of the right atrium, and causes functional closure of the flap over the foramen ovale. The ductus arteriosus closure is completed within 3–10 hours after birth. These changes in the circulation, with the initiation of ventilation after birth, result in the changes in arterial blood gases illustrated in Figure 1.

Pulmonary Adaptation

Establishment and maintenance of a stable lung volume on delivery of the fetus require the clearance of fluid from the respiratory tree, a potential alveolar surface adequate for oxygen and carbon dioxide exchange, an ample pulmonary capillary bed, the normal circulatory changes at birth, and, most importantly, a mature surfactant system of the lung. Pulmonary surfactant is a lipoprotein complex, synthesized in the Type II cells of the alveoli. It is secreted onto the alveolar surface, lowering alveolar surface tension, and thus protecting the alveolus against atelectasis. This material is used up and cleared from the alveolar surface by alveolar macrophages. Recent studies suggest that the entire surfactant lining must be replaced

FIGURE 1 Blood Gas Changes after Birth.

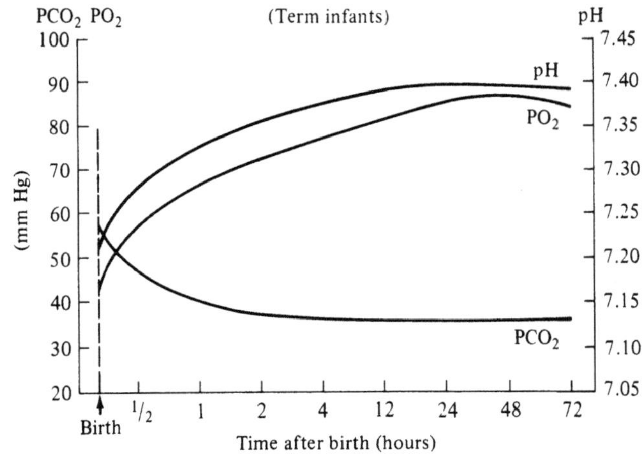

approximately every seven hours. Rapid respiratory rates increase surfactant consumption and shallow breathing may decrease the rate of surfactant secretion or retard its spreading over the alveolar surface. In addition to its primary function, the surfactant lining of the alveolus is thought to resist fluid leakage into the alveolus (e.g., prevent pulmonary edema) and protect the alveolar lining cells from direct exposure to oxygen in the inspired air.

Although surfactant appears in the fetal lung tissue as early as 16–18 weeks of gestation, its secretion onto the lung surface in quantities and at a rate sufficient to stabilize the lung does not occur until late in the third trimester of pregnancy. However, the time in gestation when surfactant is secreted at a rate sufficient to stabilize the lung surface varies greatly from fetus to fetus. It has recently become possible to monitor the state of fetal lung development prior to delivery by analysis of amniotic fluid for the major phospholipid component of surfactant. Since there is a constant flow of fluid from the alveoli of the fetal lung into the amniotic cavity, carrying with it suspended surfactant, analysis of amniotic fluid for surfactant by the lecithin/sphinogomyelin ratio or the amniotic fluid (foam) surfactant test should reveal a close correlation between the amniotic fluid surfactant titer and fetal lung maturity. In clinical practice, these tests have proven highly predictive (see Table 1).

PATHOPHYSIOLOGY OF NEONATAL RESPIRATORY FAILURE

Almost all forms of neonatal respiratory failure occur from one of four basic abnormalities in lung physiology: (a) interstitial lung disease (increase in distance for O_2 diffusion from alveolus into pulmonary capillaries and/or decrease in pulmonary blood flow), (b) obstructive airway disease (intraaluminal, congenital narrowing, compression of a large airway, diffuse intraaluminal obstruction of small airways, or hypoplasia of one or several small airways), (c) restrictive lung disease (intrapleural compression,

TABLE 1 Clinical Significance of the Amniotic Fluid Tests of Fetal Lung Maturity

	L/S TITER	FOAM TEST TITER	RISK OF RDS[a]
Positive	≥ 2	$\geq 1:2$	Low
Intermediate	1.5–2	1:1–$<$1:2	Uncertain
Negative	<1.5	Negative	High

[a] There is risk of respiratory distress syndrome if the infant is delivered within 24 hours after test performed.

congenitally small or deformed chest cavity, or immobility of rib cage or diaphragm), and (d) abnormal central control of ventilation (lack of sustained central ventilatory drive due to prematurity, metabolic disturbance, or sedatives given to the mother).

There is a miscellaneous group of disorders resulting from systemic toxicity due to sepsis, diminished oxygen carrying capacity (reduced red blood cell volume), or increased viscosity of blood and reduced pulmonary blood flow.

Many of these disorders are associated with intrapartum or neonatal asphyxia complicates the underlying physiologic abnormality. Figure 2 demonstrates the unfavorable effect of reduced pH on pulmonary vascular resistance in the newborn. When acidosis is associated with moderate hypoxia, with arterial oxygen tension P_aO_2 of <50 mm Hg, the pulmonary vascular resistance rises exponentially regardless of the severity of the acidosis. When the pH falls below 7.20, the PVR is greatly elevated when the P_aO_2 is in the normal range, and the myocardium and bronchial smooth muscle fail to respond to endogenous and exogenous catecholamines, leading to reduced myocardial contractility (decreased cardiac output) and bronchospasm.

Continuous intrapartum monitoring of fetal heart rate and intrauterine pressure can identify the fetus with asphyxia from umbilical cord compression or uteroplacental circulatory insufficiency (Table 2). Measurement of the pH of blood drawn from the scalp of the fetus can determine the severity and chronicity of fetal asphyxia. Use of these procedures has led to a more aggressive approach to delivery of the "distressed" fetus. Although the frequency of cesarean sections has increased in hospitals utilizing

FIGURE 2 Effect of changes in P_aO_2 and pH_a on pulmonary vascular resistance (PVR) in the newborn (Rudolph and Yuan).

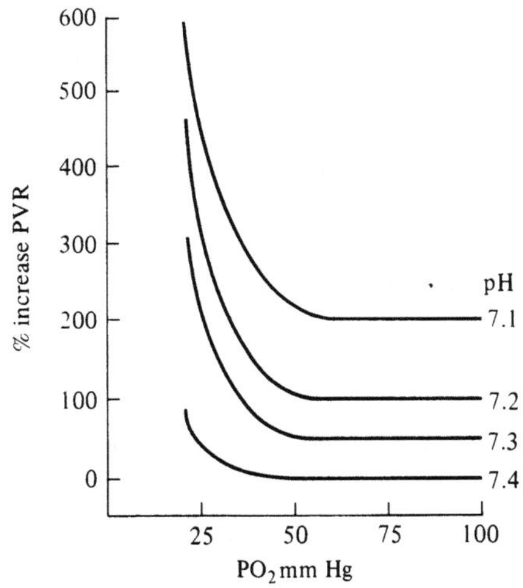

intrapartum monitoring, there has been a significant reduction in the stillbirth rate and incidence of neonatal morbidity in these institutions. Intrapartum monitoring is indicated when there is vaginal passage of meconium, a fetal heart rate of >160 beats/min or <100/min, and bradycardia persisting for more than 30 sec after the end of a uterine contraction.

While intrapartum asphyxia can lead to neonatal congestive heart failure, compromised ventilation, and metabolic acidosis as described above, it also provokes respiratory failure by compromising alveolar Type II cell metabolism, reducing surfactant secretion so that the neonate will be unable to establish and/or maintain an adequate lung volume for oxygen and carbon dioxide exchange on delivery. If this occurs, progressive neonatal atelectasis of the lung will ensue. The premature infant is at a particular high risk for this sequela of perinatal asphyxia because:

1. Lung maturity is often marginal (an intermediate amniotic fluid lecithin-sphingomyelin ratio or surfactant test).
2. The premature infant tends to have an average alveolar diameter only 40% of the adult and thus must exert greater effort to maintain alveolar size if there is an adequate surfactant lining of the lung as:

$$\text{Pressure (to maintain alveolar size)} = \frac{2\ \text{(surface tension)}}{\text{alveolar radius}}.$$

3. The chest wall of the premature neonate is more elastic than the lung, tending to collapse when the infant makes vigorous inspiratory effort.

As atelectasis becomes progressive, intrapulmonary shunting occurs since the blood flowing through airless lung tissue is not oxygenated and does not release carbon dioxide. This leads to further hypoxia and acidosis, resulting in pulmonary vasoconstriction, decreased pulmonary blood flow, and an increased right–left shunting of blood, through the following pathways: (a) lungs, as atelectasis progresses, (b) foramen ovale as right-arterial pressure again rises above that of the left due to increasing PVR, and (c) ductus arteriosus, which requires a normal arterial oxygen tension to remain in spasm and functionally close. These changes in circulation are associated with a redistribution of systemic blood flow away from the lungs, kidneys, viscera, muscles, and skin, but with preservation of vital blood flow to the heart and brain. Pulmonary parenchymal ischemia and alveolar cell and capillary endothelial damage occurs. Plasma leaks from the pulmonary capillaries into the alveoli, forming hyaline membranes.

With aspiration syndromes, the basic pathophysiologic picture outlined above is modified, the initial event being major airway obstruction with patchy atelectasis ensuing as oxygen is absorbed from the obstructed airways. Therefore, aspiration pneumonitis is an asymmetrical lung disease,

TABLE 2 Fetal Heart Rate Patterns

TYPE		SIGNIFICANCE	TREATMENT
Early deceleration	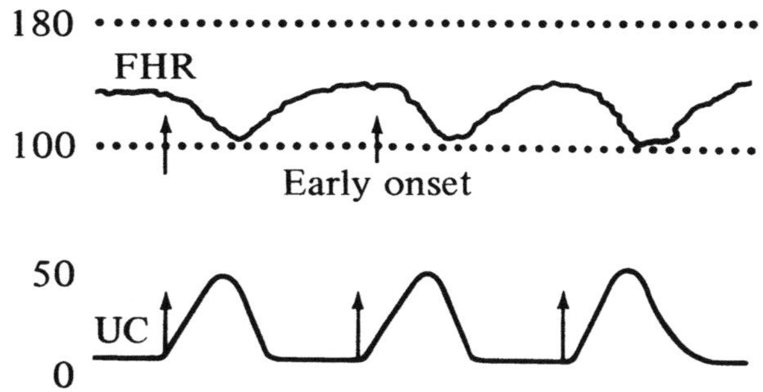	Head compression	None
Late deceleration	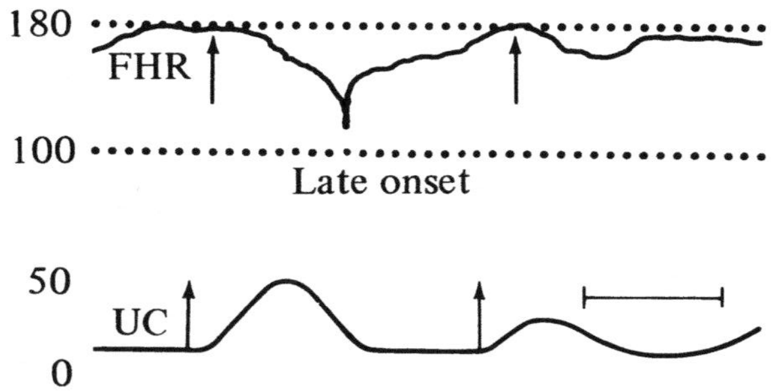	Uteroplacental circulatory insufficiency and fetal hypoxia	Prompt delivery

Variable deceleration	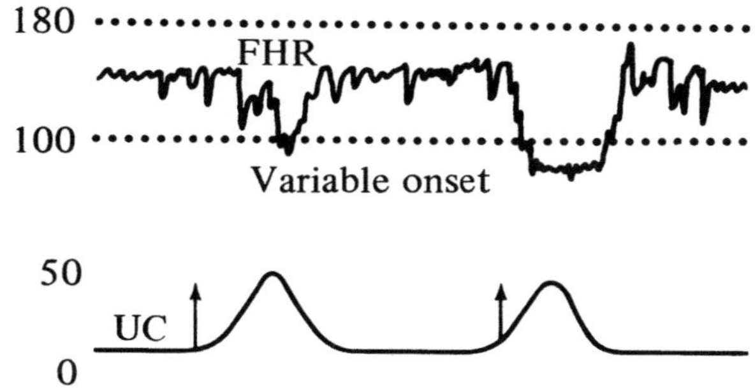	Cord compression	Change the mother's position from one side to the other and give oxygen if no improvement

FHR—Fetal heart rate
UC—Uterine contraction

overdistended units coexisting with atelectatic units. Pneumothorax and pneumomediastinum frequently complicate this condition, further restricting ventilation. The asphyxiated infant is frequently anemic at birth as acidosis and hypoxia cause generalized fetal vasoconstriction, a reduction in the size of the systemic vascular bed so that as much as 40% of the blood volume of the infant may remain in the placenta. This reduction in the oxygen-carrying capacity resulting from anemia can significantly increase hypoxia.

DIFFERENTIAL DIAGNOSIS OF NEONATAL RESPIRATORY DISTRESS

Table 3 outlines the major causes of respiratory insufficiency and failure in the newborn infant. The clinical presentation may be very variable, ranging from mild tachypnea and grunting to apnea. Selecting one or two prime diagnoses requires a careful physical examination and several laboratory studies. Nasal flaring, expiratory grunting, intercostal retractions, and cyanosis, although characteristic of the respiratory distress syndrome, are found in neonatal asphyxia and other disorders of which alveolar instability and atelectasis are major components.

TABLE 3 Respiratory Failure in the Newborn

INTERSTITIAL LUNG DISEASE

- Respiratory distress syndrome
- Transient tachypnea of the newborn
- Shock, hypovolemia
- Congestive heart failure
- Pneumonia
- Pulmonary hemorrhage

OBSTRUCTIVE LUNG DISEASE

- Aspiration syndromes
- Choanal atresia
- Vascular ring syndromes
- Lobar emphysema

RESTRICTIVE LUNG DISEASE

- Pneumothorax
- Diaphragmatic hernia
- Pleural effusion
- Asphyxiating thoracic dystrophy

TABLE 3 (*Continued*)

- Neuromuscular disorders (e.g., myesthenia gravis, Werdnig-Hoffman disease)

CENTRAL CONTROL OF VENTILATION

- Apnea neonatorum
- Intracranial hemorrhage
- Hypoglycemia
- Hypo- and hyperthermia
- Medication (mother)
  - Sedatives
  - Analgesics
  - Narcotics
  - Ethanol

MISCELLANEOUS

- Sepsis
- Necrotizing enterocolitis
- Anemia
  - Failure to receive placental transfusion
  - Fetomaternal transfusion
  - Twin–twin transfusion
  - Hemorrhage
  - Hemolysis (e.g., erythroblastosis fetalis)
- Hypertransfusion

Important Diagnostic Considerations

1. When meconium is in the amniotic fluid, it will also be found aspirated into the trachea in approximately 65% of the cases.
2. Inspiratory stridor is found in extrathoracic airway obstruction.
3. If a neonate cannot handle his respiratory secretions a radioopaque nasogastric tube should be placed into the infant's stomach and a roentgenogram taken to rule out esophageal atresia.
4. Chest roentgenograms (AP and lateral films) are also helpful in establishing the diagnosis of respiratory distress syndrome, aspiration pneumonia, pulmonary hemorrhage, congenital heart disease, lobar emphysema, and all forms of restrictive lung disease.
5. Other bedside and laboratory studies important in the initial evaluation of the distressed neonate are: (a) blood pressure and temperature, (b) hemoglobin–hematocrit, (c) arterial blood gases (see treatment), (d) dextrostik, serum blood sugar, (e) serum calcium,

(f) serum sodium, potassium, (g) ECG findings, and (h) total serum solutes.

MANAGEMENT OF NEONATAL CARDIOPULMONARY EMERGENCIES

It is advisable to have an area in the delivery suite, central to all delivery rooms, which is designated for neonatal resuscitation and where all resuscitation equipment and supplies are stored (Table 4). This area should be kept at 80–85°F. It is essential to develop a well-trained team for resuscitation of the neonate with a clearly written policy defining the responsibility of each team member. It is also of great importance to list those maternal and fetal conditions associated with a high risk of neonatal asphyxia, for which the team should be alerted and present at delivery (Table 5).

The asphyxiated or apneic neonate must be resusciated immediately on delivery as there exists a linear relationship between the depth and duration of asphyxia, the time for initiation of breathing, and long-term neurologic sequelae. The latter is predicted on the basis of the evidence of persisting cardiopulmonary and neurologic depression after birth by the 5-min Apgar score.

Resuscitation Procedures

1. Immediately after delivery the infant should be dried with a warm towel to prevent evaporative heat loss, weighed, and placed in a neutral thermal environment to minimize oxygen consumption. This is most satisfactorily accomplished in a radiant warmer with the skin temperature set to 36–36.5°C.

TABLE 4 Delivery-Room Resuscitation-Area Equipment

Heart rate, respiratory rate, blood-pressure monitor
Infant ventilator (Baby Bird or Bourns)
Two intravenous infusion pumps. Although one pump may be a roller type, the second pump must be piston-operated
Oxygen analyzer (IMI)
Olympic oxygen hoods
Heated nebulizer
Infant scale calibrated in kg
Surgical equipment necessary for umbilical arterial or peripheral arterial cutdown, chest-tube placement, and other minor surgical procedures
Hematocrit centrifuge

TABLE 5 Major Factors Contributing to Fetal and Neonatal Asphyxia

Premature Parturition
Premature Rupture of Membranes
Reduction of Placental Perfusion or Fetal Circulation
Toxemia of pregnancy
Postmaturity
Umbilical-cord compression (tight cord, true knots, prolapsed cord)
Uterine Bleeding Secondary to:
Abruptio placenta
Placenta praevia
Rupture of marginal sinus
Uterine Dysfunction
Prolonged labor
Precipative labor
Abnormal Presentation
Breech
Occipito posterior
Transverse lie
Cephalopelvic Disproportion
Illness of Mother
Hypertension
Cardiovascular disease
Endocrine disease
Diabetes mellitis
Thyroid disorder
Urinary-tract infection
Tuberculosis
Multiple Pregnancy
Maternal Medications
Sedatives
Drug addiction
Severe Isoimmunization
Rh incompatibility
ABO blood type

2. Table 6 lists the appropriate steps for the resuscitation of the distressed infant. Note that the resuscitative procedures are selected according to the severity of the asphyxia (as determined by the 1-min Apgar score, see Table 7).

TABLE 6 Guidelines for Resuscitation

APGAR SCORE (1 MIN AFTER BIRTH)	HEART RATE (BEATS/MIN)	TREATMENT
5–7	100	Suction pharynx and trachea Bag and mask inflation of lungs with oxygen Stimulate soles of feet
3–5	100	Suction pharynx and trachea Administer oxygen by positive pressure with bag and mask. If no response, intubate trachea and inflate lungs with oxygen
0–3	Absent or below 100 at birth	Suction pharynx and trachea Intubate trachea and inflate lungs with oxygen by positive pressure Closed-chest cardiac massage. If no heart beat, 120 compressions per min with lung inflations every 2–3 sec Infuse sodium bicarbonate through umbilical vein 3 meq/kg at rate of 1 meq/min Administer aqueous epinephrine 1:10,000 1–2 ml into heart or through umbilical vein

If there is meconium in the amniotic fluid: (a) immediately insert an endotracheal tube (before inflating the infant's lungs with a bag and mask), (b) apply mouth-to-tube suction while withdrawing the tube to remove meconium from the trachea, (c) connect patient to a cardiac monitor during the procedure and give oxygen, without positive pressure, if the heart rate falls below 100 during suctioning, and (d) reinsert endotracheal tube and repeat suctioning in a similar manner until trachea is cleared of meconium (~0.5–5 ml of meconium may be recovered).

If a diaphragmatic hernia is suspected, an endotracheal tube should be placed in the trachea immediately after delivery to avoid inflation of the intrathoracic bowel with air and further compression of lung tissue.

If esophageal atresia is suspected, a Replogle or orogastric tube should be placed and connected to suction drainage to prevent further aspiration of

TABLE 7 APGAR Score

SIGN	VALUE 0	1	2
Heart rate	Absent	<100/min	>100/min
Respiratory effort	Absent	Weak cry, hypoventilation	Good strong cry
Muscle tone	Limp	Some flexion of extremities	Well-flexed extremities
Reflex activity (response to stimulation of feet)	No response	Some motion	Crying
Color	Blue, pale	Body pink, extremities blue	Completely pink

fluid from the blind-pouch esophagus into the trachea and the pediatric surgeon should be summoned (to perform a gastrostomy).

Continue the resuscitation procedure as follows:

1. Catheterize umbilical artery with catheter at the level of the fourth lumbar vertebrae (confirmed by abdominal roentgenogram) in order to obtain arterial blood for blood-gas analysis.
2. Administer oxygen by hood in order to maintain an arterial oxygen tension of 50–60 mm Hg: (a) the FI_{O_2} should be increased or decreased by 10% increments to maintain this arterial oxygen tension and (b) the arterial blood gases should be measured 10 min after each change in FI_{O_2}.
3. Correct metabolic acidosis (a base deficit of >5) with sodium bicarbonate, meq of sodium bicarbonate:

$$(NaHCO_3) = (\text{weight, kg}) \times (\text{base deficit}) \times (0.3).$$

4. If there is a reduced hematocrit (<50%) or if there is a fall in blood pressure below the normal range after correction of metabolic acidosis, infuse colloid, albumisol 1 g/kg, plasma 10 ml/kg, whole blood 10 ml/kg, or *preferably* packed red blood cells 10 ml/kg through the umbilical artery, vein, or a peripheral vein.
5. Start infusion of 10% dextrose in water 80–100 ml/kg/24 hr infusion pump to prevent hypoglycemia and satisfy fluid requirements: (a) measure blood sugar and dextrostik at birth and 1 and 2 hr after birth

and (b) if true blood glucose is below 30 mg% in full-term infants and <20 mg% in low-birth-weight infants, give 1–2 cc/kg emergency dose of 25% glucose intravenously, followed by IV maintenance of 10–15% dextrose in water; use infusion pumps to eliminate blood-glucose fluctuations.

6. Start CPAP if the P_aO_2 falls below 50 mm Hg while the infant is inhaling an oxygen concentration of 0.6.
7. Administer continuous ventilation if the infant is apneic, the pH falls below 7.20 without a base deficit, or the P_aO_2 falls below 50 when the CPAP is 16 mm Hg and the FI_{O_2} is 1.0.

Selected Readings

Avery, M. E. (1968). The lung and its disorders in the newborn infant. Philadelphia: Saunders.

Avery, M. E., and **Mead, J.** (1959). Surface properties in relation to atelectasis and hyaline membrane disease. *Am. J. Dis. Child. 97:*517.

Beard, R. W., Morris, E.D. (1967). pH of foetal capillary blood as an indicator of the condition of the foetus. *J. Obstet. Gynaec. Brit. Commonwealth 74:*812.

Blystad, W., Landing, B. H., and **Smith, C. A.** (1951). Pulmonary hyaline membranes in newborn infants. *Pediatr. 8:*5.

Campbell, R. E. (1970). Intrapulmonary interstitial emphysema: A complication of hyaline membrane disease. *Am. J. Roentgenol. CX.*

Clements, J. A. (1957). Surface tension of lung extracts. *Proc. Soc. Exper. Biol. Med. 95:*170.

Clements, J. A., Platzker, A. C. G., et al. (1972). Assessment of the risk of the respiratory distress syndrome by a rapid test for surfactant in amniotic fluid. *New Engl. J. Med. 286:*1077–1081.

Donald, I. R., Freeman, R. K., et al. (1973). Clinical experience with the amniotic fluid lecithin/sphingomyelin ratio. *Am. J. Obstet. Gynec. 115:*547.

Downs, John B., et al. (1974). An evaluation of steroid therapy in aspiration pneumonitis. *Anesthesiol. 40:*129.

Freeman, Roger K. (1974). The clinical value of antepartum fetal heart rate monitoring. In: *Modern Perinatal Medicine,* Chicago: Year Book.

Gluck, L., Kulovich, M. O., and **Borer, R. C., Jr.** (1971). Diagnosis of the respiratory distress syndrome by amniocentesis. *Am. J. Obstet. Gynec. 109:*440.

Gooding, C. A., and **Gregory, G. A.** (1971). Roentgenographic analysis of meconium aspiration of the newborn. *Radiol. 100:*131.

Gregory, G. A., Kitterman, J., et al. (1971). Treatment of the idiopathic respiratory distress syndrome with continuous positive airway pressure. *New Engl. J. Med 284:*1333.

Gregory, G. A., Gooding, G., Phibbs, R., and **Tooley, W. H.** (1974). Meconium aspiration. *J. Pediatr. 85:*848.

Gregory, G. A., Tooley, W. H. (1970). Intrauterine meconium aspiration (abstr.). *Clin. Res. 18:*218.

Harries, J. T., and **Fraser, A. J.** (1968). The acidity of the gastric contents of premature babies during the first days of life. *Biol. Neonate 12:*186.

Harrison, V. C., Heese, H., and **Klein, M.** (1968). Significance of grunting in hyaline membrane disease. *Pediatr. 41*:549.

Hon, E. H. (1974). Fetal heart rate monitoring. In: *Modern Perinatal Medicine,* Chicago: Year Book.

Husain, O. A. N., and **Sinclair, L.** (1971). Studies on the cytology of amniotic fluid and of the newborn infant's skin in relation to maturity of the infant. *Proc. Roy. Soc. Med. 64*:1213.

Kattwinkel, J., Fleming, D., et al. (1973). A device for administration of continuous positive airway pressure by the nasal route. *Pediatr. 52*:131.

Kitterman, J., Phibbs, R., and **Tooley, W.** (1969). Aortic blood pressure in normal newborn infants during the first 12 hours of life. *Pediatr. 44*:959.

Lauweryns, J. M. (1970). Hyaline membrane disease in newborn infants. Microscopic, radiographic, and light and electron microscopic studies. *Human Path. 1*:175.

Leonidas, J. (1973). Pneumoperitoneum associated with chronic respiratory disease in the newborn. *Pediatr. 51*(5).

Morrison, J. C., Morrison, D. L., and **Lovett, F. A.** (1974). Nile blue staining of cells in amniotic fluid for fetal maturity. Part II. In complicated obstetric cases. *Obstet. Gynec. 44*:362.

Nelson, N. M. (1970). On the etiology of hyaline membrane disease. *Pediatr. Clin. N. Am. 17*:943.

Northway, W. H., Jr., and **Rosan, R. C.** (1968). Radiographic features of pulmonary oxygen toxicity in the newborn. *Radiol. 91*:49.

Saling, E., and **Schneider, D.** (1967). Biochemical supervision of the foetus during labour. *J. Obstet. Gynaec. Brit. Commonwealth 74*:799.

Schwarcz, R. L., Belizan, J. M., and **Cifuentes, J. R.** (1974). Fetal and maternal monitoring in spontaneous labors and in elective inductions. *Am. J. Obstet. Gynec. 120*:356.

Tsai, S., et al. (1972). Bronchopulmonary dysplasia associated with O_2 therapy in infants with respiratory distress syndrome. *Radiol. 105* (October).

Weller, W. H. (1973). Roentgenographic course and complications of hyaline membrane disease. *Pediatr. Clin. N. Am. 20*:381.

Wilson, M., and **Mikity, O. G.** (1960). A new form of respiratory distress in premature infants. *Am. J. Dis. Child. 99*:489.

Wolfson, S. L., French, R., and **Hewitt, C.** (1969). Radiographic diagnosis of hyaline membrane disease. *Radiol. 93*:339.

Impedance Reduction in Therapy of Power Failure of the Heart

H. J. C. SWAN, M.D., PH.D.
Department of Cardiology, Cedars-Sinai Medical Center, Los Angeles, and the University of California Los Angeles, Department of Medicine, Los Angeles, California

For the purposes of this chapter, the term "heart failure" is used to designate the level of cardiac output that is insufficient to satisfy the normal metabolic demands of the body organs and tissues at rest [12]. While the underlying pathophysiological processes in heart failure may affect primarily the right ventricle (e.g., pulmonary embolus), primarily the left ventricle (e.g., acute myocardial infarction), or both cardiac chambers to an equivalent degree, impedance reduction alters the performance of the left ventricle dominantly and the performance of the right ventricle in a secondary manner.

With the availability of effective and safe hemodynamic monitoring applicable at the bedside [13,14] it is now possible to optimize many of the important determinants of cardiac output. Thus, it may be shown that an inappropriate bradycardia relative to cardiac output may be the primary cause of cardiac failure, and electrical pacing of the atrium to increase the heart rate from, for example, 60 beats/min to 90 or 105 beats/min may totally correct the hemodynamic abnormality. In like manner, it is possible to optimize the filling pressure (preload) of the left ventricular at a value of 15–18 mm Hg. The Starling relationship between left-ventricular filling pressure and cardiac performance pertains at left-ventricular filling pressures of <12–14 mm Hg. Pulmonary congestion, dyspnea, and ultimately pulmonary edema occur at filling pressures of 20–25 mm Hg. By appropriate therapeutic manipulation—fluid loading or diuresis—the left-ventricular preload may be optimized so as to produce maximal cardiac output without pulmonary congestion and associated symptoms. While pulmonary venous pressure is the principal determinant of pulmonary capillary transudation and hence of interstitial and alveolar fluid accumulation, it is by no means the only such determinant, and alterations in capillary permeability and autonomic dysfunction as well as lymphatic capacitance are important additional factors. Nevertheless, in the majority of patients with low cardiac output, optimization of left-ventricular filling pressures at 14–18 mm Hg will result in the maximal cardiac output without pulmonary congestion effects.

Traditionally, the most important element in heart-failure therapy has been the use of drugs that enhance the contractile state of the myocardium. These drugs increase the velocity and magnitude of shortening of the contractile elements of the heart and, therefore, they increase the degree of emptying with, in many instances, improved geometry and a relief of symptoms. However, all of the interventions indicated above and particularly the use of inotropic agents also substantively increase myocardial oxygen demand. Reduction in preload may cause decrease in oxygen consumption of the myocardium. The increase in myocardial oxygen consumption caused by inotropic agents is equally important although variable between the different pharmacological agents. In certain cardiac states—particularly ischemic cardiac disease—there are regional differences regarding the relative adequacy of coronary blood flow, and more rapid destruction of regionally underperfused myocardium may be caused by the positive metabolic effects of inotropic agents. The underperfused myocardium, which is primarily affected by the pathophysiological process, may be unable to respond to inotropic effects and thus the overall cardiac performance is limited to the contribution of the remaining healthy myocardium, which is already performing at a normal or perhaps supernormal level.

IMPEDANCE REDUCTION

Many experimental observations have conclusively demonstrated that while the mammalian heart is an effective volume pump, it is a poor pressure pump. Progressive aortic constriction causes a progressive decrease in cardiac ejection despite the physiologic and inotropic stimulation [11]. On the other hand, the mammalian heart is capable of pumping large volumes of blood provided its geometric capacity is not exceeded and that impedance to ejection from the left ventricle remains low. Clearly, in the presence of serious myocardial dysfunction these physiological constraints are even more applicable. Since the basic hemodynamic disorder in heart failure is inadequacy of volume flow to the body tissue, it is intuitively obvious that for a given state of depression of cardiac function the heart will eject better under conditions of lowered impedance at the aortic valve. Impedance to ventricular ejection may be lowered by increasing the elastance of the aortic receiving chamber, by decreasing the resistance to outflow from it, or by altering both factors. Impedance is thus a complex mechanical property of the vascular bed, but it has been subjected to considerable theoretical and experimental analysis [8].

PHARMACOLOGIC AGENTS

The pharmacologic agents currently used to induce impedance reduction in clinical states have the common property of causing relaxation of the smooth muscle of blood vessels [9]. Largely they act by a primary direct effect on the contractile properties of muscle. By reducing the tone of vascular smooth muscle, the total systemic peripheral resistance is decreased and the total capacitance of the venous vascular bed is increased. The distensibility of the aorta may be increased if normal aortic smooth muscle has not been destroyed by arteriosclerosis. Thus, a reduction in total peripheral resistance with an increase in aortic elastance will decrease the impedance to ejection from the left ventricle with a lower diastolic blood pressure and a lower rate of pressure-rise in the aorta relative to instantaneous volume displacement. For a given state of myocardial function, these changes permit more complete emptying of the left ventricle with appropriate alterations in its chamber geometry. The actual level of pressures in the aortic conpartment will be partially restored by a larger ejection of blood from the ventricle. Hence, as a consequence of the balance between the passive properties of the arterial tree combined with the dynamic action of the left ventricle, a new equilibrium state is achieved. This is characterized by a substantively lower total peripheral arterial resistance, a slightly lower aortic pressure, and an improved cardiac performance with improved tissue perfusion. The dilated venous bed accepts substantive amounts of the intravascular volume, thereby diminishing the pressure throughout the venous bed, including the left atrium and pulmonary veins. Although redistribution of the intra- and extravascular fluid volumes would theoretically nullify this beneficial effect, in practice there appears to be a more prolonged beneficial effect.

The pharmacologic agents currently employed for impedance reduction include nitroglycerin, isosorbide dinitrate, sodium nitroprusside, phentolamine, and other agents with activity on vascular smooth muscle. The clinical experience presented in this chapter concerns sodium nitroprusside, which has a profound action on both arteriolar and venous smooth muscle. Nitroglycerin and isosorbide dinitrate appear to have lesser effect on arteriolar than on venous smooth muscle. The effects of these agents on elastance of the aorta has not been studied in man. The introduction of such concepts [3] into clinical practice has been greatly facilitated by the availability of effective and relatively safe procedures for the hemodynamic monitoring of important functional parameters in the critically ill.

Mitral Regurgitation

The acute effect of impedance reduction by means of sodium nitroprusside infusion was studied in a group of patients with mitral insufficiency of both rheumatic and nonrheumatic origin [2]. All had severe heart failure with low cardiac output and end diastolic left-ventricular pressures of 25–40 mm Hg. In this group of patients the V-wave amplitude in the left atrium was 35–70 mm Hg. All were severely disabled with the symptoms of fatigue and dyspnea. After 25 min of sodium nitroprusside infusion, the total peripheral vascular resistance diminished by 40%, the left-ventricular filling pressure by 35%, and the V-wave magnitude by 40%. The cardiac index (forward flow) had increased by 30%, and the regurgitant volume had decreased by 25%. The diastolic arterial blood pressure had fallen by 4–10 mm Hg, and the systolic arterial blood pressure by 8–15 mm Hg. All of the patients spontaneously reported marked improvement of breathing, and there were objective signs of improved peripheral circulation.

These short-term data suggested a number of practical applications of impedance reduction therapy in patients with mitral regurgitation. These included the long-term management of patients for whom mitral-valve replacement was considered inadvisable and those with symptoms of severe dyspnea, and the preoperative preparation of patients with severe heart failure associated with mitral regurgitation, particularly acute mitral regurgitation due to papillary muscle dysfunction associated with acute coronary disease. In addition, it was noted that the calculated pulmonary vascular resistance markedly diminished in certain patients with mitral regurgitation. Therefore, this therapy may benefit patients with severe pulmonary hypertension and for whom surgery is contemplated. Hence, it is suggested that impedance reduction be routinely employed for perhaps a week or more prior to mitral-valve replacement in patients with severe mitral regurgitation. The practical application of impedance reduction in the long-term therapy of patients considered unsuitable for operation will be considered in the discussion of chronic congestive heart failure and the administration of isosorbide dinitrate or Nitrol paste.

Acute Myocardial Infarction

As in mitral regurgitation, impedance reduction caused substantive improvement in cardiac performance in patients with acute myocardial infarction [1,5]. In a study of 83 such patients, all showed a consistent fall in left-ventricular filling pressure. In those patients with essentially normal initial dynamics, the stroke volume and cardiac index were either unchanged or decreased and an increase in heart rate was common. In patients with more profound hemodynamic alterations, cardiac index and stroke volume usually increased. The proportionate increase was the greatest in the patient with the least initial cardiac index. As in the patients with mitral insufficiency, in these patients intravenous sodium nitroprusside or phentolamine caused the reduction in systemic vascular resistance of 25–35%. In 43 of the most seriously ill patients, left-ventricular filling pressure was reduced from an average of 28 mm Hg to 18 mm Hg, while cardiac index increased from 1.7 to 2.2 $l/min/m^2$. In the intermediate group of patients with a lesser degree of cardiac dysfunction, filling pressure was reduced from 22 mm Hg to 14 mm Hg, while cardiac index improved from 2.6 to 3.0 $l/min/m^2$. These dynamic changes were consistently associated with an improvement in cardiac symptoms and physical signs. Of particular importance, those patients with the most severe depression of cardiac performance had significant improvement in peripheral temperature, restoration of urine flow and resolution of congestive findings throughout the lungs.

In these 83 patients there was a profound improvement in the expected mortality with 100% survival in the least affected group, 90% survival in those patients with congestive findings but intermediate levels of depression of cardiac infarction, and a 58% survival in the most affected group, in which many patients exhibited the signs of clinical shock and the remainder were in the preshock state. In these patients, impedance reduction was continued for differing periods from 3–4 hr to several days. Usually, hemodynamic improvement after 24 hr was such that the patient could be weaned from the sodium nitroprusside medication. After an appropriate period of medical treatment, such patients were discharged from the hospital. However, long-term follow-up of this group of patients was not encouraging [4]. None of the least affected patients succumbed in a follow-up period extending to 24 months. An additional 15% of the intermediate group died for a total mortality at 24 months of 25%. However, in those patients most grievously ill and who experienced a 42% hospital mortality, there was a further substantial mortality over the ensuing months, so that the survival at 24 months was less than 20%. In many instances this represented the expected mortality in elderly patients or in those with extensive heart disease, cardiomegaly, and chronic heart failure. In others, however, particularly in the younger age group, severe angina with acute myocardial infarction or sudden death occurred. This suggests that for patients without severe cardiomegaly, those who develop angina pectoris subsequent to hospital discharge, or those in the younger age category, intensive study with cardiac catheterization and coronary arteriography is essential to determine where surgical correction might prove feasible.

Chronic Congestive Heart Failure [6]

The effect of sodium nitroprusside was studied in 18 patients with chronic congestive heart failure due to multiple causes [7]. All patients had severely elevated left-ventricular filling pressures averaging approximately 30 mm Hg and were symptomatic with fatigue and dyspnea dominating the clinical picture. On the average, left-ventricular filling pressure was reduced by 12 mm Hg, while stroke volume increased by 35–40%. There was symptomatic improvement commensurate with these changes. After discontinuance of the sodium nitroprusside infusion, symptoms returned in periods of minutes to hours. Since sodium nitroprusside can only be given by intravenous infusions with continuous monitoring, it is unsuitable for chronic therapy. Accordingly, sublingual isosorbide has been tested and appears to have a relatively sustained beneficial effect. In a subgroup of the above, long-term sublingual isosorbide has resulted in a marked and relatively sustained amelioration of symptoms with improved functional tolerance. In those few patients who were restudied, a decrease in left-ventricular filling pressure and a more adequate level of cardiac output commensurate with the clinical improvement were noted. Nitroglycerin in a lanolin base absorbed through the skin also was proven beneficial for long-term use [7].

COMPLICATIONS OF IMPEDANCE-REDUCING AGENTS

In our experience, complications associated with impedance reduction are uncommon. The most frequent and symptomatically unpleasant is the occurrence of hiccup, which can be refractory to the ordinary forms of therapy and may require discontinuance of the impedance-reduction intervention. Of somewhat greater importance is the unexpected and relatively severe transient hypotension. In three patients whom we observed, these complications occurred after several hours or, in one instance, days, of therapy. Two were associated with sodium nitroprusside and one with sublingual isosorbide In the case of sodium nitroprusside, the complications probably were due to transient venous obstruction with accumulation of a relatively large quantity of infusate in a segment of the venous circulation with acute release into the general circulation, resulting profound hypotension. Methemoglobinemia, cyanosis, and adverse effects on thyroid-gland function had not been identified by us.

The development of tachyphylaxis in regard to sodium nitroprusside has been reported by others. Usually, this has occurred in patients with profound depression of cardiac function who have little or no residual functional myocardium. Our experience in a failure to improve cardiovascular function at a dose level of sodium nitroprusside of 75–100 μg/min bears a grave prognostic implication. The tachyphylaxis reported by others may represent more the total failure of the circulation than the inability of the drug to affect vascular smooth muscle when it has reached to end organs, although the pharmacologic responsiveness of vascular smooth muscle will be affected by the metabolic state of the responsive end organ. In those patients who favorably respond to impedance reduction, progressive improvement in cardiovascular function without increasing levels of drug administration is the rule rather than the exception. Thus, cardiac output will progressively rise over several hours or even days with blood-pressure levels in the normal range despite diminished peripheral vascular resistance. It is possible that this represents a readjustment of cardiac function on the basis of an altered geometry associated with more complete emptying of the left ventricle, improved perfusion of the subendocardial layers of the myocardium, and restoration of normal fluid and electrolyte relationships within the myocardial cell and in its external environment.

Seriously ill patients with profound hypotension may present difficult management decisions if application of impedance reduction is to be considered. While the perfusion pressure necessary during diastole to maintain blood flow through the coronary circulation is not known with precision, diastolic perfusion pressures of <70 mm Hg may be inadequate to perfuse the regional bed beyond a significantly obstructive coronary lesion. In addition, pressures above this value may be necessary to perfuse collateral circulatory channels. Hence, in patients with lower blood pressure, impedance reduction is employed with great caution. Left-ventricular filling pressure must be maintained at levels of 15–18 mm Hg and if necessary, by volume loading, as impedance reduction proceeds. When facilities are available, intra-aortic balloon counterpulsation or external cardiassist [10] may be a valuable adjunct to therapy in such patients with profound depression. However, it must be recognized that terminal heart failure may not be favorably effected after massive destruction of left-ventricular muscle, extensive fibrosis, and serious cardiomegaly. The level of cardiac performance, even under optimal conditions of ejection impedance, left-ventricular filling pressure, contractile state and heart rhythm and rate, may not be adequate. In such instances, the critical needs for perfusion of body tissues cannot be fulfilled.

Summary

Impedance reduction offers a rational adjunct to optimizing the performance of the heart. Normal physiological responses to decreases in cardiac output due to disease include maintenance of arterial blood pressure, frequently achieved by a relative increase in total systemic vascular resistance. Hence, although the blood-pressure level is maintained, this is accomplished by mechanisms which worsen the performance of the already burdened left ventricle. Impedance reduction may permit a more complete emptying of the ventricle and favorable adjustment to valve abnormalities. Impedance-reducing agents per se have no significant effect on the contractile properties of myocardium. Nevertheless, the reduced impedance to ventricular ejection may allow a reestablishment of an equilibrium state at conditions of more favorable geometry and performance that may be sustained for considerable periods of time in suitable cases. This intervention may play a profound role in the future management of many forms of power failure of the heart.

References

1. **Chatterjee, K., Parmley, W. W., Ganz, W., Forrester, J., Wolinsky, P., Crexells, C.,** and **Swan, H. J. C.** (1973). Hemodynamic and metabolic responses to vasodilator therapy in acute myocardial infarction. *Circulation 48:*1183.
2. **Chatterjee, K., Parmley, W. W., Swan, H. J. C., Berman, G., Forrester, J.,** and **Marcus, H. S.** (1973). Beneficial effects of vasodilator agents in severe mitral regurgitation due to dysfunction of subvalvar apparatus. *Circulation 48:*684.
3. **Chatterjee, K.,** and **Swan, H. J. C.** (1974). Vasodilator therapy in acute myocardial infarction. *Mod. Concepts Cardiovasc. Dis. 43:*119.
4. **Chatterjee, K., Swan, H. J. C., Kaushik, V. S., Jobin, G., Magnusson, P.,** and **Forrester, J. S.** (1976). Vasodilator therapy for severe pump failure in acute myocardial infarction—intermediate and late prognosis. *Circulation 53:*797–802.
5. **Franciosa, J. A., Guiha, N. H., Limas, C. J., Rodriguera, E.,** and **Cohn, J. N.** (1972). Improved left ventricular function during nitroprusside infusion in acute infarction. *Lancet 1:*650.
6. **Franciosa, J. A., Mikulic, E., Cohn, J. N., Jose, E.,** and **Fabie, A.** (1974). Hemodynamic effects of orally administered isosorbid dinitrate in patients with congestive heart failure. *Circulation 50:*1020.
7. **Gray, R., Chatterjee, K. Vyden, J. K., Ganz, W., Forrester, J. S.,** and **Swan, H. J. C.** (1975). Hemodynamic and metabolic effects of isosorbide dinitrate in chronic congestive heart failure. *Am. Heart J. 90:*346–352.
8. **McDonald, D. A.** (1974). *Blood Flow in Arteries.* Second Edition, London: Edward Arnold.
9. **Nickerson, M.** (1970). Vasodilator drugs. In: Goodman, L. S., and Gilman, A. (eds.), *The Pharmacological Basis of Therapeutics.* New York: Macmillan, pp. 745–763.
10. **Parmley, W. M., Chatterjee, K., Charuzi, Y.,** and **Swan, H. J. C.** (1974). Hemodynamic effects of noninvasive systolic unloading (nitroprusside) and diastolic augmentation (external counterpulsation) in patients with acute myocardial infarction. *Am. J. Cardiol. 33:*819.
11. **Sonnenblick, E. H.,** and **Downing, S. E.** (1963). Afterload as a primary determinant of ventricular performance. *Am. J. Physiol. 204:*604.
12. **Stead, E. A.** (1949). The role of the cardiac output in the mechanisms of congestive heart failure. *Am. J. Med. 6:*232.
13. **Swan, H. J. C.** (1975). The role of hemodynamic monitoring in the management of the critically ill. *Crit. Care Med. 3:*83.
14. **Swan, H. J. C., Ganz, W., Forrester, J. S., Marcus, H. S., Diamond, G.,** and **Chonette, D.** (1970). Catheterization of the heart in man with use of a flow-directed balloon-tipped catheter. *New Engl. J. Med. 283:*447.

V
RENAL AND METABOLIC CRISES

Acute Life-threatening Fluid and Electrolyte Abnormalities

ARTHUR GORDON, M.D.
Clinical Professor of Medicine
University of California, Los Angeles
Los Angeles, California

Crucial to the effective diagnosis and management of critical fluid and electrolyte abnormalities is a high index of suspicion. Potentially lethal abnormalities of sodium, potassium, calcium, and magnesium metabolism are all acutely reversible if recognized and treated appropriately. The significance of these electrolytes in osmotic regulation and/or neuromuscular function accounts for the predominance of neurologic and neuromuscular symptoms. Changes in sensorium, encephalopathic symptoms, weakness, paralysis, muscular disturbances, and electrocardiographic abnormalities usually dominate the clinical picture. The primary goal of emergency therapy is the rapid reversal of the life-threatening circumstances. Such therapy may be nonspecific and ordinarily requires only partial correction of the serum concentration toward normal. Thereafter, less urgent and more specific therapy can be undertaken to gradually restore normal electrolyte concentrations and prevent recurrence of the emergency states.

SODIUM

There are three prime determinants of the serum sodium (Na_S) concentration: (a) total exchangeable body sodium (Na_E), (b) total exchangeable body potassium (K_E), and (c) total body water (TBW). Their relationships are expressed in the formula

$$Na_S \sim \frac{Na_E + K_E}{TBW}$$

Most abnormalities of serum sodium concentration relate to disturbances in the relationships between exchangeable sodium and total body water; abnormalities in potassium balance may contribute but are rarely the sole cause of sodium concentration aberrations. From the following table it is readily apparent that abnormalities in the serum sodium concentration may reflect a wide variety of alterations (increase or decrease) in these interrelationships. Thus, from the serum sodium concentration alone, it is impossible to conclude which of these abnormalities exist; it merely indicates that the normal relationships between body sodium and water have been distorted. Since, in the absence of severe hyperglycemia or azotemia, sodium and its attendant anions are the major determinants of serum osmolality, abnormalities in serum sodium concentration accurately reflect alterations in serum osmolality. The serum sodium determination is an indirect measure of serum osmolality and *not* a measure of sodium balance.

Na_S	Na_E	TBW	CLINICAL EXAMPLES
↓	↓	Normal or ↑	Sodium loss with water intake, Addison's disease
↓	N	↑	Inappropriate ADH, drugs
↓	↑	↑	Heart failure, cirrhosis, nephrosis
↓	N	N	Hyperglycemia
↓	N	N	Pseudohyponatremia due to hyperlipedemia or hyperproteinemia
↑	↑	N↑or↓	Sodium poisoning
↑	N or ↓	↓	Unreplaced free-water losses

Normally osmolality is delicately balanced within the normal range of 280–300 mosmole/l by mechanisms of thirst, antidiuretic hormone (ADH) secretion, and the response of well-perfused nephrons to ADH. Abnormalities in serum osmolality must result from disturbances in one or more of these mechanisms. Hyponatremia reflects a hypoosmolar state. Exceptions to this are: (a) the hyponatremia caused by hyperglycemia, which causes a hyperosmolar state and shifts intracellular water to the extracellular space, thereby "diluting" the serum sodium concentration and (b) pseudohyponatremia, which is an artificial lowering of the serum sodium due to hyperlipidemia or hyperproteinemia. The concentration of sodium in serum water is normal.

Hyponatremia

Causes. Inability to excrete water load and maintain normal osmolality characterizes this condition and occurs due to the following: (a) persistent nonosmotic stimulus for ADH secretion (pain, stress, hypovolemia, heart failure, certain malignancies, cerebral and pulmonary disorders, and certain drugs such as morphine and other anesthetics, chlorpropamide, and cholinergic and beta-adrenergic agents and (b) abnormalities of renal perfusion or function (oliguric renal failure, prerenal reduction in renal plasma flow, and increased tubular reabsorption of sodium and water).

Symptoms and signs. There are threatening symptoms due to hypoosmolality with resultant cerebral edema, progressive symptoms of cerebral dysfunction culminating in a stupor and/or seizures, and symptoms of associated disorders. These signs and symptoms are related to rapidity of change as well as severity (95–125 meq/l).

Treatment. Administration of osmotically active solute is indicated only in most severe circumstances and should not exceed doses sufficient to correct life-threatening symptoms (i.e., do not strive for normal Na_S). The dosage formula is:

$$\text{Normal } Na_S - \text{observed } Na_S \times \text{TBW } (60\% \text{ body weight in kg}) = \text{total meq } Na^+ \text{ (to be given as } 3\% \text{ or } 5\% \text{ saline).}$$

Attempts should be made to achieve negative free water clearance. Renal blood flow may be improved by correcting plasma volume depletion, correcting congestive heart failure, and correcting hypoalbuminemia. Nonosmotic ADH stimuli should be eliminated, severe potassium depletion corrected, and free water intake restricted. Further measures include the administration of furosemide or ethacrynic acid for diuresis and renal dialysis.

Hypernatremia

Causes. This condition almost invariably reflects inability to sense or respond to thirst due to: (a) unreplaced body-fluid losses, either sensible or insensible, (b) unreplaced urinary losses (high-protein tube feedings, recovery from reversible renal failure, or glycosuria), (c) absence of thirst sensation (hypothalamic disorders, tumors, cerebral hypernatremia, or reset osmoreceptor), (d) peritoneal dialysis, and (e) salt poisoning.

Symptoms and signs. The hyperosmolality of this condition causes cerebral dehydration, resulting in lethargy progressing to coma, irritability in children, and cerebral bleeding, with convulsions. This may occur in the treatment phase and may produce permanent damage.

Treatment. The main objective is water replacement, and the formula for this is

$$\frac{\text{Observed } Na_S - \text{normal } Na_S}{\text{Normal } Na_S} \times \text{TBW (60\% body weight in kg)}$$

$$= \text{volume of electrolyte free water to correct to normal.}$$

Administer as 5% dextrose/water and correct gradually, not too rapidly or completely.

POTASSIUM

Although potassium is predominantly an intracellular cation and only a fraction of total body potassium is contained in extracellular fluid, life-threatening emergencies arise from abnormalities in the serum potassium concentration and relate to alterations in the ratio of intracellular and extracellular potassium concentration.

Hypokalemia

Causes. In this condition there is potassium loss well in excess of 300–400 meq and serum potassium is usually below 2.5 meq/l. Gastrointestinal losses are due to diarrhea, vomiting, N-G suction, fistulae, laxative and enema abuse, and villous adenomas. Renal losses are due to kaliuretic diuretics, tubular renal diseases, aldosterone or other mineralocorticoid excess (including licorice), osmotic diuretics, diuresis following acute renal failure, successful renal transplant, and relief of obstructive uropathy, alkalosis, and adaption to HCl losses. Metabolic changes include alkalosis and glycogen deposition (high glucose loads, hyperalimentation).

Symptoms and signs. These are muscular weakness, primarily in the legs, but ultimately involving the respiratory muscles and the diaphragm. Arrhythmias may be present and enhanced digitalis effects may precipitate digitalis intoxication. Electrocardiographic findings include U, T, and ST wave changes. Postual hypotension, impaired glucose tolerance, paralytic ileus, and impaired urine concentration are also symptomatic.

Treatment. Administer potassium chloride intravenously. The maximum rate should be 10–20 meq/hr except under the most extraordinary circumstances, when up to 60 meq/hr may be given with ECG monitoring. Eliminate source of potassium loss, correct alkalosis, and compensate for sodium and chloride depletion.

Hyperkalemia

Causes. This usually occurs without major increases in total body potassium, and almost always in oliguric (acute or end-stage), renal failure. It is rare in chronic renal failure except with excess potassium intake, potassium-retaining diuretics (spironolactone or triamterene), and primary hypoaldosteronism, especially in diabetics. Hyperkalemia is aggravated by (a) acidosis, with each 0.1 decrement in plasma alkalinity raising serum potassium level by approximately 0.5 meq/l (intracellular–extracellular shift), (b) catabolic or hypoxic states, and (c) extensive tissue trauma, hematomas, and gastrointestinal bleeding. There may be mineralocorticoid deficiencies, with panhypoadrenalism (Addison's disease) or primary hypoaldosteronism.

Symptoms and signs. Characteristic are progressive muscular paralysis, and serial ECG abnormalities, including: (a) peaked T waves (7–8 meq/l), (b) prolonged P–R interval, (c) disappearance of P wave, (d) widening of QRS intervals, and (e) sine wave, fibrillation, or standstill (9–10 meq/l). The changes in (c) and (d) resemble idioventricular rhythm.

Treatment. Immediate measures must be taken to counteract pH and blood-sugar imbalance (extracellular–intracellular shift) and cardiotoxicity and to restrict potassium intake. Correct acidosis or induce alkalosis with intravenous sodium bicarbonate; 7.5% $NaHCO_3$ provides 44 meq/50 ml and dose should be administered to tolerance level until critical ECG changes are reversed. For diabetic patients, give glucose ± regular insulin in dose of 1 unit/2 g glucose and for nondiabetic patients, give 1 unit/4 g glucose. For cardiotoxicity, administer calcium gluconate intravenously with repetitive 1-g doses of 10% solution up to tolerance level until critical ECG changes are reversed. Digitalis is rarely used. Avoid potassium intake and drugs such as potassium penicillin, spironolactone, and triamterene, and attempt to remove potassium from the body by: (a) dialysis (peritoneal method preferable since it can be immediately instituted and protects against excessive sodium, alkali, and calcium loads), (b) potassium-exchange resins (Kayexelate, 5–10 g orally with 30 cc of Sorbitol to prevent obstruction or Kayexelate retention enemas, 25 g; 1 g Kayexelate adsorbs 1–2 meq K^+ and liberates 1–2 meq Na^+), (c) potassium-purging diuretics in patients capable of responding to them (furosemide IV, 40–1000 mg), and (d) steroids in case of adrenal insufficiency. Correct catabolic and hypoxic states and evacuate hematomas or gastrointestinal blood reservoirs.

DIVALENT CATIONS

Life-threatening abnormalities of divalent cation concentrations are less common than sodium and potassium abnormalities and are also less often suspected or detected. Any critically ill patients with cerebral or neuromuscular symptoms not otherwise well explained should have serum calcium and magnesium analyses.

Hypercalcemia

Causes. These include: (a) hyperparathyroidism, (b) PTH-like substances due to metastases of certain types of malignancy (bronchi, kidney, ovary, colon, but *not* breast), effects of therapy (e.g., hormonal, breast), (c) vitamin D excess (sarcoidosis), (d) milk–alkali syndrome, (e) immobilization, (f) hyper- or hypothyroidism, adrenocortical insufficiency, and (g) recovery from renal failure.

Symptoms and signs. The chief symptoms are vomiting, dehydration, confusion, unconsciousness, and kidney malfunction or failure. There may be associated chemical changes such as hypokalemia, hypomagnesemia, alkalosis, and hyperchloremia. The ECG picture may show shortened QT and nonspecific ST–T changes.

Treatment. This consists mainly of: (a) hydration and diuretics (furosemide), (b) intravenous (or oral) inorganic phosphate (50 mmole (1.5 g) phosphorus in 6–8 hr; do not repeat within 24 hr), (c) sodium sulfate infusions (38.9 g) sodium sulfate decahydrate per liter H_2O; 3 liters/9 hr, (d) oral cellulose phosphate (10–20 g/day), (e) mithramycin (inhibits RNA synthesis and bone resorption), (f) peritoneal or hemodialysis (preferably with calcium-free dialysate), (g) calcitonin (not yet available), and (h) parathyroidectomy, as an emergency measure. One should also restrict calcium intake, correct the underlying disorder, and administer steroids (except in hyperparathyroidism). In high or prolonged doses, inorganic phosphate can be lethal if there is excessive calcium fall, especially with renal insufficiency. It acts by decreasing bone resorption with deposition of calcium in bone and soft tissue. Sodium sulfate acts by enhancing urinary calcium excretion; it may aggravate hypokalemia and hypomagnesemia. It may also cause congestive heart failure or hypernatremia.

Hypocalcemia

Causes. Low blood-calcium levels result due to: (a) hypoparathyroidism (true or pseudo), (b) hyperphosphatemia (renal failure, IV phosphate), (c) alkalemia, (d) osteoblastic or calcitonin producing neoplasms (lungs, breast, prostate; medullary thyroid), (e) acute pancreatitis, (f) magnesium or vitamin D (dietary malabsorption) deficiencies, and (g) EDTA, citrate, glucagon, or mithramycin administration.

Symptoms and signs. These are weakness and fatigue; twitching, tetany, and convulsive seizures, ectodermal lesions, and ECG picture showing prolonged Q–T interval.

Treatment. When correcting acidosis or alkalinizing a hypocalcemic patient, treat hypocalcemia first. Administer calcium gluconate: (a) 10% intravenously (about 10% of this is elemental calcium); 1 g Ca gluconate = 100 mg Ca^{++}; do not exceed 2 ml/min or (b) 100 cc 10% calcium gluconate (10 g = 1 g Ca^{++}) in 500–1000 cc fluid over 4–24 hours. Remember that calcium gluconate cannot be mixed with $NaHCO_3$ and also that it markedly enhances digitalis activity.

Hypermagnesemia

Causes and symptoms. Elevated magnesium level in the blood arises virtually only in renal insufficiency and with excessive magnesium ingestion (laxatives and antacids). Symptoms are peripheral vasodilatation, heat sensation (thirst at 3–5 meq/l), and drowsiness (delirium at 5–7 meq/l), followed by coma, paralysis, respiratory depression (at 10–15 meq/l), and cardiac arrest (at 15–20 meq/l), preceded by prolonged QT interval and depressed atrioventricular and intraventricular conduction.

Treatment. Stop all magnesium intake, increase urine output with IV fluids and diuretics. Administer hemo- or peritoneal dialysis, and remember that such reduction augments digitalis activity.

Hypomagnesemia

Causes and symptoms. Efficient renal and gastrointestinal conservation protects against excessive magnesium loss, except in severe and prolonged starvation, protein-caloric malnutrition, and parenteral nutrition. In the gastrointestinal tract, this loss may be reflected in malabsorption and dehydration. Oral phosphate or sodium sulfate treatment of hypercalcemia, diuretics, mineral–corticoid excess (primary aldosteronism, severe diabetes), hypercalcemia may also result in Mg loss. Hypoparathyroidism or surgical removal of the parathyroid glands can lead to severe depletion of blood magnesium. Alcoholism and hypercalcemic states are a general combination of all of the above. Symptoms are weakness, neuromuscular irritability, and irritable and aggressive behavior, followed by convulsions. Frequently associated are calcium abnormalities and low-voltage ECG, with nonspecific ST–T changes.

Treatment. Begin with intravenous magnesium sulfate (maximum rate = 2 meq/kg body weight/4 hr) and 1 g hydrated $MgSO_4 \cdot 7\ H_2O = 8.12$ meq Mg^{++}. After the acute state is reversed, start intramuscular $MgSO_4$ (0.25–0.50 meq/kg/day in equal doses every 6 hr).

Metabolic Causes of Arrhythmias in the Critically Ill Patient

STEPHEN M. AYRES, M.D.
Professor and Chairman, Department of Medicine
St. Louis University, St. Louis, Missouri

Continuous electrocardiographic monitoring with prompt interpretation and therapeutic response remains one of the most important techniques in the care of the critically ill patient. Although originally recommended for patients with acute myocardial infarction, experience has shown that such monitoring is an effective and sensitive method for identifying abnormalities in a wide variety of clinical situations. A recent patient followed in our intensive care unit emphasizes the value of such monitoring.

A 25-year-old man recovering from a drug overdosage was ventilated by a volume-cycled ventilatory. Alveolar ventilation was completely dependent on the mechanical ventilator because of severe respiratory center depression. Routine arterial blood gases obtained at 7 P.M. on November 6 were essentially normal (see Table 1). At about 10:45 A.M., the next morning, the patient suddenly became pulseless, blood pressure was unobtainable, and the electrocardiogram revealed ventricular standstill. The lack of effective electrical activity was immediately transmitted to the central ECG monitoring station and resuscitative action was begun within 1 min. Intracardiac calcium and isoproterenol, together with manual ventilation by means of a self-filling breathing bag, led to a restoration of cardiac

TABLE 1 Blood Gases in a Drug-Overdose Patient[a]

	11/6: 6:55 P.M.	11/7: 10:30 A.M.
P_{O_2}	200 mm Hg	60 mm Hg
P_{CO_2}	37 mm Hg	90 mm Hg
H_{CO_3}	23.9 meq/liter	26.2 meq/liter
pH	7.43 units	7.10 units

[a] *See text for discussion.*

action. Subsequent investigation revealed a large rent in the inspiratory tubing of the ventilator.

Routine blood-gass studies had been obtained at 10:30 A.M. that day but the results had not yet been returned to the unit. The blood-gas data detailed in Table 1 implicate acute hypercapnia with acidosis as the responsible factor. The precipitous fall in pH from 7.43 to 7.10 in response to a rise in P_{CO_2} from 37 mm Hg to 90 mm Hg reveals the vulnerability of the normal body buffer stores to sudden increments in P_{CO_2}. Although the logarithmic pH notation of Sorenson is useful for clinical interpretation, the pH drop from 7.43 to 7.10 actually reflects an increase in hydrogen-ion concentration from 38 to 80 nmole/l, a doubling in hydrogen-ion concentration not immediately apparent from inspection of the pH. A quantitatively similar abnormality in the other direction, a 50% decrease in hydrogen-ion concentration, would only occur if pH rose from 7.4 to 7.7 units. From any consideration of homeostasis, a 100% alteration is significant. Consider raising potassium from 4 meq to 8 meq/l, for example, or reducing calcium from 10 mg to 5 mg/100 ml.

This case reveals a number of important points. First, the pH notation may occasionally be misleading. The curvilinear relationship between pH and hydrogen-ion concentration makes a similar pH change more severe on the acid side of neutrality. Raising the pH from 7.4 to 7.6 decreases the hydrogen ion concentration by 16 nmole/l. Decreasing the pH from 7.4 to 7.2 increases it by 21 nmole/l, while decreasing pH from 7.2 to 7.0 increases it by a striking 37 nmole/l more. Second, electrocardiographic monitoring is an important aspect of monitoring in all patients on ventilators, even in young people with presumably normal hearts. Third, arrhythmias in the critically ill patient should not be mindlessly treated by pouring in quantities of antiarrhythmic drugs. Instead, metabolic abnormalities must be identified and, if present, promptly corrected.

Electrocardiographic monitoring may be viewed as a continuous biochemical biopsy of the myocardium; in fact, more information is probably present in recording electrical activity than in analysis of specific cellular components. Electrical stability of myocardial cells is tightly coupled to oxygen availability and hydrogen-ion concentration. An energy-dependent sodium–potassium pump maintains optimal transmembrane gradients for potassium and sodium, generating a transmembrane resting potential. Myocardial hypoxia leads to a depletion of high-energy phosphates. The sodium–potassium pump fails, sodium leaks in, and the transmembrane potential approaches threshold levels. In contrast to skeletal muscle, the myocardium is highly aerobic. The isoenzyme of lactic dehydrogenase found in the myocardium favors the conversion of lactate to pyruvate rather than the reverse reaction (pyruvate to lactate), which is necessary for the anaerobic replenishment of oxidative enzymes. Anaerobic metabolism fails even when substrate is available, because glycolytic enzymes such as phosphofructokinase are extremely sensitive to hydrogen ions.

It is difficult to separate the effects of myocardial ischemia from acidosis. As reduced substrate accumulates, intracellular concentration of hydrogen ions rises, decreasing the electrical threshold and increasing the irritability of myocardial cells. Increased hydrogen-ion concentration also decreases myocardial contractility, presumably by competing with intracellular binding sites for calcium.

The overall myocardial response to hypoxia and acidosis is complicated by the associated neurohumoral–circulatory adaptive responses. Bradycardia and a decrease in atrioventricular conduction are common in hypoxia because of increased vagal tone mediated by hypoxic stimulation of chemoreceptors. The final episode of ventricular standstill in the patient described above may be due to the combined effects of vagal depression of contractility and blood pressure, direct effect of hypoxia on cellular metabolism, and accumulation of hydrogen ions. In other situations, catecholamine release in response to hypoxic stress may lead to ventricular irritability and fibrillation. A central problem directly relating to the urgency for treatment is the realization that the neurohumoral–circulatory–regulatory system evolved over centuries of prehistoric existence and is frequently at a disadvantage in modern atheromatous man. Apparently, coronary artery disease was not anticipated when the genetic templates for a control system were first laid down; a few localized areas of vascular obstruction can derail the entire organism. The response of the diseased coronary vascular bed is relevant because a high proportion of Americans over the age of 40 have coronary artery disease. While the patient with pulmonary disorders was once thought to be somewhat immune from the development of coronary arterial disease (recent autopsy studies have revealed that as many as 25% of patients dying with acute respiratory failure have morphologic evidence of acute myocardial infarction).

We recently published a report on a series of patients with cardiac arrhythmias unresponsive to antiarrhythmic drugs [1]. Prompt correction of underlying metabolic abnormalities in these patients led to correction of the cardiac arrhythmia. Metabolic and respiratory acidosis, hypoxia, and alkalosis are all capable of producing cardiac irritability. Respiratory alkalosis due to unintentional mechanical hyperventilation was first shown by Flemma and Young [2] to produce myocardial irritability. Both rightward shifts of the oxyhemoglobin-dissociation curve with decreased oxygen unloading at the cellular level and shifts in potassium presumably contribute to ventricular irritability in alkalosis. Many of the patients described in our publication had either acute or chronic coronary artery disease.

An understanding of the liability placed on the myocardium by a diseased coronary vascular bed aids in the design of an adequate treatment program for individual patients. An illustration of the importance of this information is the question of the rate of bicarbonate administration in patients with metabolic acidosis. Soon after the lethal property of acidosis was recognized, the rapid administration of bicarbonate was advocated and a group of replacement schedules based on body weight and distribution volumes were developed. The disadvantages of too rapid administration were soon recognized. Posner and Plum [3] showed that rapid administration of bicarbonate to patients with diabetic acidosis could lead to coma, presumably because of the delayed response of brain tissue and extravascular bicarbonate concentrations. Others showed that metabolic alkalosis commonly followed the overenthusiastic administration of bicarbonate, while others emphasized that an ampoule containing 45 meq of bicarbonate also contained 90 mosmole of solute in 50 ml of water and could aggravate the hyperosmolarity common in the critically ill patient.

Hydrogen-ion excesses should be rapidly corrected when they occur in patients with compromised coronary vascular beds. A pH of 7.3 represents a 25% increase in hydrogen-ion concentration and is readily tolerated by most individuals. Bicarbonate administration is probably not necessary in the young diabetic with ketoacidosis because prompt administration of insulin leads to metabolism of ketone bodies and disappearance of excess hydrogen ions. In contrast, lactic acidosis secondary to anaerobic metabolism will not reverse itself until adequate amounts of oxygen are available, an unlikely situation in most patients with circulatory collapse. Rapid restoration of buffer stores to at least 18–20 meq/l bicarbonate concentration is indicated in this situation. Our own practice is to administer bicarbonate whenever we believe myocardial integrity to be jeopardized. Rather than calculate bicarbonate deficits, we prefer to administer divided doses of 45 meq each, monitoring the response with frequent measurements of bicarbonate concentration and carbon dioxide tension.

In general, the myocardium is a tough, well-defended organ, protected against most of nature's unkind stresses. This knowledge should not generate a cavalier attitude in physicians caring for the critically ill patient. Agents promoting ventricular irritability, such as isoproterenol and aminophylline, should be used with caution. The physician must suppress his impulse to treat each run of ventricular premature contractions with a syringe-full of lidocaine and seek instead to identify and correct abnormalities such as hypoxemia, hypercapnia, acidosis, and hypokalemia. Continuous ECG monitoring of the patient with serious respiratory disease becomes as important as frequent analysis of arterial blood gases. Observation of a few salvos of ventricular premature contractions may lead to the discovery of increasing atelectasis, pneumothorax, or an errant endotracheal tube ventilating only one lung. Viewed in this light, metabolically induced electrical instability becomes an omen of serious trouble and could be considered a useful index of myocardial oxygenation.

References

1. **Ayres, S. M.,** and **Grace, W. J.** (1969). Inappropriate ventilation and hypoxemia as causes of cardiac arrhythmias: The control of arrhythmias without antiarrhythmic drugs. *Am. J. Med. 46:*495–505.
2. **Flemma, R. J.,** and **Young, W. G., Jr.** (1964). Metabolic effects of mechanical ventilation and respiratory alkalosis in postoperative patients. *Surgery 56:*36.
3. **Posner, J. B.,** and **Plum, F.** (1967). Spinal-fluid pH and neurologic symptoms in systemic acidosis. *N. Engl. J. Med. 227:*605.

Nutrition of the Critically Ill and Traumatized Patient: Parenteral Alimentation

WILLIAM SCHUMER, M.D.
Professor and Chairman, Department of Surgery, University of Health Sciences/The Chicago Medical School, Chicago, Illinois

The human organism responds to trauma or disease by stimulating the hypothalamus, the pituitary gland, and the adrenal cortex. The hypothalamopituitary complex secretes somatotropic, adrenocorticotropic, thyrotropic, and antidiuretic (ADH) hormones. This endocrine response has two major consequences: (a) the combined effect of ADH and adrenal mineralocorticoid hormones conserving water to maintain blood volume and (b) the pituitary–adrenal axis secreting glucocorticoids to mobilize amino and fatty acids for sugar production, stimulating the adrenal medulla to secrete epinephrine for the catabolism of glycogen to sugar, and aiding the induction of lipid and protein catabolism. This accelerated breakdown of fats and proteins is the main cause of weight loss during disease and trauma. The secretion of somatotropic hormones, which usually begins on the third day of disease or trauma, increases the serum concentration of glucose by mobilizing additional fats and proteins. At the same time, the stimulated thyroid accelerates metabolism and the utilization of glucose.

GLUCONEOGENESIS DURING STRESS

Glucose is the principal molecule for energy formation. The cytosol, or cell sap, contains enzymes that catalyze the anaerobic metabolism of glucose intermediates; the mitochondria contain enzymes that complete the aerobic metabolism of glucose. Adenosine triphosphate (ATP), the energy molecule, is produced in the mitochondria by the electron-transport system. This molecule stores the energy released by the oxidation of glucose as potential chemical energy and fuels the molecular reactions that build proteins and maintain the integrity of the cellular membrane.

Glucose can be stored in glycogen molecules in liver and muscle; however, during stress such as surgery, these stores are rapidly dissipated. Other molecules are needed that can be converted either to glucose or to intermediates of the energy cycles, and these are available as fats and proteins. Fats are oxidized to fatty acids and converted to the intermediates of the energy cycles, glycerol and acetyl coenzyme-A. Proteins are catabolized to glycogenic amino acids, which can also be converted to energy-cycle intermediates.

There are many examples of the effect of stress on gluconeogenesis. Bacterial endotoxin administered parenterally has been shown to induce marked disturbances in carbohydrate metabolism. In the mouse, rat, and monkey, these disturbances appear as rapid depletion of hepatic glycogen, hypoglycemia, and an inability of the liver to synthesize glycogen and sugar from glucogenic amino and fatty acids [5]. McCallum and Berry [7] demonstrated that endotoxemia depressed the activity of the liver enzymes responsible for gluconeogenesis. LaNoue, Mason, and others [6] showed that endotoxin poisoning reduced the rate of glucose production in the liver. Williamson, Refino, and others [9] showed that endotoxemia depressed lactate metabolism in the liver. Lactate is one of the main precursors of sugar production in the hepatic Cori cycle. Thus, these alterations reflect endotoxin induced changes in the level of blood sugar necessary for peripheral cellular metabolism. In our laboratory we have seen similar effects in intact endotoxified rats and primates. Most significant was the fact that the primates died in hypoglycemia after 5–8 hours of endotoxemia [5]. This indicated that in these animals endotoxin had a profound effect on the production and perhaps the utilization of sugar.

Preliminary study seems to indicate that the hypovolemic animal also undergoes a depression of hepatic gluconeogenesis. Apparently, this inability to produce sugar from gluconeogenic precursors is an essential disturbance of liver glucose metabolism in the hypovolemic and the septic animal. Thus, when the glycogen stores of liver and muscle are insufficient to supply the long-term glucose needs and the process of gluconeogenesis is inhibited, the shock-stressed organism needs an exogenous source of sugar.

HYPERALIMENTATION

The efficacy of administering glucose as a substrate in traumatic and hypovolemic shock has been shown experimentally. Buonous, Sutherland, and associates [2] have shown that glucose protects the anoxic bowel segment, especially its mucosal function. Drucker, Pindyck, and associates [3] have recently reported that when highly concentrated glucose was administered to hypovolemic and traumatic shock patients, the function of vital organs—specifically the heart and the kidney—was improved. The studies by Baue [1] showed that the administration of ATP-magnesium protects the shocked animal and also reinforced the concept that glucose administration is necessary to fulfill the energy requirements of the stressed organism.

There is a secondary advantage to nutritional therapy in the stressed patient. We recorded the serum amino acids and the serum nonessential fatty acids in 20 patients who underwent gastric resection. Fatty and amino acids increased three- to fourfold in the 10 patients who did not receive glucose. In those patients who received 25% glucose intravenously, the serum fatty and amino acids remained within normal limits. This indicated that the infused glucose decreased the catabolism of proteins and fats and thus decreased the amino- and fatty-acid components of stress-induced metabolic acidosis.

Parenteral alimentation has a protein-sparing effect on the total organism. The infusion of glucose and amino acids obviates the need for endogenous protein and fat stores, resulting in decreased catabolism, more positive nitrogen balance, and less weight loss. The conservation of muscle protein allows the patient increased activity. Hyperalimentation decreases the energy deficit, increases protein synthesis, and promotes wound healing. Moreover, hyperosmotic parenteral solutions act as osmotic diuretics during the antidiuretic phase of trauma, protecting the kidney against acute insufficiency. The overall result is a significant shortening of the convalescent period.

Glucose. There are many kinds of energy-producing molecules, but the most important component of any formula is glucose. It is a 6-carbon molecule, which yields a significant amount of energy when systematically oxidized. One molecule completely degraded yields 288,800 calories to promote essential biochemical reactions. Glucose is the main energy source, but any molecule that can be transformed into the intermediates of the energy pathway is capable of producing ATP. For example, fructose, mannitol, or xylitol can be used as a glucose substitute. All tissues, however, cannot utilize them. The brain does not metabolize fructose or mannitol, and the liver reacts adversely to xylitol [8]. Glucose, therefore, remains the most desirable energy molecule.

Insulin and potassium. Sugar in high concentrations requires insulin to be completely metabolized. In muscle, adipose tissue, and liver, insulin facilitates the intracellular transport of glucose and amino acids, a function that requires phosphate and potassium ions. Therefore, most hyperalimentation formulas include insulin and potassium, according to the patient's individual needs.

Amino acids. Another component of the hyperalimentation formula is amino acid, which yields 4 cal/g. There are two types of amino acid: (a) nonessential, which cannot be synthesized in the human tissue cell and (b) essential, which can be synthesized. Essential amino acids include tryptophan, phenylalanine, lysine, threonine, valine, methionine, leucine, and isoleucine. Their natural structures are primarily L-forms; that is, the amine (NH_2) radical is in the *levo-* (left) configuration. Protein hydrolysates must contain these essential amino acids, since no others can be efficiently metabolized by the body. Not all amino acids can be changed into energy-cycle intermediates; those that can be converted are referred to as glycogenic amino acids. This designation cannot be attributed to any particular configuration of their structure; but, interestingly, all glycogenic amino acids are of the essential type.

Of the nonglycogenic amino acids, histidine is usually included in protein hydrolysate infusions because after numerous reactions it can be converted to pyruvic or glutamic acids, both of which are intermediates of the energy cycles. Some essential amino acids such as leucine are ketogenic, since they can be converted to fatty-acid structures. They contribute to the glyconeogenic scheme by augmenting the conversion of fatty acids to energy intermediates. Thus, protein hydrolysate or amino acid solution both provide the patient with the essential amino acids for tissue repair and add calories for direct energy formation.

Vitamins. The fourth component of the hyperalimentation formula is vitamin. The vitamin B complex is essential for the proper functioning of the energy pathways. The coenzyme thiamine plays an integral role in the conversion of the energy pathways from anaerobic to aerobic function. Riboflavin and nicotinic acid are integrants of the two main components of the electron transport system. Pantothenic acid in coenzyme-A is involved in the conversion of fatty acids into energy-cycle intermediates. Pyridoxine is a component of the coenzyme that either deaminates or transaminates amino acids to glucose skeletons for entrance into the energy pathways. Lipoic acid takes part in the specific oxidation of pyruvate and succinate in the aerobic energy cycle. Vitamin B_{12}, or cyanocobalamin, is vital for the maturation of red blood cells and yields hydrogen ions, which are important in the formation of the specific amino acids required for the production of hemoglobin. Its deficiency results in the formation of immature red blood cells.

The precise role of vitamin C is unknown, but it apparently supplies both the hydrogen ions essential in the production of mature collagen and the

OH^- radicals necessary for the hydroxylation of proline into hydroxyproline, an integral amino acid in collagen.

Minerals. Several minerals are necessary for the efficient functioning of the energy cycles. Potassium supports the enzymatic activity needed for protein synthesis as well as the transport of glucose across the cellular membrane. Magnesium is the catalyst for the enzymes of the glycolytic energy cycles. Sodium and probably chloride are important ions in the maintenance of osmolarity. The trace elements—copper, cobalt, manganese, zinc, and iodine—are associated with important enzyme functions. These elements are added to the parenteral formula when the patient is to receive hyperalimentation for more than 2 weeks.

Fat Emulsions

Although glucose and amino acids are the mainstay of parenteral hyperalimentation the use of intravenous feedings of fats has increased [4]. Their advantage is that they produce 9 calories per gram, more than either glucose or amino acids. One liter of 15% fat emulsion provides more than 1350 calories, as compared to 1 liter of 6% ethanol or 5% glucose, which yield only 420 and 200 calories, respectively. Lipomul was an early form of fat emulsion made from cotton seed. Patients who received daily infusions of this preparation developed fever, jaundice, epigastric pain, gastrointestinal bleeding, and loss of appetite. It is no longer available in the United States, but it and several similar preparations are currently in use in Europe. Lypofundin, a cottonseed oil and soybean phosphatide emulsion, is popular in Germany; and Intralipid, a soybean oil and lecithin emulsion, is used in Sweden and the United States.

These emulsions contain palmitic, oleic, and linoleic acids and small amounts of linolenic acid, all of which enter the bloodstream as particulate fats or chylomicrons. The particles are composed of triglycerides (fatty acids plus glycerol) linked with cholesterol and traces of protein. When directly infused into the bloodstream, they may be degraded to glycerol and fatty acids or transported as intact triglycerides to the receptive cells in the liver, muscle, brain, and kidney. Chylomicrons containing greater amounts of protein are referred to as lipoproteins. The clearing factor, lipoprotein lipase, works in both the cell and the blood to hydrolyze the triglyceride to fatty acid and glycerol, which can then be converted to intermediates of the glycolytic and oxidative (Krebs) cycles.

Unfavorable Effects of Hyperalimentation

There have been reports of unfavorable physiological and biochemical alterations caused by parenteral hyperalimentation [10]. High-volume infusion for 2–3 days can cause excessive water loss and increase the serum level of chlorides. We have not seen any untoward clinical effect resulting from this increased concentration, but if hyperosmotic hyperalimentation is continued, a true dehydration can occur secondary to high urine output—osmotic diuresis. This condition can be prevented by the careful monitoring of glucose excretion in the urine and the replacement of water by an additional intravenous infusion of 5% glucose either in water or in Ringer's solution.

Cases of hyperosmolar diabetes have developed with the use of hyperalimentation, usually in patients having blood-sugar levels above 500 mg% [10]. They may gradually become disoriented, lethargic, apathetic, and stuperous, exhibiting an electrolyte imbalance of high sodium, high chloride, and high blood urea nitrogen. Serum glucose may increase to as much as 1500 mg%, and there is often a normal concentration of acetone in the serum associated with a high urinary output of 2–4 l daily. A history of diabetes mellitus may or may not be present. In these cases hyperalimentation must be terminated at once and high doses of insulin (100–200 units) with large volumes of 5% glucose in water must be administered.

Another abnormality occurring during hyperalimentation is increased serum alkaline phosphatase. The cause is unknown, but the condition disappears when hyperalimentation is decreased. Recent studies have indicated that all forms of hyperalimentation can produce a colistatic hepatitis characterized by increased liver enzymes, bilirubin, and alkaline phosphatase. The obviation of this complication is the use of a cyclic hyperalimentation regime as described by Blackburn [1A]. Some allergic reactions to amino acids may also occur. They may be relieved by the concomitant administration of an antihistamine or possibly by the substitution of the synthesized L-amino-acid preparation.

Summary

We have presented the biochemical, physiologic, and pharmacologic principles supporting the use of hyperalimentation in disease or trauma. Although there have been reports of untoward biochemical and immunologic reactions, hyperalimentation remains an important nutritional therapy, which significantly shortens the convalescence of diseased and traumatized patients.

References

1. **Baue, A. E.** (1974). Adenine nucleotides: Who needs them? In: Zeppa, R. (chairman), *Pre- and Postoperative Care*. Postgraduate Course, 60th Annual Clinical Congress, American College of Surgeons, p. 19.

1A. **Blackburn, G. L., Maini, B., Bistrien B. R., Flatt, J. P., Page, J. G., Bothe, A., Benotti, P.,** and **Rienhoff, H.** (1976). Cyclic hyperalimentation and optimal technique for preservation of visceral protein. *J. Surg. Res. 20:* 515–525.

2. **Buonous, G., Sutherland, G., McArdle, A. H.,** and **Gurd, F. N.** (1967). The prophylactic use of an "elemental" diet in experimental hemorrhagic shock and intestinal ischemia. *Ann. Surg. 166:*312.
3. **Drucker, M. R., Pindyck, F., Brown, R. S., Elwyn, D. H.,** and **Shoemaker, W. C.** (1974). The interaction of glucagon and glucose on cardiorespiratory variables in the critically ill patient. *Surg. 75:*487.
4. **Hallberg, E., Holm, I., Obel, A. L., Schuberth, O.,** and **Wretlind, A.** (1967). Fat emulsion for complete intravenous nutrition. *Postgrad. Med. 42:*A-71.
5. **Holtzman, S., Schuler, J., Earnest, W., Erve, P. R.,** and **Schumer, W.** (1974). Carbohydrate metabolism in endotoxemia. *Circ. Shock 1:*99.
6. **LaNoue, K. F., Mason, A. D., Jr.,** and **Daniels J. P.** (1968). The impairment of gluconeogenesis by gram-negative infection. *Metabol. 17:*606.
7. **McCallum, R. E.,** and **Berry, L. J.** (1973). Effects of endotoxin on gluconeogenesis, glycogen synthesis, and liver glycogen synthase in mice. *Infect. Immuni. 7:*642.
8. **Schumer, W.** (1971). Adverse effects of xylitol in parenteral alimentation. *Metabol. 20:*345.
9. **Williamson, J. R., Refino, C.,** and **LaNoue, K. F.** (1970). Effects of *E.* coli lipopolysaccharide B treatment of rats on gluconeogenesis. In Porter, R., and Knight, J. (eds.), *Energy Metabolism in Trauma. A Ciba Symposium.* London: Churchill, p. 145.
10. **Wyrick, W. J., Jr., Rea, W. J.,** and **McClelland, R. N.** (1970). Rare complications with intravenous hyperosmotic alimentation. *J. Am. Med. Assoc. 211:*1697.

Metabolic Crises in the Neonate: Thermoregulation and Hypoglycemia

BETTY BERNARD, M.D.
Associate Professor of Pediatrics
Los Angeles County/University of Southern California
Medical Center, Los Angeles, California

Next to successful neonatal resuscitation, the two most critical life-support systems essential for the neonate's ultimate survival and potential are those concerned with thermoregulation and glucose homeostasis. To minimize the stresses of adaptation to an extrauterine life from the maternal source of heat and energy, a well-organized program of management must be instituted in the delivery room and continued in the nursery. The smaller or the more compromised the neonate, the more critical is the need for protocol, personnel, and equipment to provide a minimum of cold stress from the moment of birth and to begin to monitor blood glucose by the first 30–60 min of life. The healthy term infant can and does benefit from such a program, with broader parameters.

Late in the 1890s a French physician, Pierre-Constant Budin, developed one of the first incubators that provided a one-way heated air-flow, and humidity–temperature monitoring of the environment. One of his students, Martin Courney, exhibited the popular "Incubator Babies" at fairs and expositions all over the United States from 1898 to 1939 [19].

In 1900 Budin reported a mortality rate of 23% in infants weighing less than 2000 grams who had normal rectal temperatures compared to a 90% mortality in those with temperatures of 32–35°C, and a 98% mortality with temperatures below 32°C [6]. The importance of the thermal environment should have been well established by these data; however, Budin's observations made little impact for over 50 years until reconfirmed by Silverman [31], in 1958, then Buetow [7] and Day [12] in 1964.

THERMOREGULATION

A "neutral thermal" environment is defined as a set of conditions in which metabolic rate (measured by oxygen consumption) is minimal when body temperature is within a normal range.

Minimal oxygen consumption for a neonate ranges within 4–7 ml O_2/kg/min and is dependent on postnatal age and gestational age. This may increase to 15 ml O_2/kg/min with cold stress in the well baby [5]. Silverman's studies show that by maintaining the abdominal skin temperature at 36.5°C oxygen consumption is minimized [30].

Heat Losses

Babies, especially small ones, sustain a greater heat loss per kilogram body weight than adults do. This is attributed to:

1. Three to four times greater surface area for body mass.
2. Lack of hair and body curvature, allowing a 20% greater heat loss.
3. Posture (arms and legs extended) that does not conserve heat.
4. Less endogenous energy supply (glycogen and fat) for increased metabolic needs during cold stress (i.e., a 1-kg baby has 10 g of fat and 4.5 g of carbohydrate, while a 3-kg baby has 560 g of fat and 34 g of carbohydrate).
5. Three to six times increased thermal conductance as related to: (a) decreased absolute thickness of body (core to surface), (b) increased heat conductivity due to lack of insulation of heat producing organs (kidney, liver, etc.) and lack of fat insulation in subcutaneous tissue, and (c) a higher skin temperature for a normal core temperature, which increases temperature gradient of skin to environment and thereby rate of heat loss.
6. Four to five times greater heat loss per unit of skin area despite fully adequate vasoconstriction.
7. A vulnerability to CNS depression (birth asphyxia, intracranial hemorrhage, and meningitis), as an intact nervous system is necessary to affect the response to cold.
8. Tenuous extrauterine cardiopulmonary adjustments, which may limit the ability to increase respiratory rate or oxygenation for maintenance of body temperature.

Heat Production

There are two mechanisms for production of extra heat in response to cold stress: (a) increased voluntary or involuntary (shivering) muscle activity and (b) nonshivering or biochemical method. Investigations reveal that the latter is the principal mechanism in the newborn. Shivering is rarely induced unless there is a severe cold stress [4].

Brown fat [10,11,28,33] has an extraordinarily rich vascular and sympathetic nerve supply. Under cold stress, brown fat may have a 20-fold increase in oxygen consumption and account for an amazingly high percentage (up to 20%) of the total cardiac output. Chemical thermogenesis is mediated via the sympathetic nervous system by norepinephrine which stimulates lipolysis of brown fat. Tryglycerides stored in this tissue are split into glycerol and nonesterified fatty acids (NEFA). About 10% of NEFA are released into the circulation, 30% are oxidized directly and 60% are reesterified and returned to brown fat. These reactions are highly exothermic and require enormous metabolic expenditure.

The localization of the brown fat around major thoracic vessels, heart, kidney, and thoracic and cervical spinal cord suggests that chemical thermogenesis is largely a local phenomenon occurring within the brown fat which allows effective warming of the blood passing through it.

Consequences of Cold Stress

Elevated plasma NEFA leads to a fall in blood glucose and may result in hypoglycemia [10,32]. Metabolic acidosis is further potentiated by shifting from glucose metabolism. Norepinephrine increases vascular resistance as does acidosis through potent pulmonary vasoconstrictor reactions. These effects favor a return to fetal circulation and further reduce the baby's ability to oxygenate [13]. Both acidosis and NEFA interfere with pulmonary surfactant production, which could prove lethal for the infant with respiratory distress [15]. Thus, a cold stress may initiate a vicious cycle of clinical deterioration.

Hypothermia predisposes to kernicterus at low levels of bilirubin because of acidosis [23] and because an excess of NEFA is a potential competitor for bilirubin-albumin binding sites [26].

Cold Injuries

While a slight drop in temperature may produce profound metabolic changes, a large drop must occur before clinical signs are seen. Clinical features are: (a) skin cold to the touch, an inappropriate red color of the skin with central cyanosis, (b) poor feeding, (c) lethargy, (d) slow shallow respirations, (e) respiratory grunt, (f) bradycardia, (g) cardiac arrhythmias, (h) edema of extremities, (i) sclerema, (j) pulmonary hemorrhage,

(k) hypoglycemia, (l) hyperkalemia, (m) elevated blood urea nitrogen, and (n) oliguria [21]. Necropsy of the cold-stressed baby reveals no distinctive pathology or unique cause of death; however, brown fat may be reduced or depleted.

Cooling the baby *does not lower* metabolic requirements—unless a rapid controlled deep hypothermia range of $<30°C$ is reached—and only shortens the time to the last gasp [5].

THERMOREGULATION IN THE DELIVERY ROOM

In utero, the normal fetal body temperature is 37.6°C and is dependent on the temperature gradient across the placenta [2]. When a wet, bare baby is exposed to an air-conditioned delivery room, the baby's skin and rectal temperatures will fall at an extremely rapid rate of 0.3°C per min and 0.1°C per min, respectively. This corresponds to a heat loss of approximately 200 cal/kg/min in the first minutes of life (adult maximum is 90 cal/kg/min). Four ways in which heat is lost and the measures needed to minimize these heat losses in the delivery room and nursery are outlined in Table 1.

In a 25°C delivery room, Dahm and James [9] demonstrated that by drying a wet baby, heat loss is reduced from 100 to 81 cal/kg/min for the first 30 min of life. Quick application of a warm, dry blanket can further reduce the loss to only 39 cal/kg/min. A radiant heat warmer placed over the wet or dried infant reduces the heat loss to only 28 and 22 cal/kg/min, respectively. Thus, the heat loss by radiation and convection was twice that lost by evaporation.

THERMOREGULATION IN THE NURSERY

A prewarmed transport incubator helps to avoid cold stress during transfer of the baby to the nursery. Recommended initial incubator temperatures for the first 24 hr of life are summarized in Table 2. Bathing should be delayed until the temperature and vital signs are stable for 3–4 hr. Radiant heat lamps, prewarmed shirts, diapers, liquid soap, and servocontrolled isolettes are other measures that are useful in the nursery to minimize initial cold stresses in sick or small neonates. These efforts to keep a baby warm are rewarded with less metabolic acidosis and higher levels of blood glucose in the first hours of life.

Infants nursed in a neutral thermal environment gain weight and increase length more rapidly than infants raised in a cool environment who have the same caloric intake per day [14]. This is not surprising since a normal growth rate in babies is associated with a caloric intake that is usually 2–2½ times the caloric value of minimal oxygen consumption (5 cal/ml O_2).

TABLE 1 Heat Losses and Environmental Conditions Related to Thermoregulation for the Neonate

HEAT LOSSES	RELATED TO	MEASURES TO MINIMIZE
Evaporation 6–25%	Heat lost both from lungs and the wet body surface—as moisture is converted to vapor—function of minute ventilation, humidity, and temperature of ambient air	Keep room warm with 50% relative humidity Dry baby with warm towels immediately Use warm humidified air or oxygen[a]
Conductance 0–10%	Heat transfer to solid objects in direct contact with baby	Prewarm mattress, towels, and blankets
Convection 0–30%	Related to air flow and air temperature	Warm room and avoid drafts Wrap baby in warm, dry blanket and leave only face exposed
Radiation 0–50%	Temperature of solid objects not in direct contact with infant (i.e., incubator walls, room wall, windows) and not related to ambient air temperature surrounding infant. This heat loss is most critical during transport by ambulance or helicopter	Warm room, as inside walls and equipment will approximate environmental temperature Use radiant heat warmer for resuscitation, x-rays, starting intravenous infusions, and blood drawings Clothe and wrap baby in a thick blanket—this is almost as effective as radiant heater For transport, a double-walled insulated incubator is needed For small infants, add a radiant heat shield inside incubator

[a] Providing humidity may increase the risk of "water bugs" (i.e., *pseudomonas*) contamination, which can be controlled by 0.5 ml of 1:10,000 silver nitrate to 1 liter of water and by a copper coil in water reservoir of incubator.

[b] Humidified oxygen or air should be passed directly through the incubator portholes and not into incubator gas connections. This avoids moisture on the air intake filter that may destroy its effectiveness, and allows bacterial contamination. Dry gases may be attached to incubator gas connections.

Rewarming. As soon as a cooled infant is placed in a positive thermal environment, his oxygen consumption falls to a low level [16,18]. Under steady conditions, the oxygen consumption directly increases when the skin to environmental temperature difference exceeds 1.5–2°C. When an incubator is used for rewarming it must be set to 1.5–2°C above skin temperature and checked every 15 min. Rapid rewarming has been associated with increased oxygen consumption and apnea. One needs to be prepared to support respiration and simultaneously monitor arterial oxygen tension, blood-sugars and acid–base balance, and to administer intravenous fluids until temperature reaches normal. Rewarming may take several hours. No specific recommendations are made at this time for use of the newer

TABLE 2 Incubator Ambient Air Temperatures for the First 24 Hours of an Unclothed Baby[a,b]

	INCUBATOR TEMPERATURES		CONVERSION THERMOMETER	
BIRTH WEIGHT	MEDIAN °C	RANGE (±)	°C	°F
750	35.5	0.5	25	77.0
1000	35.0	0.5	26	78.8
1500	34.3	0.5	27	80.6
2000	33.5	0.5	28	82.4
2500	33.2	0.8	29	84.2
3000	33.0	1.0	30	86.0
3500	32.8	1.2	31	87.8
4000	32.6	1.4	32	89.6
			33	91.4
			34	93.2
			35	95.0
			36	96.8
			36.5	97.7
			37	98.6
			37.2	99.0
			38	100.4
			39	102.2
			40	104.0
			For interpolation (1.0)	(1.8)

[a] Recommended incubator temperatures are likely to maintain normal body temperatures. The condition of the infant and the thermal environment of the nursery must be taken into consideration if hypothermia or hyperthermia is encountered.

[b] Adapted and modified from published data of Scopes [29] and Oliver [24].

radiant-heat units. One must be aware that radiant heaters may increase insensible water loss up to 3–4 ml/kg/hr, which increases metabolic expenditure [34].

Hyperthermia. Hey and Katz [17] noted a sweating threshold of approximately 37.2°C rectal temperature in babies. A preterm baby whose sweat response has not developed may become hyperthermic more easily. Hyperthermia also increases oxygen consumption and must be suspected when a shallow and irregular respiration is observed. While considering infection in the hyperthermic infant, the environmental requirements are that: (a) thermostats in incubators and radiant-heat equipment be checked and regulated, (b) the servocontrol thermistor be attached to the baby in the epigastric area, and (c) the incubator not be in sunlight.

Normal body temperature does *not* determine whether a baby is in a neutral thermal environment. Abnormal body temperatures serve as an index to situations in which the thermal stress has been so severe that normal thermoregulatory mechanisms have been overpowered. By maintaining the infant's upper abdominal skin temperature about 1–2°C less than a normal rectal temperature, the effect of the variables determining heat exchange between the baby and its thermal environment can be overcome. If the majority of the recent advances in neonatology have been the eradication of iatrogenic disease, then it is with some trepidation that I have presented thermoregulation as is practiced today. We have lessened metabolic stresses and improved survival, but we have still to perfect the physical environment to provide the "ideal" thermal environment for the newly born infant's optimal physical, neurological, and adaptive development.

HYPOGLYCEMIA

The newborn infant balances precariously between a relatively high obligatory glucose requirement of 240–360 mg/kg/hour—80% for the brain—and his ability to maintain this supply during caloric deprivation following birth. Several factors may contribute to hypoglycemia in the neonate [20, 27]. Since glucose is constantly supplied from the mother, the enzymatic capability for gluconeogenesis may be poorly developed or sluggish to respond [1]. The fetal liver synthesizes and deposits glycogen when an abundant glucose supply is available. This process increases to a maximum toward the end of gestation, except in the undergrown or premature babies who are ultimately deficient in glycogen stores. Following parturition, glycogen stores are rapidly depleted and the ability to mobilize other gluconeogenic substrates may be delayed.

Previously, Cornblath [8] defined hypoglycemia as less than 30 mg%. More recently, Pagliara, Karl and others [25] defined hypoglycemia in newly born infants to be a plasma glucose concentration of less than 40 mg per 100 ml because significant findings have been reported to occur when blood glucose levels were less than 40 mg per 100 ml of blood.

Lubchenco [20] reported the incidence of hypoglycemia, defined as $<$30mg%, as follows (Table 3):

Clinical manifestations. Signs of hypoglycemia are less obvious in the neonatal period and may be either overlooked or absent [8,22]. Manifestations include: (a) episodes of tremor, (b) apnea, (c) cyanosis, (d) limpness, (e) twitching, (f) hypothermia, (g) weak cry, (h) refusal to

TABLE 3 Relationship between Gestational Age, Weight, and Signs of Hypoglycemia

	SMALL FOR GA*	APPROPRIATE FOR GA	LARGE FOR GA
Pre-term	67%	15%	38%
Term	25%	10%	4%
Post-term	18%	5%	7%

* Percentage of infants with signs of hypoglycemia.

feed, (i) eye rolling, (j) aimless sucking on upper lip, (k) coma, and (l) convulsions. Prophylaxis of neuronal damage from hypoglycemia first demands a high index of suspicion. The conditions which increase the risks of neonatal hypoglycemia are summarized in Table 3.

Monitoring. Any high-risk infant is monitored with Dextrostix. If the Dextrostix is <45 mg/dl, it is confirmed by a laboratory blood glucose

TABLE 4 Classification of Neonatal Hypoglycemias

HYPERINSULINISM TYPE	DEFICIENT SUBSTRATE	IDIOPATHIC
Infant of diabetic mother	Small for gestational age	Infants of mother with toxemia
Erythroblastosis	Prematurity	Sepsis
Abrupt cessation of intravenous glucose	Smaller of twins	Meningitis
Sulfonylurea drugs to mother	Enzymatic defects	Cold stress
Islet-cell adenoma	Defects in hormonal regulation	Asphyxia
Beckwith's syndrome	Addison's disease	Alcohol
Islet hyperplasia	Congenital adrenal hyperplasia	Congenital CNS defects
Leucine sensitivity	Thyroid deficiency	Polycythemia
	Adrenal hemorrhage	
	Inborn errors of amino-acid metabolism	
	Diarrhea	
	Cessation of intravenous glucose	
	Late feeding of neonate	

determination. For the hyperinsulinism type of hypoglycemia, monitoring must be initiated during the first hour of life and followed at 30–60-min intervals as necessary for the first 4 hr of life. Continue to follow at 2–6-hr intervals until blood sugar stabilizes and the baby takes formula feeding well. Other types of hypoglycemia may be monitored at 2–4 hr intervals and preferably prior to a feeding. Any change in symptoms warrants immediate Dextrostix screening and laboratory determination of blood glucose levels. It is wise to monitor blood glucose for the first 2–3 hr following cessation of an intravenous glucose infusion so as to detect reactive hypoglycemia.

Treatment. All infants with a blood glucose <40 mg/dl need treatment to maintain levels above 40 mg/dl. For a specific episode of hypoglycemia, administer 2–4 ml. of 25% glucose in water by slow intravenous push and follow with an intravenous infusion of a 10–25% glucose solution to run at 300–1200 mg of glucose/kg/hour. Continue to monitor blood glucose closely, as hypoglycemia may occur even while a glucose infusion is in progress. On the other hand, use the minimum necessary to keep blood glucose >40 mg/dl and <200 mg/dl. Beware of inducing a significant hyperglycemia, which may cause an osmotic diuresis, dehydration, acidosis, and intracranial hemorrhage, especially in premature infants. Taper strength and/or rate of glucose infusion before discontinuing intravenous administration. Selection of other forms of treatment depend upon the etiology of the hypoglycemia: (a) glucagon, 300 μg/kg administered as a single dose in the delivery room to macrosomic infants of diabetic mothers (not to be used in babies small in size due either to prematurity or in relation to gestational age) (b) hydrocortisone 5 mg/kg/day orally or intravenously in divided doses every 8 hours for 2–4 days, (c) ACTH, 4μ/kg/day intramuscularly in divided doses every 12 hours to stimulate glucogenesis, glucagon, and NEFA release, (d) pancreatectomy for intractable hypoglycemia, and (e) diazoxide 10–15 mg/kg/day in permanent hyperinsulinism associated with Beckwith's syndrome, or leucine sensitivity (but this is not presently recommended for neonates).

Prevention. Initiation of early formula feedings at 3–4 hr of life is the most efficacious combatant of neonatal hypoglycemia. Most high-risk infants (see Table 4) will do better if an intravenous infusion of 10% glucose at 3–4 ml/hr is promptly begun for fluid therapy and glucose homeostasis.

Summary

The thermoneutral zone or the critical temperature is described as the environmental temperature and conditions at which the oxygen consumption and energy needs are at their lowest with a normal body temperature. In the sick or premature infant, adequate thermoregulation and energy (glucose) supply can minimize the stresses of adaptation and increase survival and decrease morbidity.

Invariably, heat is rapidly lost in the first minutes of life by the wet naked neonate even with the most prompt attention to the thermal environment. This inevitable mild cold stimulus may play an important role in the onset of breathing. However, hazards of cold stress dramatically increase directly with the diminishing size, gestational age, or health of the newly born infant. Clinical hazards of cold stress in addition to a significant decrease in survival include increased oxygen and caloric requirements, an increase in norepinephrine and plasma nonesterified fatty acids, hypoglycemia, metabolic acidosis, an increased pulmonary vascular resistance, a predisposition to kernicterus at relatively low levels of bilirubin, a bleeding diathesis, and sclerema.

For initial thermoregulation management, dry the infant and place him on a warm, dry surface in a room with no drafts. Wrapping the healthy term baby in a warm, dry blanket may be all that is necessary. Delivery room resuscitation or procedures in the nursery require a radiant heat warmer with an abdominal skin temperature monitor to allow ready accessibility and observation of the unclothed baby.

Neonatal hypoglycemia (<40 mg/dl) is found most frequently in the small-for-date, premature infant, or infant of a diabetic mother. Any infant who has had a prolonged fast (>6 hr) before a milk feeding can develop hypoglycemia. Increased glucose needs and hypoglycemia may be found in infants who have erythroblastosis, Beckwith's Syndrome, or whose mothers are diabetic. Glucose needs may range from a *minimum* of 0.3 gm/kg/hr to 1.2 gm/kg/hr. In high risk neonates, early recognition is assured by monitoring every 1–2 hr with dextrostix and confirmed by the laboratory when blood glucose decreases to <45 mg/dl. Early feeds of colostrum or formula at 0–4 hr and prompt intervention utilizing a 10–25% glucose infusion with or without a preceding bolus of 0.5 to 1.0 gm/kg can ameliorate the damage that a glucose dependent nervous system might otherwise suffer.

All hospitals who have neonatal patients must also have adequate facilities for thermoregulation and energy support.

References

1. **Adam, P. A.** (1971). Control of glucose metabolism in the human fetus and newborn infant. *Adv. Metabol. Disor. 183*:270.
2. **Adamson, K., Jr.** (1966). The role of thermal factors in fetal and neonatal life. *Pediatr. Clin. N. Am. 13*:599.
3. **Adamson, K., Jr., Gandy, G. M.,** and **James, L. S.** (1965). The influence of thermal factors upon oxygen consumption of the newborn human infant. *J. Pediatr. 66*:495.

4. **Bruck, K.** (1961). Temperature regulation in the newborn infant. *Biol. Neonat. 3*:65.
5. **Bruck, K.** (1970). Heat production and temperature regulation. In: Stave, U. (ed.), *Physiology of the Perinatal Period*. New York: Appleton-Century-Crofts, pp. 493–557.
6. **Budin, P.** (1900). Le nourisson. In: *Alimentation et Hygeine Des Enfants Debiles—Enfants nes a Terme*, Paris: Octave Dion (ed.).
7. **Buetow, K. C.**, and **Klein, S. W.** (1964). Effect of maintenance of "normal" skin temperature on survival of infants of low birth weight. *Pediatr. 34*:163.
8. **Cornblath, M.**, and **Schwartz, R.** (1976). Hypoglycemia in the neonate. In: Schaffer, A. J. (ed.), *Disorders of Carbohydrate Metabolism in Infancy*. Philadelphia: Saunders, Vol. III, 2nd edition, pp. 155–205.
9. **Dahm, L. S.**, and **James, L. S.** (1972). Newborn temperature and calculated heat loss in the delivery room. *Pediatr 49*:504.
10. **Dawkins, M. J.**, and **Hull, D.** (1964). Brown adipose tissue and the response of newborn rabbits to cold. *J. Physiol. 172*:216–238.
11. **Dawkins, M. J.**, and **Scopes, J. W.** (1965). Non-shivering thermogenesis and brown adipose tissue in the human newborn infant. *Nature 206*:201.
12. **Day, R. L., Caliguri, L., Kamenski, C.**, and **Ehrlich, F.** (1964). Body temperature and survival of premature infants. *Pediatr. 34*:171.
13. **Gandy, G. M., Adamsons, K., Jr., Cunningham, N., Silverman, W. A.**, and **James, L. S.** (1964). Thermal environment and acid base homeostasis in human infants during the first few hours of life. *J. Clin. Invest. 43*:751.
14. **Glass, I., Silverman, W., and Sinclair, J.** (1968). Effects of the thermal environment on cold resistance and growth of small infants after the first week of life. *Pediatr. 41*:1033.
15. **Gluck, L., Kulovich, M. V., Eidelman, A. I., Cordero, L.**, and **Khazin, A. F.** (1972). Biochemical development of surface activity in mammalian lung. IV. Pulmonary lecithin synthesis in the human fetus and newborn and etiology of the respiratory distress syndrome. *Pediat. Res. 6*:81–99.
16. **Hey, E.** (1969). The relation between environmental temperature and oxygen consumption in the newborn baby. *J. Physiol. 200*:589.
17. **Hey, E.**, and **Katz, G.** (1970). The optimum thermal environment for naked babies. *Arch. Dis. Child. 45*:328.
18. **Hey, E.**, and **O'Connell, B.** (1970). Oxygen consumption and heat balance in the cot-nursed baby. *Arch. Dis. Child. 43*:335.
19. **Liebling, A. J.** (1939). Patron of the premies. *New Yorker Magazine* (June 3): 20–24.
20. **Lubchenco, L. O.**, and **Bard, H.** (1971). Incidence of hypoglycemia in newborn infants classified by birth weight and gestational age. *Pediatr. 47*:831.
21. **Mann, T. P.**, and **Elliot, R. I. K.** (1957). Neonatal cold injury due to accidental exposure to cold. *Lancet 1*:229.
22. **Milner, R. D. G.** (1972). Neonatal hypoglycemia—a critical reappraisal. *Arch. Dis. Child. 47*:679.
23. **Odell, G. B.**, and **Cohen, S.** (1960). The effect of PH on the protein binding of bilirubin. *Am. J. Dis. Child. 105*:525.

24. **Oliver, T. K., Jr.,** and **Karlberg, P.** (1963). Gaseous metabolism in newly born human infants. *Am. J. Dis. Child. 105:*427.
25. **Pagliara, A. S., Karl, I. E., Haymond, M.,** and **Kipnis, D. M.** (1973). Hypoglycemia in infancy and childhood (part I). *J. Pediatr., 82:*365.
26. **Polacek, K., Novak, M.,** and **Melichar, V.** (1965). Influence of free fatty acids on the distribution of bilirubin and its clinical significance in the newborn. *Rev. Czech. Med 11:*161.
27. **Raivio, K. O.,** and **Hall, N.** (1968). Neonatal hypoglycemia. *Acta Pediatr. Scand. 57:*517.
28. **Schiff, D., Stern, L.,** and **Leduc, J.** (1966). Chemical thermogenesis in newborn infants: Catechomine excretion and the plasma non-esterified fatty acid response to cold exposure. *Pediatr. 37:*577.
29. **Scopes, J. W.,** and **Ahmed, I.** (1966). Range of critical temperatures in sick and premature newborn babies. *Arch. Dis. Child. 41:*417.
30. **Silverman, W.,** and **Agate, F.** (1964). Variations in cold resistance among small newborn animals. *Biol. Neonat. 6:*113.
31. **Silverman, W. A., Fertig, J. W.,** and **Berger, A. P.** (1958). The influence of the thermal environment upon the survival of newly born infants. *Pediatr. 22:*876.
32. **Stern, L.** (1970). The newborn infant and his thermal environment. *Curr. Probl. Pediatr. 1:*3.
33. **Stern, L., Lees, M. H.,** and **Leduc, J.** (1965). Environmental temperature, oxygen consumption, and catecholamine excretion in newborn infants. *Pediatr. 36:*367.
34. **Wu, P. Y. K.,** and **Hodgman, J. E.** (1974). Insensible water loss in preterm infants: Changes with postnatal development and non-ionizing radiant energy. *Pediatr. 54:*704.

VI

PLANNING AND OPERATIONS

The "Stat" Laboratory

SYBIL MICHAELS, B.A.
Chief Laboratory Technologist
University of Southern California Center for the Critically Ill
Los Angeles, California

The critical care environment demands immediate response from the laboratory to aid the physician in the management of the patient who is in a crisis condition and whose immediate survival is threatened by failure of respiratory, cardiac, or metabolic function. These are the circumstances that have prompted the development of the "stat" laboratory.

Ideally, this "stat" laboratory should be adjacent to the bedside. In our center it lies midway between the intensive care, coronary care, and dedicated observation units and adjacent to the critical care ward. It is staffed 24 hours a day, 7 days a week.

Twenty-three measurements are made on each blood sample brought to the laboratory (Table 1). Arterial blood gas predominates over all other procedures, since the effectiveness of gas exchange and the metabolic consequences of circulatory failure are promptly identified. These guide the decisions for intubation and mechanical ventilation, the use of alkali to reverse acidosis, and the options of sedation and analgesia.

Whole blood hemoglobin and hematocrit, calculation of bicarbonate and base excess or deficit, and estimates of total plasma proteins complement the basic blood pH, P_{CO_2}, and P_{O_2}. The independent measurement of oxygen

TABLE 1 Measurements on Single Blood Sample

DIRECT MEASUREMENTS		
Whole Blood	Plasma	DERIVED MEASUREMENTS
Hct	Osmolality	P_{O_2}, P_{CO_2}, pH (Pt. temp.)
Hb, COHB, S_{O_2}	COP	S_{O_2}
P_{O_2}, P_{CO_2}, pH	Protein (calc.)	HCO_3^-, STD. HCO_3^-
Lactate	Na, K, Cl	Base excess (H^+)
8	6	9

saturation, together with P_{O_2}, provides indications of major shifts in the oxygen-dissociation curve. Carboxyhemoglobin is measured for diagnosis of a form of selective hypoxemia which may otherwise escape clinical detection. Colloid osmotic pressure, as described by Da Luz (p. 195), constitutes a critical guide for volume loading of an order of importance equal to that of physiological measurement of pulmonary artery wedge pressure (PAWP) with a Swan–Ganz catheter. Arterial blood lactate is the best reference for quantitation of perfusion failure and the identification of shock, as described by Shubin et al (p. 101).

Additional routines have been evolved in our center so as to provide a broad laboratory survey complementing blood-gas measurements for purposes of immediate care. These include measurements of plasma osmolality for immediate diagnosis of hyperosmolar states such as (a) diabetic acidosis, nonketotic hyperosmolar coma, alcohol intoxication, or dehydration or (b) water intoxication. Measurement of plasma potassium, sodium, and chloride are used for the assessment of electrolyte balance. A single determination of urine osmolality supplies a remarkable wealth of information on renal status, particularly when related to plasma osmolality.

Within 11 min after the blood specimen is received by the technician, these 23 measurements have been completed and reported back to the physician. In a recent report [1], the value of both whole blood osmolality and blood pH and P_{CO_2} to aid in titrating the dosage of sodium bicarbonate during cardiac resuscitation has been documented. We have arranged our procedures so that the results of these two measurements, together with those of P_{O_2}, are available within 3 min after the specimen arrives in the laboratory.

For routine purposes a blood sample is brought to the laboratory in an iced heparinized syringe and utilized following the scheme in Table 2. Measurements requiring manual treatment of the sample are processed first.

One-tenth (0.1) ml whole blood, measured with a disposable micropipet,

TABLE 2 Blood-Sample Utilization Scheme

4.0 ml heparinized blood arterial and/or venous in syringe	0.05 ml	Hematocrit
	0.10 ml	Lactate
	2.0 ml	Plasma (≈ 1 ml)
	1.0 ml	Blood gases & pH
	0.5 ml	Co-oximeter
	3.65 ml	

is added to a premeasured 0.9-ml perchloric acid for the protein free filtrate necessary for the lactate determination.

The hematocrit is drawn by capillary action from the syringe. Two milliliters of whole blood are ejected into a sample cup for spinning in order to have sufficient plasma for measurement of colloid osmotic pressure, osmolality, estimated protein, and electrolytes.

Measurements utilizing whole blood directly are next on the menu. The blood-gas electrodes pH, P_{O_2}, P_{CO_2}, and the Co-oximeter are utilized.

While the blood gas electrodes are equilibrating, the technician has a few moments to begin centrifuging the hematocrit, the filtrate, and the whole blood. Two microhematocrit centrifuges are used as a time-saving device. The filtrate and the whole blood require 2.5 min of centrifuge time while the hematocrit must spin for 5 minutes. Centrifuging begun, the technician returns to the blood-gas analyzer.

The electrodes having reached equilibrium as indicated on the strip chart recorder, the technician records the measured values for pH, P_{O_2}, and P_{CO_2}. We routinely record the output of our blood gas and pH electrodes. Without this, the technician fails to detect drift, which results in clinically significant inconsistencies between technologists. As soon as the output has zero slope, a straight line, we read the values on our standard meter.

Next we read the Co-oximeter for O_2 saturation, and levels of hemoglobin and carboxyhemoglobin. We have independently evaluated the validity of the O_2 saturation as well as hemoglobin and find a remarkably close correlation with reference methods of O_2 content and standard spectrophotometric methods of hemoglobin measurement. On the other hand, the validity of carboxyhemoglobin is less secure since no easy method for its day-to-day calibration is available. However, the carboxyhemoglobin measurement has proven to be sufficiently reliable for clinical purposes when calibrated against standards at 3-month intervals.

The sample cup containing the lactate filtrate is placed directly on the autoanalyzer wheel. The start button is pushed and the lactate is totally automated beyond this point. With the aid of a digital computer, the output of the autoanalyzer is reported on a teletype.

Next we turn to the measurement of plasma colloid osmotic pressure. Two-tenths (0.2) ml of plasma is deposited in the colloid osmotic sample chamber. Colloid osmotic pressure is now an important measurement for the differential diagnosis of low protein states and the likelihood of pulmonary edema. The principle of this measurement involves the detection of pressure changes in a pressure transducer when 0.2 ml of plasma is placed at the top of a semipermeable membrane with pressure developed in reference to an isotonic solution on the other side of the membrane.

Three-tenths (0.3) ml of plasma is sampled for osmolality and two drops for the refractometer for estimating total protein. If the osmolality falls outside of normal limits, electrolytes are measured routinely without necessitating a specific order from the physician.

The technician then calls for the blood gas program at the computer keyboard and enters the measured P_{O_2}, P_{CO_2}, pH, patient temperature, hemoglobin, and hematocrit. Within 0.5 min, the teletype printout is available with the measured values corrected for patient temperature and the O_2 saturation, bicarbonate, standard bicarbonate, base excess, and (H^+) concentration, including a statement that serves as an interpretation of the data (Fig. 1).

The 23 measurements, direct and derived on a single sample, are now complete and the report is en route to the bedside (Fig. 2). All abnormal laboratory values are brought to the immediate attention of the physician either by the technician directly or through the nurse. The physician may confer with the laboratory personnel at any time regarding the results.

For purposes of completeness let me also mention the other measurements that are performed on a routine basis in our "stat" laboratory in addition to the 11-min blood panel (see Carrington, p. 340).

FIGURE 1 Teletype printout of patient arterial blood gas measurements.

```
ARTERIAL BLOOD GAS INPUT FOR K.W.
SAMPLE TIME:002/0819          ARTERIAL BLOOD GAS RESULTS
BREATH MIX= 30                PO2= 108
VENTILATOR:MA-1               PH= 7.36
TEMPERATURE 38.0              PCO2= 29
HEMOGLOBIN= 6.8               O2 SAT(DER)= 97.5
HEMATOCRIT= 20.0              P50= -0.0
O2 SAT(MEAS)=100.0            H-ION CONC= 44
PO2= 101                      HCO3= 16.5
PH= 7.37                      STD HCO3= 18.2
PCO2= 28                      BASE EXCESS= -8.3

ARTERIAL OXYGENATION IS ADEQUATE
OVER-VENTILATION HAS PRODUCED HYPOCAPNEA, BUT THE ACIDEMIA AND NEGATIVE
BASE EXCESS INDICATE AN ASSOCIATED METABOLIC ACIDOSIS.
```

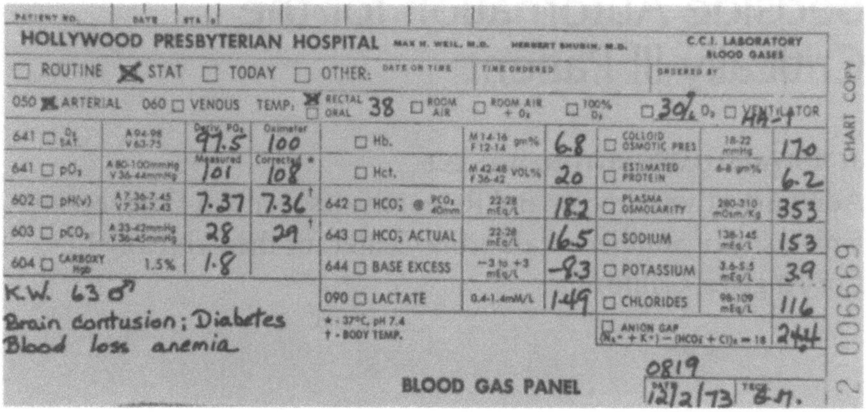

HOLLYWOOD PRESBYTERIAN HOSPITAL MAX H. WEIL, M.D. HERBERT SHUBIN, M.D. C.C.I. LABORATORY BLOOD GASES

☐ ROUTINE ☒ STAT ☐ TODAY ☐ OTHER: DATE OR TIME | TIME ORDERED | ORDERED BY

050 ☒ ARTERIAL 060 ☐ VENOUS TEMP: ☒ RECTAL ☐ ORAL 38 ☐ ROOM AIR ☐ ROOM AIR + O_2 ☐ 100% O_2 ☐ 30% O_2 ☐ VENTILATOR HA-1

641 ☐ O_2 SAT	A 94-98 V 63-75	Deriv. PO_2 97.5	Oximeter 100	☐ Hb.	M 14-16 F 12-14 gm%	6.8	☐ COLLOID OSMOTIC PRES	18-22 mmHg	17.0
641 ☐ pO_2	A 80-100 mmHg V 36-44 mmHg	Measured 101	Corrected * 108	☐ Hct.	M 42-48 F 36-42 VOL%	20	☐ ESTIMATED PROTEIN	6-8 gm%	6.2
602 ☐ pH(v)	A 7.36-7.45 V 7.34-7.43	7.37	7.36 †	642 ☐ HCO_3^- @ PCO_2 40mm	22-28 mEq/L	18.2	☐ PLASMA OSMOLARITY	280-310 mOsm/Kg	353
603 ☐ pCO_2	A 33-42 mmHg V 36-45 mmHg	28	29 †	643 ☐ HCO_3^- ACTUAL	22-28 mEq/L	16.5	☐ SODIUM	138-145 mEq/L	153
604 ☐ CARBOXY Hgb	1.5%	1.8		644 ☐ BASE EXCESS	−3 to +3 mEq/L	−8.3	☐ POTASSIUM	3.6-5.5 mEq/L	3.9
				090 ☐ LACTATE	0.4-1.4 mM/L	1.49	☐ CHLORIDES	98-109 mEq/L	116
							☐ ANION GAP $(Na^+ + K^+) - (HCO_3^- + Cl^-) = 18$		24.4

K.W. 63 ♂
Brain contusion; Diabetes
Blood loss anemia

* = 37°C, pH 7.4
† = BODY TEMP.

BLOOD GAS PANEL

0819
DATE 12/2/73 TECH

CHART COPY
2 006669

FIGURE 2 Measurements from teletype printout entered on patient's bedside chart.

1. Urine osmolality is measured every 8 hr on all patients in ICU, CCU, and DOU to help the physician in his assessment of his patient's kidney function and fluid balance. Urine electrolytes are measured on request.
2. Blood volumes are measured as the incidence of hypovolemic shock is relatively high. The "stat" lab is equipped to measure both plasma volume and red-cell mass using radioactive isotope techniques. The laboratory does an average of 30 blood-volume studies a month.
3. Although cardiac output measurements are routine in our critical care ward, the laboratory provides talent and mobile equipment for performance of both standard dye-dilution measurements and ear-piece dye curves for assessing cardiovascular and hepatic function utilizing indocyanine green dye. More recently, thermal dilution techniques have also been adopted.
4. The laboratory also has responsibility for the calibration and maintenance of the equipment used for intravascular pressure measurements for patients outside the critical care unit and at other than prime shifts for routine 13 lead electrocardiograms.

Reference

1. **Mattar, J. A., Weil, M. H., Shubin, H.,** and **Stein, L.** (1974). Cardiac arrest in the critically ill. Hyperosmolal states following cardiac arrest. *Am. J. Med. 56*:162–168.

Bedside Automation for the Critically Ill Patient

J. HOWARD CARRINGTON, B.A., P.E.
Administrative Director and Research Associate in Engineering
University of Southern California Center for the Critically Ill
Los Angeles, California

During the past decade there has been a great proliferation of devices for bedside monitoring and treatment of the critically ill patient. While providing a potential for enhancing patient care, such devices also pose a problem to bedside personnel insofar as they necessitate additional time and attention and create a potential barrier to easy patient access. In an effort to reduce these demands in our clinical service, major efforts have been made to automate bedside procedures.

Pressure measurements. Intravascular blood pressures are measured by pressure transducers connected to catheters in the patient's vessels. Transducer outputs are amplified and delivered to a computer for calculation, analysis, and display or are preserved on an analog recorder. Calibration of the pressure amplifiers is accomplished using internal servo loops (Fig. 1). Pressing switches on the amplifier causes control valves to open the system to reference pressures that are applied to the transducers. A reference pressure of zero is translated into a zero-voltage output and a reference pressure of 200 mm Hg is translated, by automatic gain adjustment, into a 4-volt output. This simplified calibration procedure secures operator-independent accuracy and reliability of pressure measurements. The am-

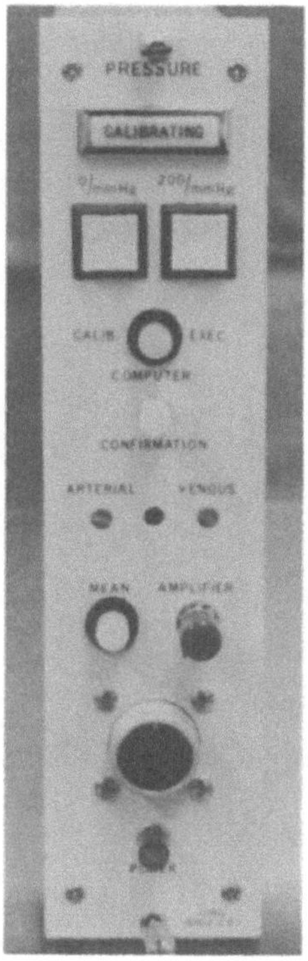

FIGURE 1 Automated Servo Amplifier.

plifier is provided with a test circuit, and an indicator light alerts the operator to failures in amplifier calibration. The amplifiers are of small size and of modular configuration in order to permit the clinical staff to interchange units readily in the event of failure during the period of clinical use.

Vascular interface system. Automated patient-care systems are limited by the interface between the affector–effector system and the patient. Routine hemodynamic and biochemical measurements require a hydraulic connection with the patient's vascular system. This prompted the development and bedside operation of a vascular interface system (Fig. 2). In the present bedside unit, provision is made for a hydraulic interface to four intravascular catheters. Provision is made also for flush solutions, automated fluid pumps and catheter flush, pressure transducers, precise pressure references for calibration, and pneumatically operated valves for automated switching of the fluid and blood pathways during sampling of blood and infusion of fluids. The vascular interface system consists of a catheter interface module, the interface plate support module, the controller, and computer controllable supply air valves and drivers [1].

The valves employed for switching fluid streams are reliable and reason-

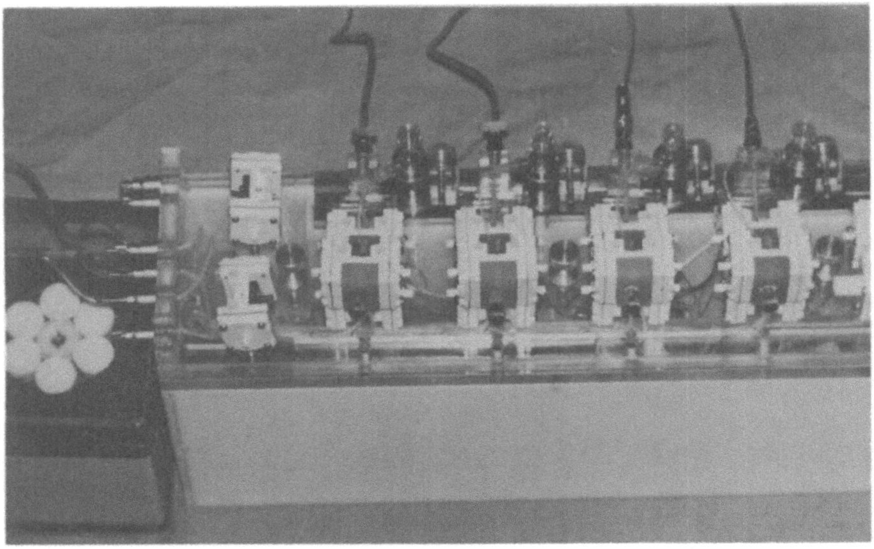

FIGURE 2 Vascular Interface System.

ably small; they are made of materials compatible with blood, permit routine gas sterilization, and provide assurance of electrical safety for patients with catheters implanted in the heart chambers. The valves are pneumatically activated but have a manual override feature. Fluid paths between valves and input–output fittings are through Teflon tubing. To minimize dead-space volume and the size of the bedside assembly, only short tubes without connectors are used.

The catheter interface module consists of 11 valves mounted on a ½″ Plexiglass plate which is coupled through "O" ring seals to a fixed base support containing the pneumatic control lines. The Plexiglass plate is removable for cleaning and sterilization. Four pressure transducers and connectors are mounted in the assembly and Luer lock connections are provided for coupling with blood volume, blood gas, cardiac output infusion pump, and other modules.

The vascular interface control system panel (Fig. 3) has 14 push-button switches, pilot lights, and one rotary switch. Provision is made to accept control signals from the computer. This panel allows for override of computer operations. In addition, logic is provided so that complex operations may be initiated by pushing a single push-button switch. For instance, an arterial, venous, or pulmonary artery blood sample may be withdrawn with ease into a syringe by simply depressing the appropriate button. On completion of sampling, a flushing mode is actuated which automatically flushes all surfaces that have come into contact with blood and then returns the unit to a normal pressure-monitoring mode.

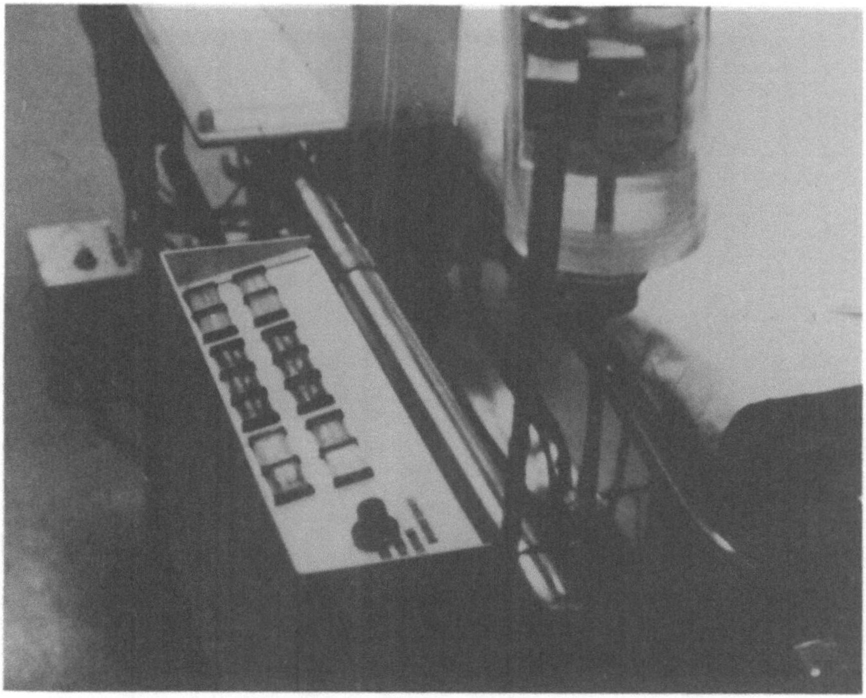

FIGURE 3 Interface Control Panel.

Cardiac output module. This module was developed as an accessory to the vascular interface unit (Fig. 4). Two pneumatic valves, three pneumatically operated syringes, and a mixing chamber are mounted on a Plexiglass plate. Provisions are made for hydraulic connections to the catheter interface module and to a separate pump, the speed of which is automatically controlled. The calibration, injection of dye, withdrawal of blood through the densitometer, and computation of cardiac output have been fully automated. A cardiac output measurement with its own dye calibration may be obtained within 2 min. An automated pump system under manual or computer control has been developed. This system delivers volumes of 0.01–30 ml/min with the precision of $\pm 2\%$ over the total range.

Temperature measurements. Thermistor probes are routinely placed in the rectum, under both large toes and at the bedside for ambient temperature [2]. An amplifier has been developed that accepts the nonlinear signals of the four thermistor probes and provides scaled linear outputs suitable for dispaly of the temperature value directly on digital voltmeters. A perfusometer unit indicates temperature differences between the higher great toe temperature and ambient temperature. Temperature differences greater

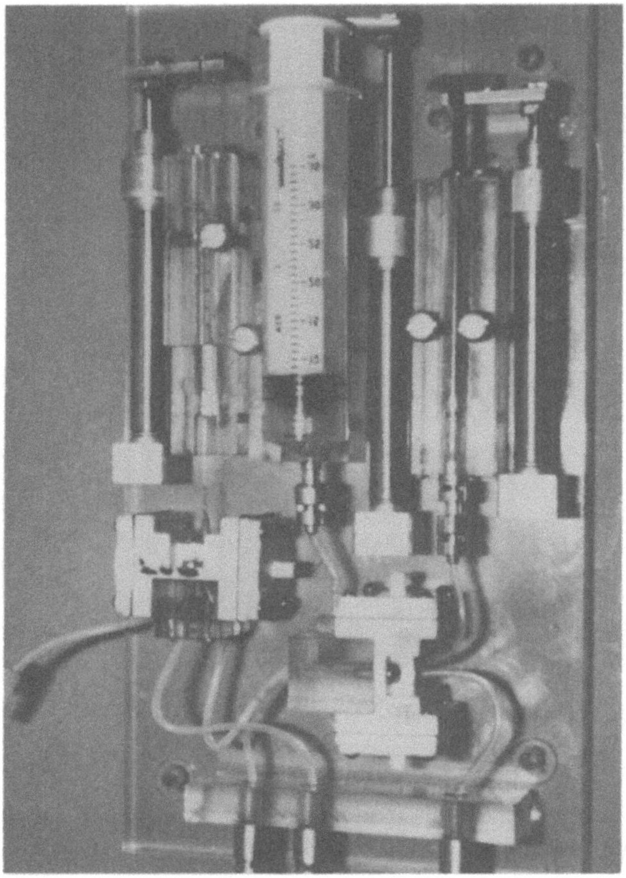

FIGURE 4 Cardiac Output Module.

than 2°C are indicated by a green light, those of 0.5–2°C illuminate the yellow light, and differences of >0.05°C illuminate the red light.

Urinometer. An automated miniature urinometer [3] (Fig. 5) has been developed and equipped with a solid-state amplifier controller mounted remotely from the congested bedside. An indwelling catheter is routinely inserted into the bladder. The urine drains into a collecting cylinder. The hydrostatic pressure in the cylinder is transmitted to a strain-gauge transducer via an air column. The output of the transducer, which is proportional to the volume of urine in the cylinder, is sampled at 1-min intervals by the computer. The change in volume between successive measurements establishes the flow rate. When the urine column in the collecting cylinder reaches

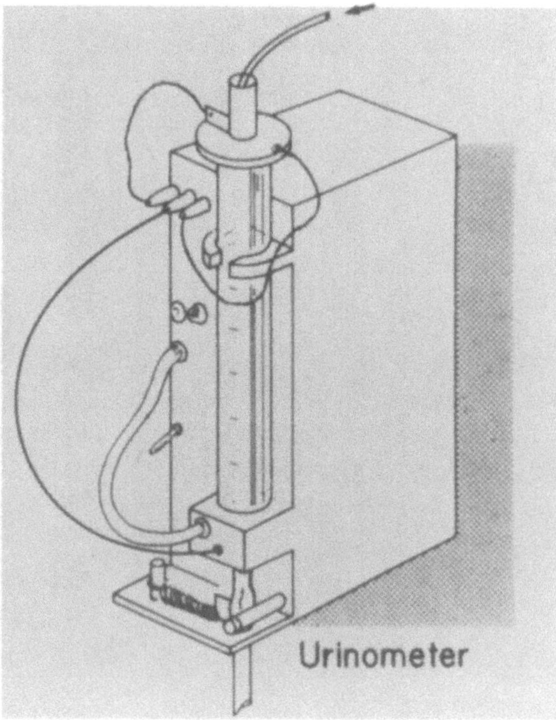

FIGURE 5 Urinometer.

a predetermined level, a valve controlled by the computer is opened and the urine empties into a reservoir. The design of amplifiers for measurement of urine flow has been modified to eliminate routine calibration. Flow rates are measured over a dynamic range of 0.2–50 cc/min.

Automated system for measurement of blood lactate. A specific enzyme method for measurement of lactate has been developed in our unit that utilizes metaphosphoric acid as the protein precipitant [4]. This method has since been adapted to the Technicon single-channel auto-analyzer system. Blood-sample size has been reduced to ≤ 100 μl and analysis time, to 6 min. A computer program has been developed that allows entry of calibration data, provides an optimum calibration curve, and types out lactate levels equivalent to peak deflections. More recently, we have implemented a system that eliminates all manual operation except loading a single standard and samples into a sample tray. On receiving an interrupt, the computer examines the output of the fluorometer, determines the optimum peak deflection, and computes equivalent lactate values which are then printed on a teletype. The results are automatically displayed on the video output above the patient's bed (Fig. 6). Continuous use of these automated

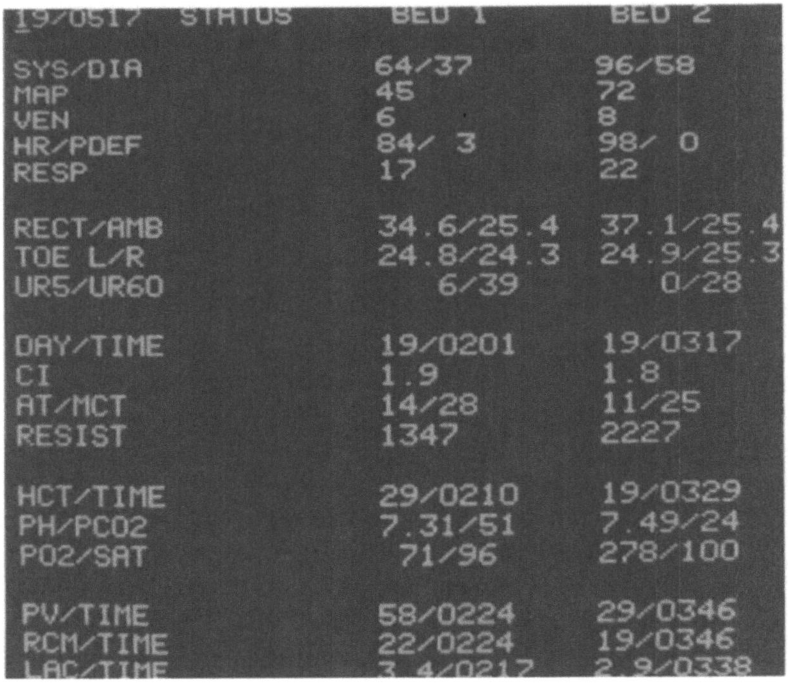

FIGURE 6 Patient Status Display.

devices at bedside over a long period of time has convinced us of their usefulness. The reasons that justify such a position include:

1. Its use makes it easier for the medical and paramedical personnel to handle their heavy work load.
2. Repetitive measurements can be made in a more regular and uniform manner.
3. Automation not only supplies bedside personnel with informative numerical data but is time saving and hence allows this personnel to devote greater attention to the patient's needs and wishes.
4. Designing for automation presents an opportunity to incorporate discreet equipment elements into a system.
5. This effort gives the designer a chance to miniaturize and redistribute components to maintain good patient access.

References

1. **Bisera, J., Weil, M. H., Carrington, J. H., Palley, N.,** and **Chaffee, M.** (1978). Vascular interface system for automation of hemodynamic monitoring and therapy. *Med. Biol. Engr. 16:*298.
2. **Joly, H. R.,** and **Weil, M. H.** (1969). Temperature of the great toe as an indication of the severity of shock. *Circulation 39:*131.

3. **Meagher, P. F., Jensen, R. E., Pearcy, M. G., Weil, M. H.,** and **Shubin, H.** (1966). Automatic urinometer for on-line monitoring of patients with circulatory shock. *Med. Res. Engr. 5:*38.
4. **Boycks, E., Michaels, S., Weil, M. H., Shubin, H.,** and **Marbach, E. P.** (1975). Continuous-flow measurement of lactate in blood: A technique adapted for use in the emergency laboratory. *Clin. Chem. 21:*113.

Electrical Safety

JOSE BISERA, M.S.
Center for the Critically Ill/Shock Research Unit,
University of Southern California
Los Angeles, California

Medical instrumentation and its relation to patient safety is attracting widespread public attention. This is true of devices that are physically connected to the patient's body and provide life support, such as artificial kidneys or monitors used in intensive and coronary care units. Public awareness will continue to grow because of the increasing need for these services, their dramatic and emotional impact, and the exceptionally high cost associated with them. It is widely agreed that Federal medical safety legislation is inevitable and necessary.

At the present time, a number of professional and industry associations such as Association for the Advancement of Medical Instrumentation (AAMI), American National Standards Institute (ANSI), National Fire Protection Association (NFPA), and Underwriters' Laboratories, Inc. have prepared safety standards and are attempting to draw up further guidelines for establishing safety and performance standards. The federal government, primarily within the Food and Drug Administration, is addressing itself to the task of enforcement.

There is widespread feeling that with the exception of users in major research hospitals, operating personnel are insufficiently sensitive to the problems of safety and lack an adequate knowledge of the technical aspects of medical instrumentation. The physicians, nurses, and technicians have both the obligation and opportunity to reduce the risk of electrical shock, through recognition of potential hazardous condition and by the manner in which line powered equipment is connected to and near the patient.

ELECTRICAL HAZARDS

Electrical hazards that arise in the hospital environment can be categorized into two types [1,3,4]. The first and most obvious type is dangerous not only to the patient but to the medical staff as well, and is caused by electrical wiring failure that allows personal contact with a live wire or surface at the full power-line voltage. Frayed power cords, broken plugs, and faulty lamp sockets all have the potential of allowing contact with electrically live parts (Fig. 1). These hazards are usually well understood and a good maintenance program generally keeps them under control.

A more subtle hazard is that of a "leakage current." Leakage current is an unfortunate name as it implies that the equipment is faulty, when actually, leakage current exists more or less in all power-line-operated equipment. "Leakage current" is an inherent flow of current from the live electrical parts of an instrument to the accessible metal casing or parts. This current normally flows through a third wire connection to ground. Although the exact range of currents capable of producing fibrillation in humans by direct application to the heart in high concentration (current density) is not well defined, the range demonstrated on humans is from 180 μA to 20 mA [1,4].

It is generally agreed that a current of 20 μA applied directly to the heart muscle is of a magnitude sufficient to override the normal sequence of

FIGURE 1 Defective components illustrating electrical hazards.

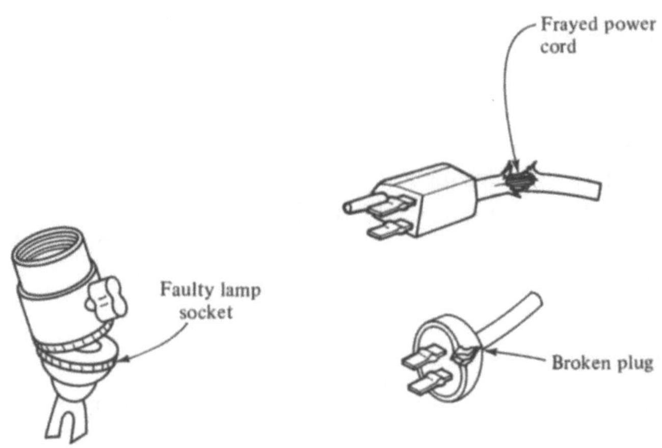

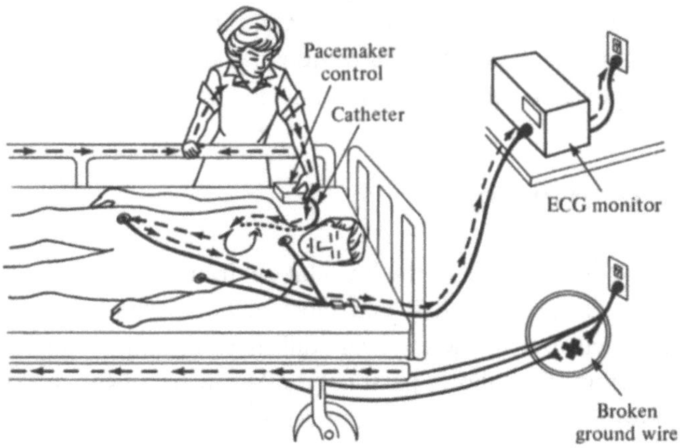

FIGURE 2 Leakage current illustrating electrical hazards.

activation [2,5]. This current can start a random out-of-sequence contraction of the heart muscle and may result in ventricular fibrillation.

Possible Hazard

When several pieces of electrically operated equipment are being used for one patient, one device may act as a "current source" and another as a "ground" with the patient as a "current path" between the two. This could happen even though only one device made actual "wired" connection to the patient, if, for example, the patient were to touch a second device, or make contact with it through another person simultaneously touching both it and the patient.

One example is an electrically operated bed with a leakage of 200 μA. This leakage current would normally return to "ground" through the "third wire." If this wire is broken or has a faulty connection, the leakage current could return to the "hospital" grounding system through the attending staff, the pacemaker, and through the ECG monitor via the right-leg ECG electrode (Fig. 2). This hazardous current may not be felt by the staff member but is almost certain to be a hazard to a catheterized patient. A clue to the presence of this type of phenomenon might be an increase in the amount of line frequency interference in the ECG trace on the monitor. Although this fault would be due to a faulty ground connection from the bed, the same kind of hazard would exist if the "ground" connection in the ECG monitor were broken instead.

Recommendations

Leakage currents cannot be eliminated, but their effects can be minimized. Personnel at the bedside as well as the patient are part of the electrical environment. While the human body may not be an efficient electrical conductor, it can serve as a path for carrying electricity.

The current consensus in minimizing electrical hazards to the patient include:

1. To provide good electrical grounding with equipment, not with the patient. A ground connection to the equipment gives any currents flowing through the equipment case or frame a safe path to "drain off." To use currently available monitors to quantitate leakage currents on a routine basis under the supervision of a qualified clinical engineer.
2. When two instruments or electrical devices are in use with or near one patient, to connect them to the same power receptable (wall outlet) if possible.
3. When adjusting instrument controls, checking electrode attachments, or handling the patient, not to touch electrical devices or their metal surfaces with the other hand.
4. To spend part of the time at the bedside to spot-check for dangling power or patient cables, loose plugs in receptables, or worn or frayed wires.
5. To report anything suspicious immediately. If faulty equipment is discovered, to remove it from service and have it checked by a properly trained person.

References

1. **Bruner, J. M.** (1967). Hazards of electrical apparatus. *Anesthesiol. 28:* 396–425.
2. **Lubin, D.** (1969). Electrical safety. *Hospital, 43:*57.
3. **Stanley, P. E.** (1967). Hospital electrical safety and shielding. *J. Assoc. Adv. Med. Instrum. 2:*8–12.
4. **Starmer, C. F., Whalen, R. E.,** and **McIntosh, H. D.** (1964). Hazards of electric shock in cardiology. *Am. J. Cardiol. 14:*537–546.
5. **Whalen, R. E.,** and **Starmer, C. F.** (1967). Electric shock hazards in clinical cardiology. *Mod. Concepts Cardiovasc. Dis. 36:*7.

The Ethics of Sustaining Life in the Infirm Aged and Critically Ill

CHAPLAIN JACK CALHOUN
Hollywood Presbyterian Medical Center
Los Angeles, California

During the last few years, the church, in particular the United Presbyterian Church, has been asked for guidance concerning the problem of technological prolongation of life—or to be more specific, the "technological prolongation of dying." As a result, it is interesting to note the following recommendation:

> "Affirms the right of older persons to stipulate that technology shall not be used to prolong biological functions when there is no medical hope of restoration of meaningful existence; and encourages older persons and their families, in consultation with their pastors, to plan for the closure of life, including appropriate measures in the treatment of terminal illness and various options for the disposition of the body."

In this presentation, we shall be considering primarily matters related to the process of dying, an event that is individually human.

These are difficult times, and they present uncertainties with regard to human life. We need to discuss at length the application of new medical knowledge, and lines of responsibility need to be established. Scientific advancement and competence have raised serious questions concerning the process of life and death such as: (a) whether the person who is dying as a result of a fatal accident should be considered primarily as a donor for various organ transplants, or simply as a person who has had a fatal accident and is dying, (b) how long an elderly person should be forced through the clinical dying process, and (c) whether there is a terminal point to this type of suffering.

In these matters there arises the question of the quality and the quantity of life. In general, our scientific competence has stressed the longevity of life as being of primary importance. The biblical perspective has emphasized quality. Our popular theology, our medical philosophy and practice, our financial arrangements for our life and death care, our social perspective and philosophy, are all areas that need to be reconsidered in terms of quality versus quantity. I believe the starting point would be with the family.

THE FAMILY

There are apparently paradoxical occasions when death is recognized by the family as both a time of sadness and a sense of joy; sadness at a human parting, but rejoicing that a life has been lived and the person has been a part of the family. This can be true whether the deceased is old, middle-aged, or young. If the illness has been a prolonged one, the process of the death event can be accepted calmly. Charles Lindbergh's death was an example of such a situation. He chose to die with dignity, without scientific prolongation of life, with no heroic measures, and not in a clinical setting. Instead he chose to die surrounded by his family and close friends in the beauty of an island he loved. His personal physician told me that there was a sense of happiness as he planned his own funeral and burial service with his family. Invariably the religious perspectives of the family group, formal or informal, are a very important factor in attitudes like this. If, through some form of religious involvement together, the family knows that death is an intrinsic aspect of life, then acceptance of death is assumed.

THE DYING PATIENT

What does the patient know about the process of dying? In what way are patients generally informed that they are in the dying process? To what degree are they prepared for this process? In what way are their wishes sought in regard to the medical procedures related to their dying? Are there opportunities for them to express their desires and beliefs about the process? Is there an interested person ready to discuss and listen, and if so, does this person have the authority to carry out the wishes of the patient?

In general, the answer to all of these questions is a very definite NO!

The dying patient has become a sort of nonperson who, because of illness, is not regarded as having very much in the way of what we have become accustomed to call "civil rights." This is why phrases like "the right to die" or "the right to die with dignity" have very little power. If we wish to use present daily social language we may well say that the millions of dying persons are a minority group completely without representation. They have absolutely no political power. No one speaks for them in Congress. They have no elected representatives in the State Assembly. Probably they will not even vote in the next election.

Hence persons in the process of dying are, in effect, nonpersons. The major decisions affecting their living or dying are taken away from them and placed in the hands of health or family organizations, hospitals, staff, physicians, insurance companies, and the frequently reluctant, and either overly guilty or overly detached, family.

Each of these groups has its own particular sense of responsibility which is very natural, human and serious, but which likely has no dimension of concern for the expectations of the dying person. In general, the health professionals and hospitals are all directed to prolongation of life. In the actual situation it seems very complicated, but in fact it is simple. The main direction and purpose of the health professionals as they are trained at present is to save life and therefore to fight death.

THE DESIRE TO DIE WITH DIGNITY

Death as an event in existence is a natural human problem. Death itself is such a mysterious event that many people develop and hold some philosophical or religious faith which helps them to face the inevitability of death. The statements of faith of various religions have continued to help people cope with the mystery of death.

Recent advances in medical knowledge and technology have in many cases made dying a very difficult human problem. This process under modern medical management can be prolonged in some cases indefinitely. Major surgical interventions take place, machines replace the work of diseased organs, nourishment is provided intravenously, elimination can be processed, and drugs can relieve pain. Such procedures are generally conducted under the rubric of the Hippocratic Oath of "do no harm." In the present practice of medicine this means the maintenance of life at all costs, and in many instances, these medical procedures, can make death a very difficult process.

These life-saving procedures were not designed to do this. They are primarily the result of new knowledge gained for the purpose of combating disease, supporting life, and relieving pain. However, when applied to the dying person the procedures frequently result in an extremely inhumane situation; a situation that many dying people dread much more than they fear the event of death itself.

In the light of these experiences in the prolongation of the dying process, phrases such as the "right to die" and "death with dignity" have come into common use. The implication is that dying persons should have the right to refuse prolongation of life through use of the techniques, knowledge and competencies of hospitals and the health professionals, and that they should have the right to decide how best they want to die. Rather than submit to a great invasion of privacy by medical procedures that strip away human dignity during the last few prolonged weeks of life, there should be a way by which decisions can be made so that they have a humane dying experience.

As we consider the new human problems introduced into the process of dying during the last two or three decades, it is clear that there is indeed no easy solution. They are really new problems, with a number of complex factors that makes them difficult. Consider for a moment the variety of people and institutions involved: the medical profession, the hospital and its staff, the patient's family and friends, the patient, and the mores of our culture and the courts that maintain them. Major emotional, economic, religious, scientific, and cultural forces are evident.

Summary

There is one factor evident throughout all of these forces that we must mention in closing, namely the evasive human element of "caring." I read some time ago—somewhere—a dying patient's comments to the medical and religious staff that no matter how effective the clinical procedures were or how efficiently the nursing staff performed—or how often the Chaplain came by for a visit—the only thing that mattered was did they care? The patient went on to say "but just believe me, if you care, you can't go wrong. Just admit that you care. This is really what we search for."

I believe that the time has come where we deal with the terminal patient as a person, ministering to them as both physician and priest.

Psychopharmacologic Management of Psychiatric Syndromes in the Critically Ill

WILLIAM F. KIELY, M.D.
Departments of Psychiatry and Medicine, University of Southern California School of Medicine, and Los Angeles County/ University of Southern California Medical Center, Los Angeles, California

Skill in the appraisal and evaluation of the cerebrocortical functions of attention, perception, conception, orientation, and memory as well as of attitudes, feelings, and behavioral tendencies of the ill or injured person is becoming part of the comprehensive-care approach of the staffs of critical care units. They have come to recognize that either extremes of overwhelming anxiety or abject depression are danger signals interacting with a precarious balance of forces in their severely ill patients[11].

Likewise, physicians and nurses are becoming increasingly aware of the importance of the patient's previous life-experience pattern, style of coping in the face of challenge, and particular strengths or vulnerabilities in the face of stress, and are taking account of such factors in their treatment planning. It has become increasingly evident that while the support systems for malfunctioning organs or organ systems may be highly impersonal and technologized to a large extent—for instance, in cardiac rhythm monitoring or assisted pulmonary ventilation—the care of a patient needs be highly personal. The mind–body relationship, or psychosomatic unity, is nowhere more evident than as exhibited by patients under the stress of critical illness.

PATTERNS OF INCIDENCE

The frequency of critical-care psychiatric syndromes varies considerably with the type of illness and differs in prevalence in the several types of intensive-care facility. The concept of an "ICU psychiatric syndrome" developed originally out of reports of a high incidence of delirium (40–70%) following open-heart surgery [2]. Some observers felt that this syndrome, developing typically between the third and fifth postoperative day, reflected the influence of the intensive care unit's environmental impact upon the patient. A combination of sleep deprivation, sensory monotony, loss of a sense of time passage and a day–night cycle were felt to be major contributing factors to the loss of reality sense [12]. Postcardiotomy delirium has subsequently been found to be highly correlated with neurological deficit and organically determined cognitive dysfunction [7] perhaps related to the duration of exposure to cardiopulmonary bypass, microemboli originating in the heart, duration of anesthesia, and depth and duration of hypothermia. Significant differences in the incidence of psychiatric disturbances following lung surgery are noted in comparison to open-heart surgery. It would appear that the incidence of such syndromes in well-organized coronary care units is considerably less than that noted in post-cardiotomy recovery rooms [8]. Intensive care units treating a wide spectrum of critically ill and injured patients, including the seriously burned, will number among their patients a majority who may suffer from renal, cardiac, or pulmonary failure, serious septic or hypovolemic shock, considerable anemia, fever, and toxemia. Such disease-related elements very probably account for the significantly different incidence of delirium and other psychiatric disorders among such patients as compared to the generally much more intact acute coronary patient or even many post-cardiotomy patients.

NEUROBIOLOGIC INTEGRATIVE PRINCIPLES

Hess [9], as early as 1925, pointed out that an animal's reaction to environmental challenge is importantly reflective of the influence of subcortical centers that coordinate autonomic, somatic, and psychic functions. He suggested that these centers were organized through reciprocally balanced systems, which he termed "ergotropic" (signifying "approach" or "go") and "trophotropic" (signifying "avoidance" or "no-go"). Highly integrated neural functions of the type underlying cognitive process, which are generally considered reflective of cortical activity, are under the modulating influence of these primitive, tonically active subcortical systems. All perceptual stimuli, be they of exteroceptive or interoceptive source, as well as memory and logical thought sequences, reveal the shaping influence of these balanced systems. Their anatomical basis, physiological interconnections, and neurochemical transmitters are distinguishable and separable [3]. Their influence is identifiable across the entire gamut of consciousness from sleep to the heights of ecstasy physiologically [5], and from stupor to catatonic excitement psychopathologically [6].

The ergotropic system integrates functions that prepare the individual for positive action. It is characterized by altering, arousal, excitement, increased skeletal muscle tone and sympathetic nervous activity, and the release of catabolic hormones. The trophotropic system, on the other hand, integrates systems that promote withdrawal and conservation of energy: raising of the stimulus barrier to perceptual input, decreased skeletal muscle tone, increased parasympathetic nervous function, and the circulation of anabolic hormones. A developing body of data indicates that the biogenic amines norepinephrine and dopamine are neurotransmitters for the ergotropic system, while 5-hydroxytryptamine (serotonin) and acetylcholine play similar roles for the trophotropic system [10].

A few basic principles play a primary role in the operation of this quite complex psychobiological process, and underly the resultant patterns of behavior. Firstly, the two systems stand in mutually reciprocal relationship and share tonic, enduring, and balanced physiologic activity. With increasing degrees of activation of the ergotropic "go" (approach) system there is a corresponding degree of inhibition of trophotropic "no go" (avoidance) system, and vice versa.

Secondly, when either system is stimulated the reactivity of both systems is altered, affecting their state of readiness, set, or tuning [4], so to speak. In moderate states of activation, or tuning, the reactivity of the various anatomic and physiologic components of the affected system is heightened, while that of the reciprocal system is correspondingly reduced. Thus in situations of moderate, but not extreme, challenge or threat the "go" system expresses itself cortically through alerting or vigilance, autonomically in a sympathetic stimulation, and behaviorally in a state of muscular readiness. At the same time, the reactivity of the several components of the "no go" system is correspondingly suppressed.

Thirdly, at maximal stimulation, the reciprocal balance between systems breaks down and both systems discharge simultaneously, a pathophysiological consequence. A clinical example is the state of anxiety wherein a variety of psychic, skeletomuscular, and visceral disturbances reflect such simultaneous discharge of opposing systems. Flooding of the cerebral cortex by afferents from both systems may be experienced as dread; weak knees may coexist with tremulous hands; and sweating, tachycardia, and hypertension may coexist with nausea, vomiting, and bowel or bladder hyperactivity.

CRITICAL CARE PSYCHIATRIC SYNDROMES

The most common syndromes encountered in critical care units are schematically characterized in Table 1. They may range from the occasionally encountered overwhelming *fear* reaction, accompanied by a paralyzing sense of helplessness in which the behavioral-avoidance grip of the "no go" system is evident, through more adaptive but sometimes physiologically stressful states of restless *tension*. In these polar opposite states of tuning, or adaptation, reciprocal suppression of the opposing system is maintained. At higher degrees of CNS arousal, maladaptive, sustained *anxiety* is encountered with simultaneous discharge to varying degrees of both "go" and "no go" systems as noted psychically, viscerally, and in skeletomuscular groups. At still higher degrees of stimulations, *anxious* or agitated *depression* reactive to the stress of crisis may be encountered. One sometimes sees examples of acute *schizophreniform psychotic disintegration* with thought disorder, delusions, or hallucinations maintained in the context of clear consciousness and without loss of orientation or memory function. Especially in patients with cardiopulmonary or renal failure, or patients in circulatory shock and particularly in the middle-aged or elderly, one frequently encounters *delirium*. Delirium is a state of cerebral insufficiency with impairment of some or all of such cognitive functions such as attention, perception, conception, logical sequence, orientation, and memory. Some degree of clouding of consciousness is characteristic of this state, not uncommonly punctuated by lucid intervals. The affect of the delirious patient may vary from apathy to irritable restlessness, and the autonomically modulated visceral concomitants may follow a corresponding spectrum.

TABLE 1 Most Common Syndromes Encountered in Critical Care Units

PSYCHIATRIC SYNDROMES	BEDSIDE CLINICAL FEATURES
Acute fear	Facial expression of terror. Body musculature limp.
	Feelings of powerlessness overwhelming.
	Parasympathetic nervous system dominance: bradycardia, hypotension, nausea or vomiting.
	Sleep disturbance minimal.
Sustained tension	Vigilant, hyperalert facies. Body musculature tense and movement patterns quickened.
	Emotional tone reflective of assertive engagement.
	Sympathetic nervous hyperreactivity: sweating, tachycardia, wide pupils.
	Difficulty in falling asleep.
Anxiety	Worried facies. Jittery, tremulous voluntary movements.
	Feelings of dread or doubt in face of great threat.

TABLE 1 (*Continued*)

PSYCHIATRIC SYNDROMES	BEDSIDE CLINICAL FEATURES
	Hyperactivity of both sympathetic and parasympathetic systems simultaneously: sweating, tachycardia, nausea or vomiting, urinary frequency.
	Restless and interrupted sleep.
Agitated depression	Saddened facies with verbal and nonverbal expressions of dejection or futility.
	Feelings of helplessness and hopelessness intermingled with dread and anxiety; maybe negativism in cooperation with nursing procedures.
	Memory, orientation, and other cognitive functions intact.
	Sleep disturbance very pronounced.
Acute schizophreniform stress reaction	Hyperalert level of awareness. Facies often expressive of bewilderment.
	Feeling tone ranging from fear over spectrum to negativistic resentment.
	Thought patterns incongruous, tangential, self-referential, maybe delusional; hallucinations, if present, are auditory rather than visual.
	Memory and orientation intact.
	Sleep disturbance very pronounced.
Acute delirium	Clouded, uneven, variable level of consciousness.
	Mood variable from apathy to excitement.
	Orientation and recent memory defective.
	May exhibit delusional ideas or hallucinations—more likely visual than auditory.
	Sleep fitful and interrupted.

PSYCHOPHARMACOLOGIC TREATMENT

Based on the neurobiological principle of balance, the disturbance of which is accompanied by psychopathology and often by very undesirable psychophysiologic visceral and behavioral concomitants in critically ill patients, one's goal in the use of psychoactive drugs should be the restoration of physiologic reciprocity between opposing ergotropic and trophotropic systems, a situation wherein clarity of cognitive function, smoothness of visceral autonomic activity, and overall behavioral control may be recovered.

TABLE 2 Psychoactive Drugs for the Critically Ill and Effective Dosage Ranges

			DAILY ADULT ORAL DOSE RANGE (mg) (reduce by ½ for I.M. use)	
DRUG CLASS	GENERIC NAME	TRADE NAME	HIGH	MODERATE
Benzodiazepine	Chlordiazepoxide	Librium	150–300	75–150
	Diazepam	Valium	30–60	15–30
	Oxazepam	Serax	75–120	45–75
	Clorazepate	Tranxene	45–90	25–45
Butyrophenone	Haloperidol	Haldol	15–60	6–15

Table 2 summarizes a fairly reliable approach to the use of a modest number of drugs, whose dosage range, site of principal CNS action, and expectable effects are fairly clear. Efficacy is claimed for literally scores of psychoactive drugs, produced under a wide variety of trade names, too numerous for the average clinician to develop personal experience with. A wise course, particularly for the physician treating acute, life-threatening illnesses of limited duration, is to master the use of a small group of drugs of antianxiety, antipsychotic, and antidepressant classes. The actions and interactions, modes of administration, dosage ranges, and potential side effects of each class of drug should be mastered.

As antianxiety agents, the benzodiazepines are preferable to the meprobamate group. Benzodiazepines, but not meprobamates, are available in both oral and parenteral forms. They are preferable to the barbiturates in not significantly depressing cerebrocortical functions in dosage ranges wherein tranquilization is feasible. The four available benzodiazepines: (a) chlordiazepoxide (Librium), (b) diazepam (Valium), (c) oxazepam (Serax), and (d) chorazepate (Tranxene) are essentially identical except for dose and duration of action, chlordiazepoxide being the longest acting and oxazepam the shortest acting of the group. In duration of action, all rank with the moderate- or long-acting barbiturates, such as phenobarbital. Although oxazepam is an active metabolite of diazepam, poorer bowel absorption necessitates a larger dose. There is pharmacologic evidence to suggest that the antianxiety effects of the benzodiazepines are the result of action in limbic forebrain and limbic midbrain areas rather than upon the recticular formation, an important site of barbiturate and nonbarbiturate sedative–hypnotic action. The interruption of serotonergic neurotransmission in limbic suppressor sites appears to block the avoidance (trophotropic) side of approach–avoidance conflict and in so doing reduces fear and tension, permitting more physiologic balance between opposing "go" and "no go" systems [14] (Table 3).

TABLE 3 Neurobiology of Psychiatric Syndromes

STATE OF TUNING	CLINICAL EXAMPLE	PHARMACOLOGIC INTERVENTION	SITE OF ACTION
Trophotropic dominance	Acute fear	Benzodiazepine agent (Librium, Valium, Serax, Tranxene)	Limbic forebrain and midbrain serotonergic suppressor sites
Ergotropic dominance	Sustained tension	Benzodiazepine agent	Limbic forebrain and midbrain noradrenergic suppressor sites
Simultaneous "T" and "E" discharge	Anxiety	Benzodiazepine agent	Limbic forebrain and midbrain noradrenergic and serotonergic suppressor sites
	Agitated depression	Benzodiazepine agent	Limbic forebrain and midbrain noradrenergic and serotonergic suppressor sites
	Acute schizophreniform stress reaction	Butyrophenone (Haldol)	Neostriatal and mesolimbic dopamine receptor sites
	Acute delirium	Butyrophenone (Haldol) or benzodiazepine agent	Neostriatal and mesolimbic dopamine receptor sites Limbic forebrain and midbrain noradrenergic and serotonergic suppressor sites

The various depressive syndromes encountered in critically ill patients are generally reactive to, or concomitants of, the overwhelming illness being treated, and more often than not are associated with considerable reactive anxiety or agitation. Since the clearest indication for the use of tricyclic antidepressants is in retarded, endogenous, or psychotic depressions, and since an average of 2–3 weeks is generally required for evidence of the clearcut efficacy of these drugs, they are best avoided in critically ill patients. One of the benzodiazepine group of antianxiety agents is often of some use in depressed patients with prominent symptoms of tension, anxiety, or somatic complaints. Controlled trials indicate that antianxiety drugs may be useful in these types of depression [13]. Because of the danger of inhibition of monoamine oxidase in critically ill patients, many of whom might require vasopressor circulatory support or sympathomimetic bronchodilator inhalation aerosols, the use of monoamine oxidase inhibitors is best avoided in the care of the critically ill.

At present, the most widely used antipsychotic agents are of the phenothiazine class, with chlorpromazine (Thorazine) the most thoroughly studied member of the class. In comparison to trifluoperazine (Stelazine) or fluphenazine (Prolixin; Permitil), it is of lower potency and has greater sedative effect. The potential of phenothiazines, particularly chlorpromazine, to block alpha-adrenergic vasopressor receptor sites, and to intensify the vasodilating and other beta-adrenergic effects of epinephrine, together with other autonomic side effects, renders this class of drug less desirable for use in the seriously ill patient than the newer butyrophenone compound, haloperidol (Haldol). This agent is rapidly and completely absorbed from the gastrointestinal tract and is available in injectable form as well. It causes little autonomic nervous system receptor blockade and has no adverse interactions with digitalis, diuretics, or other cardiovascular drugs. For the elderly, for those with cardiovascular disease, and for the deliriously excited patient it may be the drug of choice when psychotic behavior and confusion require pharmacologic treatment [1].

Summary

Management of psychopathology in the critically ill patient by means of psychoactive drugs is best achieved when based on clear conceptual understanding of the neurobiologic basis underlying the various forms of psychiatric maladaptation. The influence of subcortical systems underlying and coordinating autonomic, somatic, and psychic patterns of adaptation in terms of arousal and excitement, as contrasted with inhibition and withdrawal, is outlined. Based on the mutually reciprocal relationship of such systems, as well as their pathologic simultaneous discharge, psychiatric syndromes of acute fear, sustained tension, acute anxiety, agitated depression, acute schizophreniform stress reaction, and acute delirium are discussed. Probable major sites of disturbed brain physiology are identified and correlated with appropriate psychopharmacologic agents known to stabilize function in such sites. The use of benzodiazepines and butyrophenone drugs are discussed together with recommended dosage ranges.

References

1. **Appleton, W. S.,** and **Davis, J. M.** (1973). *Practical Clinical Psychopharmacology*. New York: Medcom.
2. **Blachly, P. H.,** and **Starr, A.** (1964). Post-cardiotomy delirium. *Am. J. Psychiatr. 121*:37.
3. **Gellhorn, E.** (1967). *Principles of Autonomic-Somatic Integrations*. Minneapolis: University of Minnesota Press.
4. **Gellhorn, E.** (1969). Further studies on the physiology and pathophysiology of tuning of the central nervous system. *Psychosomat. 10*:94–104.
5. **Gellhorn, E.,** and **Kiely, W. F.** (1972). Mystical states of consciousness: neurophysiological and clinical aspects. *J. Nerv. Ment. Dis. 154*:399–405.
6. **Gellhorn, E.,** and **Kiely, W. F.** (1973). Autonomic nervous system in psychiatric disorder. In: Mendels, J. (ed.), *Biological Psychiatry*. New York: Wiley.

7. **Gilman, S.** (1965). Cerebral disorders after open-heart operations. *New Engl. J. Med. 272:*489–494.
8. **Hackett, T. P., Cassem, N. H.,** and **Wishnie, H. A.** (1968). Coronary-care unit: appraisal of its psychologic hazards. *New Engl. J. Med. 279:*1365–1367.
9. **Hess, W. R.** (1958). *The Functional Organization of the Diencephalon.* New York: Grune and Stratton.
10. **Kety, S.** (1971). Brain amines and affective disorders. In: Ho, B. T., and McIsaac, W. M. (eds.), *Brain Chemistry in Mental Diseases.* New York: Plenum.
11. **Kiely, W. F.** (1974). Psychiatric aspects of critical care. *Crit. Care Med. 2:*139–142.
12. **Kornfeld, D. S., Zimberg, S.,** and **Malm, J.** (1975). Psychiatric complications of open-heart surgery. *New Engl. J. Med. 273:*282–287.
13. **Raskin, A., Schulterbrandt, J. G., Reatig, N. Crook, T. H.,** and **Odle, D.** (1974). Depression subtypes and responses to phenelzine, diazepam, and placebo. *Arch. Gen. Psychiatr. 30:*66–75.
14. **Wise, C. D., Berger, B. D.,** and **Stein, L.** (1972). Benzodiazepines: anxiety-reducing activity by reduction of serotonin turnover in brain. *Science 177:*180–183.

Index

R

FSC
www.fsc.org
MIX
Papier aus verantwortungsvollen Quellen
Paper from responsible sources
FSC® C105338

If you have any concerns about our products,
you can contact us on
ProductSafety@springernature.com

In case Publisher is established outside the EU,
the EU authorized representative is:
Springer Nature Customer Service Center GmbH
Europaplatz 3, 69115 Heidelberg, Germany

Printed by Libri Plureos GmbH
in Hamburg, Germany